Biochemistry for Sport and Exercise Metabolism

Biochemistry for Sport and Exercise Metabolism

Don MacLaren
James Morton
Liverpool John Moores University, UK

WILEY-BLACKWELL

A John Wiley & Sons, Ltd., Publication

Library of Congress Cataloguing-in-Publication Data

MacLaren, Don, 1947–
Biochemistry for sport and exercise metabolism / Don MacLaren and James Morton.
        p. cm.
    Summary: "This book will provide them with the basics of the subject presented in a clear, accessible style placed firmly within a sporting context" – Provided by publisher.
    ISBN 978-0-470-09184-5 (hardback) – ISBN 978-0-470-09185-2 (paper)
    1. Human mechanics. 2. Biochemistry. 3. Sports–Physiological aspects. 4. Exercise–Physiological aspects.
    5. Energy metabolism. 6. Muscles–Metabolism. I. Morton, James, 1982– II. Title.
    QP303.M23 2012
    612.7′6 – dc23

                                                                                    2011030216

A catalogue record for this book is available from the British Library.

This book is published in the following electronic formats: ePDF: 9780470091869; ePub: 9781119967828; Mobi: 9781119967835

Typeset in 10/12pt Times-Roman by Laserwords Private Limited, Chennai, India

First Impression 2012

Contents

Preface

Ever since I started lecturing, firstly as a biologist (1973–1980) and then as a sport scientist (1980–2010), I always encouraged my students to keep in mind the questions 'how' and 'why' – in other words, how does that happen and why does that happen? In essence, I wanted them to possess an enquiring mind and not to be satisfied with a superficial understanding of the subject matter if possible – especially if the subject is one in which they wish to specialize.

As a young lecturer in exercise physiology in 1980, I was fortunate enough to possess the wonderful '*Textbook of Work Physiology*' by Astrand and Rodahl, and so get my teeth into a new subject area. As a biologist with a passion for sport, this really was exciting and novel to me. Having an opportunity to lecture in this field with my world-renown colleague, Tom Reilly, I couldn't have wished for a better start. However, there was a problem. In order to understand the 'how' and the 'why' of energy production for muscle contraction and exercise, it was imperative to have a knowledge and understanding of biochemistry.

I was fortunate enough to have undertaken some modules in biochemistry as an undergraduate at Liverpool University, but the sports science students also required this knowledge. In the early years, this was achieved by placing them with the biology and biochemistry students. Unfortunately, it didn't really work out, because the emphasis was not (at least initially) on relating to sport and exercise. The same was said of the statistics modules – too pure, too detailed and not applied enough.

So what did I do? I decided to run the biochemistry modules myself for our own students. The end result was greater satisfaction from the student cohorts and a greater interest by myself in what was necessary and to what depth. I was not intent on producing biochemists, but rather enabling sport science (physiology) students to gain a better grasp on aspects of biochemistry and metabolism as relating to sport and exercise.

Did I (and thereby my students) have recourse to any useful biochemistry texts for support? The answer was a qualified 'yes'. I was also fortunate enough to buy another wonderful textbook, '*Biochemistry for the Medical Sciences*' by Newsholme and Leech. This was a rather large tome to get through, but it did present much of the material I felt was needed for our students and, because the *late* Eric Newsholme had a passion for running, it related to aspects of sport. To gain further understanding, I encouraged my students to read other biochemistry textbooks (which were for students on biochemistry degree courses) that were available in the library. Over the years, I presented my adapted versions from such texts, since nothing else was suitable. Of course, more recently, a number of biochemistry textbooks have been written for sport and exercise science students, and what is interesting to note, in general, is how traditional black and white texts have become more colourful (and perhaps more interesting).

In May 2002, a young, eager second year student came to see me about getting on my level 3 'Muscle Metabolism' module. A prerequisite for this module was to undertake my level 2 'Biochemistry for Sport' modules. Being a science and football student and not a sports science (physiology) student, he had not had the opportunity to take this module. I tried to put him off, but he was quite insistent. So I gave him a biochemistry text to read over the next four weeks and to come back and see me. I had hoped it would turn him off. Fortunately, he kept coming back for tutorials to get a clear grasp of various concepts. I realised that this guy was not for turning and I allowed him to enrol on my level 3 module. He completed the module with a clear first class mark, obtained a first class degree overall, and went on to successfully undertake a PhD (with myself on his supervisory team) in exercise metabolism. His name? Dr James Morton – my co-author.

Since first arriving in Liverpool ten years ago, James has developed a passion for research and teaching exercise biochemistry and metabolism. He has helped me enormously. When I was asked to write this book, I agreed to do so on the basis that he would help me. Thankfully he agreed. We both feel that we needed to provide a textbook dedicated to sport and exercise science students who want to gain a solid (not necessarily comprehensive) understanding of key aspects in biochemistry – particularly those relating to energy metabolism. That is our mission in this text. We hope that the way we have approached and organized the work is interesting and makes you want to continue. Although not a superficial text, this book is not a comprehensive biochemistry treatise, but rather one which should 'tickle your fancy' and want you to read more and develop yourself.

We have organised the book into three parts. The first part encompasses some rather basic information for you to get to grips with. This includes an overview of energy metabolism (hopefully to gain your interest), some key aspects of skeletal muscle structure and function and some simple (but necessarily basic) biochemical concepts. The second part of the book really gets to grips with the three macromolecules which provide energy and structure to skeletal muscle – carbohydrates, lipids, and protein. The third and final part moves beyond biochemistry to examine key aspects of metabolism, i.e. the regulation of energy production and storage. To this end, we have a chapter on basic principles of regulation of metabolism, followed by three chapters exploring how metabolism is influenced during high-intensity, prolonged and intermittent exercise by intensity, duration, and nutrition. We also provide some pointers towards an understanding of fatigue when undergoing these activities. This is, after all, how we teach and progress our biochemistry and metabolism modules, and so we want to share this with you.

Dear reader, I hope you enjoy the journey into biochemistry and muscle metabolism as much as I have over many years. Sadly, I have come to the end of my career, but am fortunate enough to pass on the mantle to my dedicated and enthusiastic colleague, James Morton. Remember to always ask the questions 'how' and 'why'.

Don MacLaren, PhD

Exercise metabolism is undoubtedly an essential component of sport and exercise science degree programmes. While many students are fascinated by this topic, they often have difficulty in grasping the underpinning biochemistry that regulates how our muscles produce energy for exercise. Students tend to focus on learning the essential facts, chemical structures and the major metabolic pathways, often neglecting the understanding of how these factors respond to the stress of exercise.

A focus on factual recall without understanding of application is, of course, not representative of a deep approach to learning. To this end, we have sought to develop a text which combines a traditional approach to biochemistry teaching but with a focus on sport, by ensuring that the material is always dominated by exercise-related questions. In our experience, students of sport and exercise science learn better when their real interest of sport and exercise dominates the conversation. If by the end of this text, you now understand how exercise mode, intensity, duration, training status and nutritional status, etc. can all affect the regulation of energy-producing pathways, then I believe we will have achieved our aim. Additionally, if you can apply this material in the real world, perhaps to develop training and nutritional programmes to maximise athletic performance, then you have successfully acquired the deep approach to learning that we strive to achieve every time we enter a lecture theatre.

In writing this text, I must acknowledge the support of several people who have played a significant role in these early years of my academic career. Firstly, I will be forever grateful to my co-author, Professor Don MacLaren. It was Don who first fuelled my passion for exercise metabolism as an undergraduate student, and who continued to provide much valued support both as a postgraduate student and as an academic member of staff. His open door approach and his ability to motivate students to ask 'how' and 'why' are just two of many traits that I have tried to replicate in my own teaching.

Liverpool John Moores University is a wonderful institution. In addition to outstanding facilities, it is really through the collective hard work of many talented people which makes it such a special place. In particular, I must thank the late Professor Tom Reilly, Professor Tim Cable and Dr Barry Drust, all of whom have been instrumental in providing me with the platform that allows me to study something I love.

With the increasing time pressures of balancing the demands of teaching, research and applied practice, much of the writing of this text was written outside of office hours. For this, I must acknowledge the understanding and patience of my partner, Natalie. Thank you for understanding that exercise science is more than just my profession, it is my hobby. Finally, I extend my sincere appreciation to my Dad, Mum, Lisa and Julie for teaching me my most important lesson – that is, when all things else are considered, it is family that really gives meaning to life.

James Morton, PhD

Part One
Basic Muscle Physiology and Energetics

1

Energy sources for muscular activity

Learning outcomes

After studying this chapter, you should be able to:

- outline the key energy sources for exercise;
- distinguish between anaerobic and aerobic sources of energy;
- describe the essential structure of ATP;
- draw and explain the components of the energy continuum;
- describe the role of PCr in ATP synthesis;
- explain how PCr is resynthesized;
- describe the involvement of carbohydrates and fats as energy sources for exercise;
- explain reasons why an athlete is unable to sprint a marathon;
- describe the amounts and sources of energy in the body and their rates of energy formation;
- discuss how amino acids can be used as an energy source during exercise.

This chapter presents a brief overview of the energy sources used by muscles in order to engage in various activities. It is a 'taster' that will (hopefully) encourage you to delve a bit more deeply into the basic biochemistry of the macronutrients which provide energy, as well as to gain an understanding of the likely regulation of the processes which produce energy. From this perspective, this chapter examines the energy-yielding processes from a superficial level in addressing issues of energy for sprinting and for more prolonged events.

Key words

adenosine diphosphate (ADP)	fatty acid
aerobic	glycogen
anaerobic	glycogenolysis
anaerobic alactic	glycolysis
anaerobic glycolytic	lipid
anaerobic glycolysis	lipolysis
anaerobic lactic	mitochondria
adenosine triphosphate (ATP)	oxidation
carbohydrate	PCr (phosphocreatine)
CK (creatine kinase)	phosphorylation
creatine	protein
dephosphorylation	protein degradation
energy continuum	protein synthesis

1.1 Adenosine triphosphate: the energy currency

In order for our muscles to contract and provide movement, energy is required. Such energy is

Biochemistry for Sport and Exercise Metabolism, First Edition. Don MacLaren and James Morton.
© 2012 John Wiley & Sons, Ltd. Published 2012 by John Wiley & Sons, Ltd.

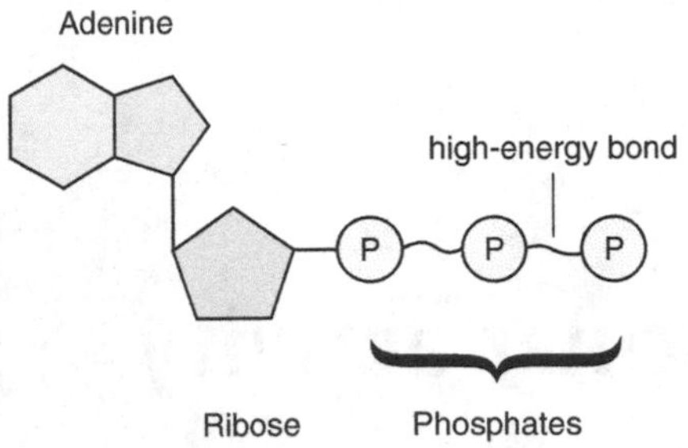

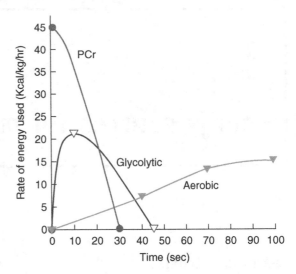

Figure 1.1 Adenosine triphosphate (ATP)

provided by **adenosine triphosphate (ATP)** and is the only energy capable of being used for muscle contraction in humans. Figure 1.1 provides the structure of an ATP molecule. As you can see from this diagram, ATP consists of a base (adenine) attached to a sugar (ribose), to which is attached three phosphate molecules. The phosphates are attached by 'high energy' bonds which, when removed, provide energy.

$$ATP \leftrightarrow ADP + P_i + Energy \quad (7.3 \, kcal \; or \; 30.5 \, kJ)$$

The process is reversible, which means that ATP may be re-formed from **adenosine diphosphate (ADP)** as long as there is sufficient energy to restore the missing phosphate molecule on to the ADP. The latter can be achieved by **phosphocreatine (PCr)** or by processes such as **anaerobic glycolysis**, and **aerobic** processes.

The stores of ATP in muscle tissue are rather limited, so there is a constant need to resynthesize it for survival, let alone movement. The amount of ATP in a muscle cell amounts to 25 mM/kg dry muscle or about 40–50 g in total, which is sufficient to enable high intense activity for around 2–4 seconds if it is the only useable source of energy available. This is not a great amount – hence the importance of resynthesis of ATP at rates sufficient to enable appropriate levels of exercise to ensue, i.e. fast rates of resynthesis for sprinting and slower rates for prolonged exercise.

1.2 Energy continuum

The major energy sources for exercise are dependent on the intensity and duration of the

Figure 1.2 Energy continuum

activity. Examination of Figure 1.2 highlights that there appears to be three such sources, i.e. PCr, glycolytic and aerobic. These energy-producing processes predominate exercise from 1–10 seconds, 10–60 seconds and beyond 60 seconds respectively.

Another way of expressing the **energy continuum** is represented in Figure 1.3, which shows the major energy sources for running events of varying distances. Note that short, highly intense sprinting bouts lasting 1–10 seconds use PCr predominantly, while events such as the 400 metres mainly use anaerobic glycolysis, and thereafter aerobic metabolism predominates.

1.3 Energy supply for muscle contraction

ATP is not stored to a great degree in muscle cells. Therefore, once muscle contraction starts, the regeneration of ATP must occur rapidly. There are three primary sources of ATP; these, in order of their utilization, are PCr, anaerobic glycolysis and aerobic processes.

Energy from ATP derives from cleaving the terminal phosphate of the ATP molecule. The resulting molecule is adenosine diphosphate (ADP). Phosphocreatine converts ADP back to ATP by donating its phosphate in the presence of the enzyme **creatine kinase** (CK), and

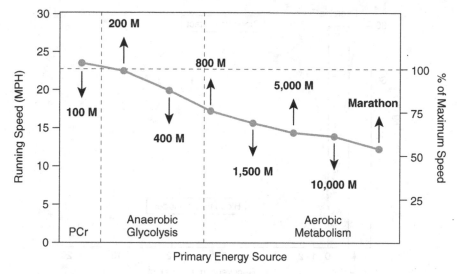

Figure 1.3   Primary energy sources for different running distances

in turn the PCr forms **creatine** (Cr), i.e. the **dephosphorylated** form of PCr.

$$ADP + PCr \underset{CK}{\Longleftrightarrow} ATP + Cr$$

The reaction of PCr with ADP to form ATP is very rapid, but is short-lived since the cell does not store high amounts of PCr (the muscle concentration of PCr is about 80 mM/kg dry muscle or 120 g in total). However, during short, high-intensity contractions, PCr serves as the major source of energy. This form of energy generation is often called **anaerobic alactic**, because it neither produces lactic acid nor requires oxygen. It is of paramount importance in sports requiring bursts of speed or power, such as sprints of 1–10 seconds.

Figure 1.4 provides a schematic to show the synthesis of ATP from ADP using PCr at the muscle crossbridge, and also the regeneration of PCr from Cr by ATP at the mitochondria.

Thus, Cr is formed from PCr during intense bouts of exercise, while Cr is re-phosphorylated to PCr by ATP produced in the mitochondria during aerobic recovery. Oxygen is needed for recovery of PCr, as can be seen in Figure 1.5, which clearly demonstrates that recovery of exercise-depleted PCr only happens when the blood supply to the exercising muscle is not occluded, i.e. there

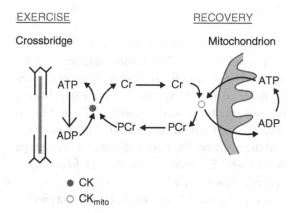

Figure 1.4   PCr shuttle

is an intact blood supply taking oxygen to the cells. If the blood supply is occluded (e.g. via a tourniquet), then PCr resynthesis fails. As a consequence, you should appreciate the need for a low level (so called active) recovery in between bouts of intense exercise.

The enzyme CK, which regulates PCr activity, exists in a number of forms known as isoforms (this will be dealt with later). Note that not only is there a CK which favours the formation of ATP from PCr, but there is also another form, CK_{mito}, which is present at the mitochondria and favours the synthesis of PCr from Cr using ATP.

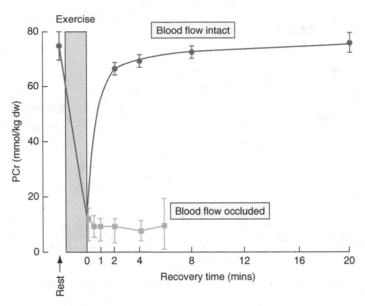

Figure 1.5   Resynthesis of PCr after exercise with and without an occluded blood supply (adapted from Hultman *et al.*, 1990)

You should also note from Figure 1.5 that there is a rapid loss of PCr during intense exercise and that it is rapidly recovered (this may even be depleted if the exercise is sufficiently intense or prolonged). Indeed, nearly 75% of PCr is resynthesized within the first minute of recovery and the rest over the next 3–5 minutes. The graph is biphasic, i.e. rapid restoration at first, then a second, slower phase.

As soon as muscle contraction starts, the process of anaerobic glycolysis also begins. Anaerobic glycolysis does not contribute as large an amount of energy as PCr in the short term, but its contribution is likely to predominate from 10–60 seconds.

During glycolysis, locally stored muscle **glycogen,** and possibly some blood-borne glucose, supply the substrate for energy generation. **Glycolysis** takes place in the cytoplasm, where no oxygen is required, so the process is called anaerobic. It may also be called '**anaerobic lactic**', since lactic acid is formed as the end product. Sufficient lactic acid formation can lower the pH of the cell (i.e. make it more acid) to the extent that further energy production may be reduced.

The major substrate for **anaerobic glycolysis** (see below equation) is glycogen, so prior hard exercise without adequate repletion of glycogen will limit further high-intensity short-term work.

$$\text{Glycogen} \rightarrow \text{Glucose-1-P} \rightarrow \text{Lactic acid} + \text{ATP}$$

Exercise beyond 60 seconds requires mainly aerobic energy sources, such as the complete **oxidation** of glucose or **fatty acids** to carbon dioxide and water. These processes necessitate oxygen and take place in the **mitochondria** of the cells. The equations below illustrate the essence of aerobic metabolic reactions:

$$\text{Glucose} + \text{Oxygen} \rightarrow \text{Carbon dioxide}$$
$$+ \text{Water} + \text{ATP}$$
$$\text{Fatty acid} + \text{Oxygen} \rightarrow \text{Carbon dioxide}$$
$$+ \text{Water} + \text{ATP}$$

We shall see more detail about these processes in Chapters 5 and 6.

Aerobic activities invariably occur at lower exercise intensities (which are those lasting

Energy expenditure
(kcal.kg^{-1}.min^{-1})

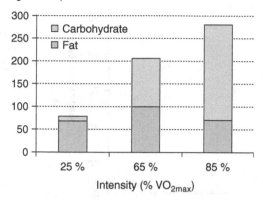

Figure 1.6   Carbohydrate and fat use at three exercise intensities (adapted from Romijn *et al.*, 1993)

longer than one minute), and the contributions of **carbohydrate** and fat at these levels of intensity can be realized in Figure 1.6. Note that fats contribute a greater percentage (and amount) of energy at 25% VO_{2max} (i.e. walking pace), around 50% of the energy at 65% VO_{2max} (i.e. steady state pace), and around 25% of the energy at 85% VO_{2max} (i.e. an intense aerobic bout with some significant anaerobic energy involved).

1.4   Energy systems and running speed

Based on world record times, humans can maintain maximum sprinting speed for approximately 200 m. The average speeds for the 100 m and 200 m world records are similar, at 22.4 mph and 21.6 mph respectively. However, with increasing distances, average speeds decline. The average speed for the marathon world record is 12.1 mph, which is 55% of the world sprint record. This is remarkable, since the marathon distance is more than 200 times the length of a 200 m race.

Although natural selection plays a crucial role in elite sprinting and marathon performance, the energy systems must also be highly trained and exercise-specific to be successful. For example,

the energy needed to maintain an average sprinting speed of 22 mph for 200 m or less, and that required for an average running speed of 12.1 mph for the marathon, are acquired by two very different systems (the predominant energy systems required for running at different speeds can be seen in Figure 1.3). The primary energy source for sprinting distances up to 100 m is PCr. From 100 m to 400 m, anaerobic glycolysis is the primary energy source. For distances longer than 800 m, athletes rely primarily on aerobic metabolism.

The rate of glycogen and fat utilization varies according to the relative running speed. Although the rate of glycogen utilization is low while running a marathon, the duration of the event increases the possibility of depleting glycogen stores. In contrast, the rate of glycogen utilization is substantially higher during a 5,000 m run, but glycogen depletion is not a concern because of the shorter duration of the event.

Maximum maintainable speed decreases by approximately 7 mph as running distance increases from 200 m to 1500 m. However, as the distance increases from 1500 m to 42.2 km, maximum maintainable speed only drops by an additional 3.5 mph. On average, a healthy, fit, non-elite, male athlete can be expected to sprint at an average speed of 16–18 mph for 100–200 m and at approximately 6–8 mph for a marathon (see Figure 1.7).

1.5   Why can't a marathon be sprinted?

Figure 1.7 clearly demonstrates the inability to sustain high running velocities for a protracted duration. So why is an athlete unable to keep up higher running speeds over a marathon distance? The different energy sources have already been noted above, but what it is necessary to understand is that each of these energy sources resynthesizes ATP at varying rates. Table 1.1 highlights the likely rates of ATP production, and you should note the hierarchy.

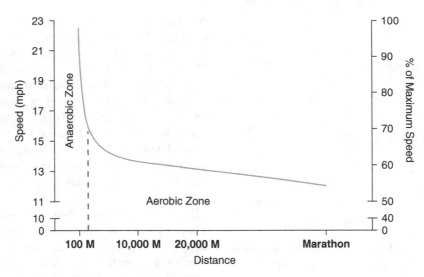

Figure 1.7 Sustainable running speed and distance run

Table 1.1 Maximum rates of energy production

Process	Maximum power
PCr → ATP	9 mM/kg/s
CHO → lactate + ATP	4 mM/kg/s
CHO → CO_2 + H_2O + ATP	2 mM/kg/s
Fat → CO_2 + H_2O + ATP	1 mM/kg/s

The PCr system is the most rapid of these ATP-producing systems. A calculated rate of 9 mM/kg dry muscle/s is more than twice as fast as ATP generation from anaerobic glycolysis which in turn is twice as fast as aerobic oxidation of carbohydrates. Furthermore, the aerobic breakdown of carbohydrates produces ATP at twice the rate of fats (i.e. 2 mM/kg/s vs. 1 mM/kg/s). It thus seems that energy processes in the cytoplasm produce ATP at a faster rate than those which require oxidation via the mitochondria, and that carbohydrates produce ATP quicker than fats.

In later chapters, we will see that whereas PCr generation of ATP is a single reaction, anaerobic glycolysis entails ten reactions, aerobic breakdown of glucose necessitates around 26 reactions (if the TCA cycle is used twice), and somewhere in the region of 90–100 reactions are required for complete fatty acid oxidation. No wonder, that there are varying rates for ATP production.

Since the muscle stores of PCr are rather limited, and the end product of the rapid ATP generation from anaerobic glycolysis produces lactic acid, it would appear that it is not possible for an athlete to keep running at a sprint pace when undertaking a marathon – they would either run out of PCr, or the pH of their muscles would be significantly reduced due to lactic acid production. In addition, there are also limited stores of muscle and liver carbohydrate (glycogen) which would seem to be problematic as a source of energy for a complete marathon, so the need to employ fatty acids is important in energy production. Fatty acids produce the slowest rates of ATP synthesis – hence the fact that when these stores are engaged, running speeds are lowered.

1.6 Energy sources and muscle

Table 1.2 highlights a number of key points in relation to energy sources for muscle. These include:

1. the total amount of the energy source, from which it is quite apparent that the faster

ATP-producing sources are limited (notably PCr and glycogen for anaerobic glycolysis);

2. the likely duration for which these energy sources will last if they are the only source of ATP production;

3. the maximal rates by which they can produce ATP.

1.7 Can muscle use protein for energy?

So far there has been little or no mention of using **proteins** for energy. Muscles are made of protein in the main, but can muscle protein provide energy? The answer is, to a limited extent, yes. A major difference between carbohydrates and fats is that they are essentially made up of carbon, hydrogen and oxygen only, whereas protein molecules also contain an amino group, (i.e. a nitrogen). The end result of carbohydrate and fat oxidation is the generation of carbon dioxide and water, whereas oxidation of proteins requires the removal of nitrogen.

Figure 1.8 illustrates the fact that amino acids (the basic structural component of proteins) can, after the removal of the nitrogen (which ends up as urea), be converted to carbohydrates,

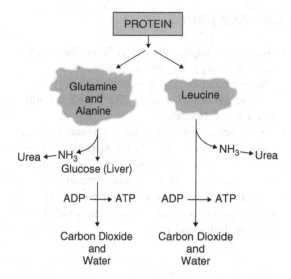

Figure 1.8 Likely use of amino acids for energy

which can then be oxidized. During prolonged exercise, the amino acids alanine and glutamine are converted to glucose in the liver, and the glucose is then oxidized by muscle. In addition, the muscle also has a limited capacity to oxidize the amino acid leucine. In total, amino acids usually accounts for 5% of the energy needed by muscle.

Table 1.2 Energy sources available to working muscle including amounts and likely duration before depletion

	ATP	PCr	Anaerobic glycolysis	Carbohydrte oxidation	Fatty acid oxidation
Total amount	40 g	120 g	350 g of CHO	500 g of CHO	15,000 g of fatty acids
Duration of exercise before depleted stores		4–6 s	1–2 min	1–2 h	>6 h
Max rate of ATP synthesis (mM/kg/s)		9	4	2	1

1.8 Key points

- Adenosine triphosphate (ATP) is the useable form of energy for muscle contraction.
- Phosphocreatine (PCr), anaerobic glycolysis and aerobic processes enable ATP to be resynthesized during exercise.
- High intensity bouts of exercise demand a faster rate of ATP generation if the activity is to proceed and this is achieved by the faster 'anaerobic' sources, i.e. PCr and anaerobic glycolysis.
- Low to moderate bouts of exercise use aerobic energy processes such as complete oxidation of carbohydrates and fats.

- ATP and PCr content are limited in muscle and hence the reduced capability to engage in very intense levels of activity for prolonged periods.
- Anaerobic glycolysis results in lactic acid formation which is considered by some research to contribute to fatigue.
- Carbohydrate sources of energy (glycogen) are limited in comparison with fat sources.
- Amino acids from protein breakdown can contribute to energy production in a limited manner.

2

Skeletal muscle structure and function

Learning outcomes

After studying this chapter, you should be able to:

- describe the gross anatomical structure of skeletal muscle;
- list the main sub-cellular components of the muscle fibre and outline their location and function;
- draw and label the sarcomere including the A-band, I-band, M-line and H-zone;
- describe the structure of the thick and thin filaments;
- define the term motor unit;
- explain the structure and function of the neuro-muscular junction;
- explain and outline the main stages involved in the process of muscle contraction;
- compare and contrast the structural, biochemical and functional properties of type I, type IIa and type IIx muscle fibres;
- explain how muscle fibres are recruited with varying exercise intensities;
- define what is meant by lengthening, shortening and isometric muscle contractions;
- highlight and explain the phases of a twitch contraction;
- describe how stimulation frequency affects contractile force and define the term tetanus;
- explain the length-tension and force-velocity relationships;
- define the terms fatigue, central fatigue and peripheral fatigue.

Key words

A-band	force-velocity relationship
actin	frequency
α-actinin	I-band
acetylcholine	isometric
ACh receptors	isotonic
ATPase	H-zone
central fatigue	latent period
concentric	length-tension
contraction phase	M-line
crossbridges	motor end plate
desmin	motor neurons
dihydropyridine receptor	motor unit
eccentric	M protein
endomysium	multinucleated
epimysium	muscle fibre
fascia	muscle glycogen
fascicles	muscle triglyceride
fast twitch	myofibrils
fatigue resistant	myoglobin

Biochemistry for Sport and Exercise Metabolism, First Edition. Don MacLaren and James Morton.
© 2012 John Wiley & Sons, Ltd. Published 2012 by John Wiley & Sons, Ltd.

myomesin	subsarcolemmal
myosin	mitochondria
nebulin	summation
perimysium	synaptic cleft
nebula	synaptic end bulbs
neuromuscular	synaptic vesciles
junction (NMJ)	
peripheral fatigue	tendons
point of origin	tetanus
point of insertion	thick filament
postmitotic	thin filament
principle of orderly	titin
recruitment	
relaxation phase	tropomyosin
ryanodine receptor	troponin
sarcolemma	troponin C
sarcomere	type I fibres
sarcoplasm	type IIa fibres
sarcoplasmic	type IIx fibres
reticulum	
satellite cells	twitch contraction
SERCA	T-tubules
size principle	Z-lines
sliding filament	
mechanism	

Skeletal muscle can be considered an organ as it is composed of cells from multiple tissues, i.e. nervous tissue, connective tissue, etc. and, of course, cells from muscle tissue itself. In this context, skeletal muscle is the largest organ in the human body, comprising 40 to 50% of total body weight.

There are over 600 muscles in our bodies, all performing common functions:

1. producing body movements;
2. maintaining posture;
3. storing and moving substances within the body; and
4. generating heat.

Skeletal muscle is so called because it primarily functions to move bones of the skeleton and as such, muscle tissue is connected to bones by connective tissue known as **tendons**. Each end of a specific skeletal muscle is attached to a bone that is essentially stationary (termed the ***point of origin***) or to a bone that is moved (termed the ***point of insertion***) during the specific muscle contraction. For example, the *biceps brachii* muscle has its points of origin and insertion in the scapula and radius bones, respectively.

2.1 Skeletal muscle structure

In Chapter 1, we provided an introductory overview of the energy sources and systems involved in producing energy for muscular activity. Given that our focus is on the provision of energy for working *skeletal muscle*, it follows that we should now develop a sound understanding of the both the structure and function of muscle itself. These topics are therefore the central theme of this chapter. Much of what will be discussed herein relates to the combined interplay between a variety of sub-cellular components and proteins involved in co-ordinating muscle contraction. For this reason, readers not familiar with general cell structure or protein function may wish to initially read sections of Chapter 4 prior to reading this chapter.

2.1.1 Gross anatomical structure

The gross anatomical structure of skeletal muscle is shown in Figure 2.1. Surrounding the entire whole muscle is a strong sheet of fibrous connective tissue known as *fascia*. Three separate layers of connective tissue then extend from the outermost layer of fascia to strengthen and protect the muscle further.

The initial layer encompassing the whole muscle is known as the *epimysium*. If we were to cut through the epimysium, we would then encounter the *perimysium*. The perimysium encloses groups of 10 to 100 muscle cells and essentially separates them into muscle cell bundles known as *fascicles*. In turn, each muscle cell within this bundle is also separated from one another by a layer of connective tissue known as the *endomysium*.

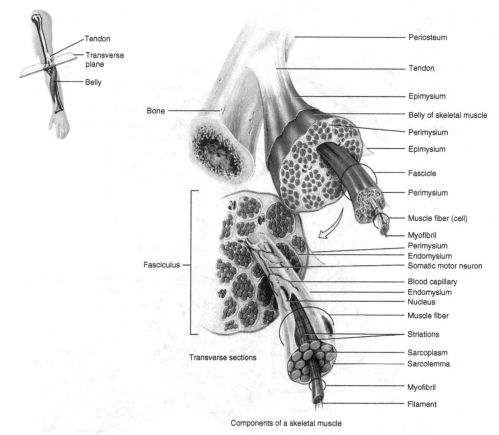

Components of a skeletal muscle

Figure 2.1   Gross anatomical structure of skeletal muscle. (From Tortora and Derrickson, *Principles of Anatomy and Physiology, Twelfth Edition*, 2009, reproduced by permission of John Wiley & Sons Inc.)

2.1.2 The muscle fibre

Skeletal muscle cells are more commonly referred to as *muscle fibres* and they differ from many other cells in the body for a number of reasons. Muscle fibres have a unique shape in that they are long and cylindrical and generally extend the entire length of the muscle itself. For example, for small muscles such as those of the eye, fibre length can be a few millimetres, whereas for those in the thigh, fibre length can be nearly 30 cm.

They are also *multinucleated* (i.e. can contain more than 100 nuclei located at the periphery of the fibre) and are *postmitotic* (i.e. they cannot undergo cell division). For this latter reason, the number of muscle fibres contained within a muscle is determined before we are born, and the

growth that occurs from childhood to adulthood occurs due to the growth of existing fibres. Most fibres range from 10 to 120 μm in diameter, and the number of fibres present in a single muscle can range from several hundred to more than a million.

Muscle cells are comprised of approximately 75% water, 20% protein and 5% of substances such as vitamins, minerals, various ions, amino acids, carbohydrates and fats. Given the extremely small size of the muscle fibre, we need to examine muscle cells under a microscope so as to learn about the ultrastructural level of skeletal muscle. A schematic illustration detailing the structure of a skeletal muscle fibre and its various cellular components is shown in Figure 2.2.

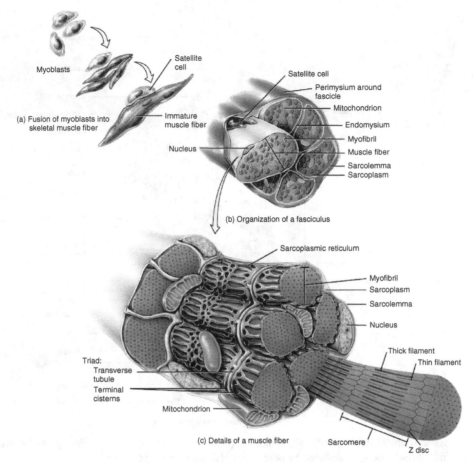

Figure 2.2 The structure of a single skeletal muscle fibre (cell). (From Tortora and Derrickson, *Principles of Anatomy and Physiology, Twelfth Edition*, 2009, reproduced by permission of John Wiley & Sons Inc.)

Sarcolemma

The plasma membrane of skeletal muscle cells is usually collectively known as the *sarcolemma*. However, the sarcolemma essentially consists of the plasma membrane (i.e. a lipid bilayer) and the basal lamina. Extending perpendicular from the surface of the sarcolemma through to the interior of each fibre are thousands of membranous channels known as transverse tubules (*T-tubules*). These channels are extremely important for the process of muscle contraction, as the action potential which propagates along the fibre membrane can subsequently travel to the interior of the fibre to activate the contractile apparatus (see Section 2.2).

Also located between the sarcolemma and the basal lamina are a pool of mononuclear undifferentiated cells known as *satellite cells*. These cells are important for skeletal muscle as they are capable of undergoing differentiation to develop into mature muscle fibres during times such as injury or indeed, muscle growth during strength training (Hawke & Garry, 2001). A pool of mitochondria is also located underneath the sarcolemma and is therefore referred to as *subsarcolemmal mitochondria*. The positions of these mitochondria are obviously advantageous as they reduce the diffusion distance for oxygen to travel from the capillaries delivering the blood supply to the site of utilization in the mitochondria.

Sarcoplasm

The *sarcoplasm* is the cytoplasm of skeletal muscle fibres and therefore contains all of the subcellular organelles (i.e. mitochondria, nuclei, etc.) and intracellular fluid. The sarcoplasm also contains vital energy stores such as *muscle glycogen* (the storage form of carbohydrate for muscle cells) and *muscle triglyceride* (the storage form of fat for muscle cells), as well as a small supply of ATP. In addition, the protein **myoglobin** is also located here, where it functions to store oxygen (similar to how haemoglobin in the bloodstream operates) until the mitochondria need it for ATP production. However, by far the largest component of the sarcoplasm are the *myofibrils*.

Myofibrils

Myofibrils are rod-like structures which run the entire length of the muscle fibre, as shown in Figure 2.3a. The number of myofibrils present within a muscle cell can vary but there are thought to be around 2000 in an adult muscle fibre (Jones *et al.* 2004). Myofibrils can be considered as the *contractile apparatus* of the muscle fibre as they contain the contractile proteins **actin** and **myosin**. Collectively, actin and myosin comprise 85% of total muscle protein, with myosin taking the lion's share (60%). The actin protein is 42 kDa in size and is often referred to as the *thin filament*, whereas myosin is referred to as the *thick filament* because it is 480 kDa.

The structure of the thick and thin filaments is shown in Figure 2.4. Note the unique shape of myosin molecules in that each molecule is shaped like two golf clubs twisted together – the myosin tail (i.e. the golf club shafts) points towards the centre of the **sarcomere** (the *M-line*). The myosin heads (often referred to as the **crossbridges**) project outward from the shaft in a spiralling fashion and extend towards one of the six thin filaments that surround each thick filament.

The main component of the thin filament is actin, where individual actin molecules are joined together to form an actin filament that is twisted into a helix-type structure. As we will cover in the next section, a major characteristic of actin filaments is that they contain a myosin binding site, where a myosin head can attach to initiate muscle contraction. In a relaxed muscle, however, myosin is prevented from binding to actin because strands of the **tropomyosin** protein cover the binding sites which in turn, are held in place, by another regulatory protein known as **troponin**.

Myofibrils can be further divided into smaller segments known as the *sarcomere*, which is the basic functional (i.e. contractile) unit of the muscle fibre (Figure 2.3b). A myofibril is therefore effectively a series of sarcomeres and, in relaxed conditions, the length of a sarcomere ranges from 2–2.5 μm.

When examined under a microscope, skeletal muscle has a striated appearance consisting of alternating light and dark bands known as the *I-band* and the *A-band* respectively. A schematic illustration and an electron micrograph of a sarcomere are shown in Figures 2.3b and 2.3c, respectively. A simple way to remember which of these contrasting bands is which is through remembering the second letter of both light (i.e. l*I*ght) and dark (i.e. d*A*rk).

The I-band predominantly contains the actin protein, whereas the A-band largely consists of the myosin protein. However, because of how actin and myosin are arranged (i.e. layers that run parallel to one another), there is also a zone of overlap. A narrow *H-zone* exists in the centre of the A-band, which contains thick filaments only. The H-zone itself is further bisected by a dark line known as the *M-line*.

Whereas approximately 85% of the protein forming the myofibrillar complex consists of actin and myosin, there are many other proteins which also play important structural and regulatory roles – for example, we have already mentioned troponin and tropomyosin, which form part of the thin filament. The M-line is composed of the structural proteins of **M protein** and **myomesin**, which essentially function to attach thick filaments to one another. Each sarcomere is also separated from each other by *Z-lines* which consist of structural proteins such as **nebulin**, **α-actinin** and **desmin**. These collectively function to bind thin filaments

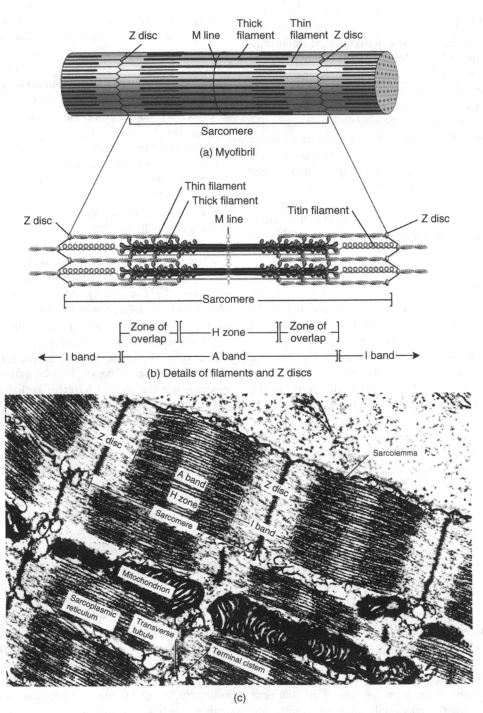

Figure 2.3 Arrangement of thick and thin filaments within a sarcomere. (From Tortora and Derrickson, *Principles of Anatomy and Physiology, Twelfth Edition*, 2009, reproduced by permission of John Wiley & Sons Inc.)

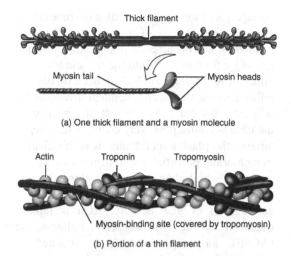

(a) One thick filament and a myosin molecule

(b) Portion of a thin filament

Figure 2.4 Structure of thick and thin filaments. (From Tortora and Derrickson, *Principles of Anatomy and Physiology, Twelfth Edition*, 2009, reproduced by permission of John Wiley & Sons Inc.)

from adjacent myofibrils together and provide overall structural integrity. **Titin** is the largest of muscle proteins and functions to stabilize myosin proteins along their longitudinal axis.

Sarcoplasmic reticulum

Surrounding the myofibril in an envelope-like fashion is a membranous network of channels known as the *sarcoplasmic reticulum* (SR) (see Figure 2.2). The SR runs parallel to the myofibrils and functions as a storage site for calcium ions in millimolar concentrations. It is the release of calcium from the SR into the sarcoplasm which is essential for muscle contraction. The SR also contains a protein pump that is known as the *sarcoendoplasmic reticulum* Ca^{2+} *ATPase* (**SERCA**) (Periasamy & Kalyanasundaram, 2007). This protein functions to 'pump' calcium back from the sarcoplasm into the SR in order to restore calcium levels back to the necessary concentration required for muscle contraction.

Neuromuscular junction

In order for muscle cells to function, they require an appropriate nerve supply. Fortunately,

skeletal muscle is well supplied with neural inputs through communication with the nervous system and, specifically, through the action of α-*motor neurons*. These cells have thread-like axons which extend out from the spinal cord to groups of muscle fibres. A *motor unit* is then defined as a single α-motor neuron and all of the muscle fibres which it innervates (see Figure 2.5). For small muscle groups such as those in the eye or the hand, a motor unit may contain only a few fibres, whereas for those motor units innervating large leg muscles there are typically a few thousand fibres.

The point of communication between the neuron and muscle fibre is referred to as the *neuromuscular junction* (**NMJ**). It is important to note that the two cells do not physically come into contact; rather, there is a small space between them known as the *synaptic cleft*. As the axons from the **motor neurons** extend towards the muscle fibre, they branch out into clusters known as *synaptic end bulbs*, in a similar fashion to how the main trunk of a tree divides into branches. Located within the cytosol of each end bulb are small, sac-like structures called *synaptic vesicles* which contains the neurotransmitter **acetylcholine** (ACh). As you will see in the next section, it is this release of ACh from the synaptic end bulbs (upon the delivery of a nerve impulse from the central nervous system) and its subsequent diffusion across the synaptic cleft which results in the necessary communication signalling the muscle fibre to contract.

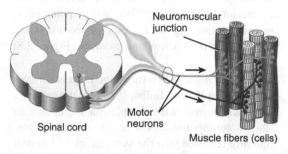

Figure 2.5 Illustration of the motor unit. (From Tortora and Derrickson, *Principles of Anatomy and Physiology, Twelfth Edition*, 2009, reproduced by permission of John Wiley & Sons Inc.)

The muscle fibre side of the NMJ is the region of sarcolemma opposite each synaptic end bulb and is known as the ***motor end plate***. It is the presence of transmembrane proteins known as ***ACh receptors*** within each motor end plate which permits this cell-to-cell communication to occur. An illustration of the NMJ and its related sub-components is shown in Figure 2.6.

2.2 Muscle contraction

Having outlined basic skeletal muscle structure, it is now appropriate to move onto the process of muscle contraction. When students begin to study this process, they often neglect the importance of the central nervous system and instead become more engrossed in the peripheral mechanisms of muscle contraction (Morton *et al.*, 2008). However, it is important to note that voluntary muscle contractions begin with a nerve impulse travelling from the motor cortex in the brain through to the spinal cord via the brain stem. As outlined in the Section 2.1, the neural impulses are then communicated to skeletal muscle fibres through the action of the motor neurons which branch out from the spinal cord (see Figure 2.7).

2.2.1 Propagation of the action potential

In order for muscle fibres to contract, an action potential needs to be generated and must propagate along the surface of the fibre and deep into the interior of the fibre. This action potential is generated according to a series of events at the NMJ, as described below and shown in Figure 2.8:

1. *Release of ACh.* When the nerve impulse arrives at the synaptic end bulbs, it causes the synaptic vesicles to fuse with the plasma membrane of the motor neuron. As a result, ACh is subsequently released into the synaptic cleft, where it can diffuse across the space between the motor neuron and motor end plate.
2. *Activation of ACh receptors and production of action potential.* The ACh receptors function as voltage-gated ion channels which become active upon binding of two ACh molecules. As soon as binding has occurred, the ion channel opens, causing a flow of Na^+ into the muscle fibre and efflux of K^+. However, Na^+ influx exceeds K^+ efflux because the electrochemical driving force is greater for Na^+. As a result, the interior of the fibre becomes positively charged, thus depolarizing the plasma membrane. It is this change in membrane potential which triggers the action potential, which then propagates along the sarcolemma and into the T-tubules.
3. *Termination of ACh activity.* ACh is rapidly degraded by the enzyme acetylcholinesterase (AChE), an enzyme which is attached to collagen fibres in the extracellular matrix of the synaptic cleft. For this reason, a continual production of muscle action potentials is needed in order for contractions to be sustained.

2.2.2 Excitation-contraction coupling

The process of excitation-contraction (EC) coupling collectively refers to those stages which connect muscle excitation (i.e. propagation of an action potential) through to muscle contraction itself (i.e. generation of force). While there are various steps in this process, the release of Ca^{2+} from the sarcoplasmic reticulum is an integral component. Calcium is stored in the SR in millimolar concentrations (at approx 10 mM), whereas its concentration in the sarcoplasm is 10,000 times lower (i.e. 0.1 μM).

The release of calcium is essentially underpinned by the conversion of an electrical signal into a chemical signal, and it requires the presence of two key membrane proteins. When the action potential has travelled into the T-tubules, it causes a conformational change in the voltage sensing type channel known as the ***dihydropyridine*** (DHP) ***receptor***. This change in DHP receptors, in turn, opens the calcium release channels in the SR, the ***ryanodine receptors (RyR)***. Calcium then flows down its electrochemical gradient, signalling the contractile apparatus to contract according to the ***sliding filament mechanism*** (see Figure 2.8).

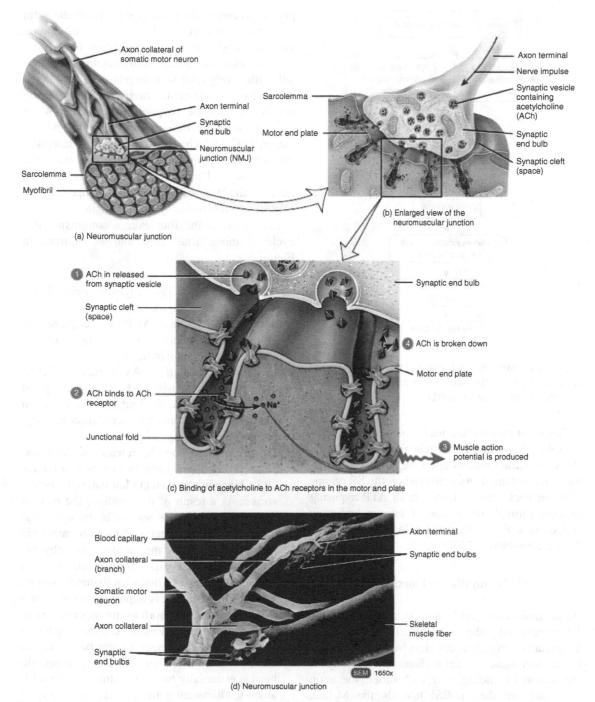

Figure 2.6   The neuromuscular junction (NMJ). (From Tortora and Derrickson, *Principles of Anatomy and Physiology, Twelfth Edition*, 2009, reproduced by permission of John Wiley & Sons Inc.)

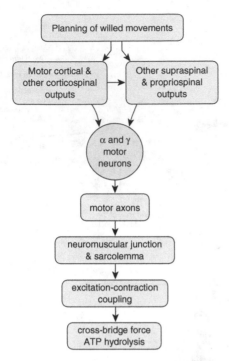

Figure 2.7 Simplified schematic of the chain of events from brain to muscle which result in force production. (adapted from Gandevia, 2001)

Note that the calcium needs to be pumped back into the SR so that it is again available to signal the contractile proteins upon the next delivery of an action potential. As noted earlier, the SR pumps calcium back into its lumen in an ATP-requiring process through the action of sarcoendoplasmic reticulum Ca^{2+} ATPase (SERCA) (Periasamy & Kalyanasundaram, 2007).

2.2.3   The sliding filament mechanism

At a molecular level, muscle contraction can be explained by the *sliding filament mechanism*. Essentially, this process involves the binding of myosin heads to actin filaments. By way of the action of sliding over each other, the actin filaments are then pulled towards the M-line. As a result, the overall length of the sarcomere shortens and hence the muscle fibre contracts.

In a relaxed muscle, however, myosin is prevented from binding to actin because the protein tropomyosin is wrapped around the actin filaments, thus covering the actin-myosin binding site. The positioning of tropomyosin is, in turn, held in place via three related proteins which we will collectively refer to as troponin (though in the instance of muscle contraction we are specifically concerned with the **troponin C** protein). When Ca^{2+} is released into the cytosol, it binds to troponin C, which then causes the troponin-tropomyosin complex to move away from the binding site. Upon exposure of the myosin binding site, the series of events comprising the *contraction-relaxation cycle* can begin.

Let's look at the four events comprising this cycle in more detail now and as outlined in Figure 2.9:

1. *ATP hydrolysis.* The myosin head binds ATP, and the enzyme myosin ATPase then hydrolyzes ATP into ADP and a phosphate group. The products of this reaction are still attached to the myosin head.
2. *Crossbridge formation.* As a result of ATP hydrolysis, the myosin head becomes energized and attaches to the binding site on the actin filament to form *crossbridges*. Upon binding, the phosphate group is released.
3. *Power stroke.* Upon the release of the phosphate group, the myosin head tilts and rotates on its hinge in a movement known as the *power stroke*. As a result of the rotation, the myosin head generates forces and pulls the actin filaments towards the centre of the sarcomere via the sliding filament mechanism, whereby the thin and thick filaments slide over one another. As a consequence of the actin filaments sliding towards the M-line, it is important to note that it is the I-band which shortens during contraction, whereas the A-band does not change length (see Figure 2.10). The stages of the power stroke can be likened to walking, in that each myosin head is essentially 'walking' along the actin filaments, ultimately getting closer and closer to the Z-disc. In turn, the actin filaments are being pulled towards the M-line.
4. *Detachment of myosin from actin.* At the end of the power stroke, the myosin then releases ADP

and myosin remains bound to actin until the next supply of ATP binds to myosin. Upon ATP binding, myosin then becomes released and the contraction cycle can begin again when ATPase hydrolyzes ATP.

In order for the above events to occur, it is important to appreciate that there needs to be a continual supply of ATP and Ca^{2+}. Depending on the particular contractile conditions (e.g. intensity and duration), the continual production of ATP can be provided from high-energy phosphates and/or the metabolism of carbohydrate, fat or protein, as introduced in Chapter 1. Part 2 will outline the basic biochemical pathways involved in these processes and, in Part 3 we will examine the regulation of these pathways during different types of sports and exercise.

2.3 Muscle fibre types

2.3.1 General classification of muscle fibres

Generally speaking, human muscle fibres can be classified into three types according to the structural, biochemical and contractile properties of the fibre. These fibres are referred to as type I (slow oxidative fibres, SO), type IIa (fast oxidative glycolytic fibres, FOG) and type IIx (fast glycolytic fibres, FG).

Much of what we now know about muscle fibres has been learned through the muscle biopsy technique, which was first applied in the sport and exercise sciences in the late 1960s. An overview of the distinguishing characteristics of these fibres are shown in Table 2.1 and discussed in the following sections.

Slow oxidative fibres

Type I fibres are referred to as slow 'twitch' oxidative fibres, largely because the isoform of myosin ATPase present in these fibres hydrolyzes ATP at a relatively slow rate. As a result, the contractions proceed at a slow pace, the maximal force produced is relatively small (compared to type II fibres) and their ATP production is mainly supported by the oxidative metabolism of carbohydrate and fat. These fibres are the smallest in diameter of all muscle fibres, and appear as red due to the presence of large myoglobin stores and the large supply of blood capillaries. The fibres contain a large amount of mitochondria and are therefore capable of producing ATP aerobically for sustained periods of time. As a result, these fibres are highly **fatigue resistant** and are active in endurance type exercise events such as marathon running, cycling, etc.

Fast oxidative glycolytic fibres

Type IIa fibres are referred to as fast oxidative glycolytic fibres, given their capacity to support ATP production by both means of aerobic and anaerobic metabolism. As such, they are often viewed as intermediary between type I and type IIx. The isoform of myosin ATPase present within these fibres is capable of hydrolyzing ATP at a faster rate (approximately 3–5 times faster) than type I fibres. They also contain a moderate amount of myoglobin and mitochondria, thus making them somewhat fatigue resistant. Given their capacity to hydrolyze ATP at a faster rate (and thus with a higher rate of contraction and relaxation), these fibres can produce greater force than type I fibres and are highly active during high-intensity activities undertaken at near-maximal or supra-maximal levels, i.e. close to maximal aerobic capacity or sprinting (e.g. 400–800 m races).

Fast glycolytic fibres

Type IIx fibres contain the least amount of myoglobin and mitochondria (and are therefore white in colour), have limited capacity for oxidative metabolism and thus are the least resistant to fatigue of all fibre types. However, the isoform of myosin ATPase present in these fibres can hydrolyze ATP at a fast rate and they are capable of both high rates and absolute levels of maximal force production. For these reasons, type IIx fibres are heavily recruited during activities which require maximal rates of force production and crossbridge formation, such as sprinting or

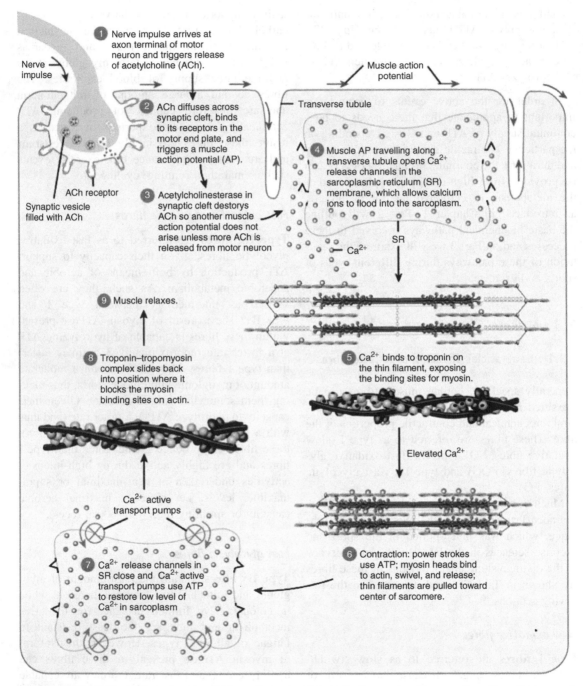

Figure 2.8   Initiation and propagation of the action potential, excitation-contraction coupling. (From Tortora and Derrickson, *Principles of Anatomy and Physiology, Twelfth Edition*, 2009, reproduced by permission of John Wiley & Sons Inc.)

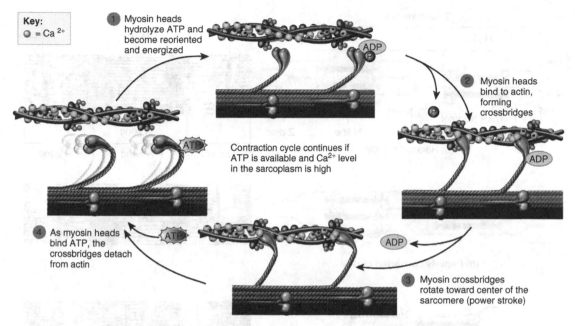

Key:
○ = Ca²⁺

1. Myosin heads hydrolyze ATP and become reoriented and energized

2. Myosin heads bind to actin, forming crossbridges

Contraction cycle continues if ATP is available and Ca²⁺ level in the sarcoplasm is high

4. As myosin heads bind ATP, the crossbridges detach from actin

3. Myosin crossbridges rotate toward center of the sarcomere (power stroke)

Figure 2.9   The contraction-relaxation cycle. (From Tortora and Derrickson, *Principles of Anatomy and Physiology, Twelfth Edition*, 2009, reproduced by permission of John Wiley & Sons Inc.)

weightlifting. ATP production is mostly supported through anaerobic metabolism via the breakdown of carbohydrates or through phosphocreatine metabolism. These fibres also have a large capacity to hypertrophy (i.e. get bigger) during strength training programmes, via the accumulation of more myofibrillar proteins which ultimately result in greater force production.

2.3.2   Muscle fibre distribution

Most of our muscles contain a mixture of all three fibre types. In sedentary men and women, the ratio is typically around 45–55% slow twitch, with the remainder equal proportions of the type II sub-fibre types. There are instances, however, in which muscles have a greater proportion of certain fibre types, depending on their function or the individual's training history, genetics, etc. For example, postural muscles such as those in the neck, back and legs tend to have a high proportion of slow twitch fibres due to the continual need for tension.

Given the distinct differences between muscle fibres' structural, functional and biochemical characteristics, it is tempting to speculate that elite athletes have a greater proportion of specific fibre types, depending on their chosen sport. There are, indeed, numerous data sets available to confirm this hypothesis.

For example, endurance-based athletes such as elite runners and cyclists tend to have a greater percentage proportion of type I fibres, and these fibres tend to be slightly larger than type II fibres (Costill *et al.*, 1976). Conversely, athletes involved in power-based sports, such as weightlifters and sprinters, have a greater proportion of type II fibres, which are also hypertrophied. A comparison of the percentage of type I and type II fibres from male sprinters, distance runners and non-athletes is shown in Table 2.2.

While the variation between fibre types can be highly distinguishable between athletes from very different sporting backgrounds, it should be noted that variation also exists between fibre type proportions within elite athletes in a given sport (Costill *et al.*, 1976). For this reason, fibre type alone is

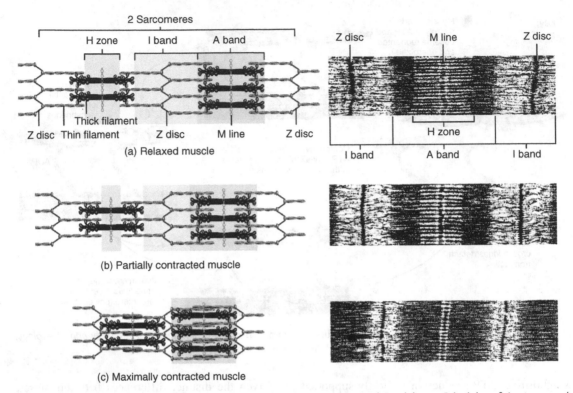

Figure 2.10 Sarcomere shortening during contraction. (From Tortora and Derrickson, *Principles of Anatomy and Physiology, Twelfth Edition*, 2009, reproduced by permission of John Wiley & Sons Inc.)

not the only determinant of sporting performance, and it is the complex interplay between a host of physiological, biochemical, biomechanical and psychological factors which underpin human performance (Joyner & Coyle, 2008).

2.3.3 Muscle fibre recruitment

Whereas most skeletal muscles contain a mixture of fibre types, the muscle fibres within a given motor unit are all of the same type. We have already outlined in Table 2.1 that there are more muscle fibres present in type IIa and type IIx motor units compared with type I motor units. For this reason, when a type I α-motor neuron is activated, there are fewer absolute muscle fibres activated compared with when a type II α-motor neuron is activated. As a result, type II fibres reach peak tension quicker and collectively they generate more force than type I fibres.

When our muscles contract, the contribution of specific fibre types towards the contractile force generated is dependent on the intensity and duration of the contraction. For example, if only small amounts of force are required, such as in walking or in light jogging, then slow twitch fibres will be most active. If the pace of jogging increases to higher-intensity running, then type IIa fibres will become active. Finally, if the exercises progresses to an 'all-out' sprint, type IIx fibres are recruited. Muscle fibres are therefore recruited in a sequential manner (i.e. type I, type IIa and type IIx), according to the increase in exercise intensity.

This sequential recruitment of fibre types is known as the *principle of orderly recruitment*, which may be explained by the *size principle* which states that the recruitment of motor units is directly related to motor neuron size. Because the type I motor units have smaller motor neurons, it is these that are recruited first as exercise

Table 2.1   Qualitative characteristics of human muscle fibre types. Description of activity of key biochemical enzymes are based on review of data cited by Spurway & Wackerhage (2006)

	Type I	Type IIa	Type IIx
Structural			
Colour	dark red	red	white
Type of myosin ATPase	slow	fast	fastest
Myoglobin content	large	medium	low
Mitochondrial density	high	medium	low
Fibre diameter	small	medium	large
Capillaries density	high	medium	low
Motor neuron size	small	medium	large
Fibres per neuron	≤ 300	≥ 300	≥ 300
Functional/contractile			
Fatigue resistance	high	moderate	low
Oxidative capacity	high	moderate	low
Glycolytic capacity	low	high	highest
Vmax (speed of shortening)	low	intermediate	highest
Specific tension	moderate	high	high
Recruitment order	first	second	third
Biochemical			
Metabolism	oxidative	oxidative/ glycolytic	glycolytic
Glycogen stores	low	medium	high
Creatine kinase activity	low	medium	high
Phosphorylase activity	low	medium	high
Phosphofructokinase activity	low	medium	high
Lactate dehydrogenase activity	low	high	highest
Citrate synthase activity	high	medium	low
Succinate dehydrogenase activity	high	medium	low
3-hydroxyacyl dehydrogenase activity	high	medium	low

intensity progresses from rest to low to moderate, after which type II motor units with larger motor neurons also contribute to force production (see Figure 2.11).

Much of what we know about muscle fibre recruitment patterns during exercise comes from research investigating muscle glycogen depletion patterns in different muscle fibre types. Typically, such research has demonstrated that glycogen depletion is greatest in type I fibres during low to moderate intensity exercise, whereas depletion is greatest in type IIa/x fibres during high-intensity activity (Gollnick *et al.*, 1974).

It can therefore be concluded that type I fibres are preferentially recruited during prolonged endurance type events where absolute exercise intensity (e.g. running speed) is relatively low, whereas type II fibres are recruited more in higher-intensity activity such as fast-paced running and sprinting, etc.

In sports characterized by alternating periods of sprinting and running/jogging/walking (e.g. soccer), it is no surprise to see glycogen depletion in all fibre types during exercise (Krustrup *et al.*, 2006). These sports are characterized by intermittent activity profiles, and we will examine

Table 2.2 Typical muscle fibre composition in elite male athletes and non-athletes. Data taken from Costill *et al.* (1976)

	Per cent slow (Type I)	Per cent fast (Type IIa/x)
Distance runners	65–75	25–35
Sprinters	20–30	70–80
Non-athletes	45–55	45–55

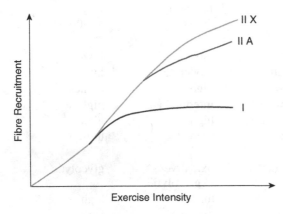

Figure 2.11 Muscle fibre recruitment as a function of exercise intensity

the bioenergetics of this type of activity in detail in Chapter 10.

2.4 Muscles in action

2.4.1 Types of muscle contraction

When a muscle produces force (i.e. tension), it can do so by contracting dynamically (often referred to as an *isotonic* contraction) via the muscle, either *shortening* (a **concentric** contraction) or *lengthening* (an **eccentric** contraction). Alternatively, the muscle can also produce force by an **isometric** contraction (often referred to as static contractions), where the muscle neither shortens or lengthens. Although the terms 'eccentric' and 'concentric' are frequently used in the literature, they are scientifically incorrect

and muscle physiologists therefore prefer to classify contractions as lengthening or shortening (Faulkner, 2003).

Examples of the different types of contractions can be considered when performing a standard bench press exercise commonly undertaken by athletes. Lowering the bar towards the chest muscles during the initial part of the exercise is an example of a lengthening contraction. Conversely, raising the bar upwards from the chest during the final part of the exercise is a concentric contraction. If you were to keep the bar raised above your chest and prevent it from eventually lowering back towards your chest due to the pull of gravity, this would be an isometric contraction, as in this case your muscle is producing tension without actual movement. Examples of isometric contractions in sport and exercise would be exerting force in tackling activities such as in a rugby scrum. Isometric contractions are also important in everyday life as they help to maintain posture and balance.

2.4.2 The twitch contraction

When the muscle fibres within a motor unit are stimulated by a single action potential, the resultant contractile force produced is known as a ***twitch contraction***. A muscle twitch can be studied in the laboratory by direct electrical stimulation of a motor neuron or its muscle fibres. The recording of the muscle contraction can be recorded on a myogram; various characteristics of the contraction, such as time to peak tension and relaxation, etc. can then be recorded. An example of a typical muscle twitch and the various sub-phases are shown in Figure 2.12.

Whereas the duration of a single action potential is very small (1–2 ms), the duration and rate of the actual twitch contraction/relaxation produced is much larger (20–200 ms) and is dependent on fibre type (for many of the reasons outlined in Table 2.1). Note that there is an initial **latent period** (a few milliseconds) between onset of the stimulus and resultant development of tension. During this phase, Ca^{2+} are released from the SR, thus signalling the contractile apparatus to undergo actin-myosin binding and crossbridge

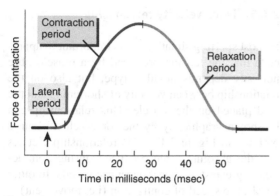

Figure 2.12 A muscle twitch contraction. (From Tortora and Derrickson, *Principles of Anatomy and Physiology, Twelfth Edition*, 2009, reproduced by permission of John Wiley & Sons Inc.)

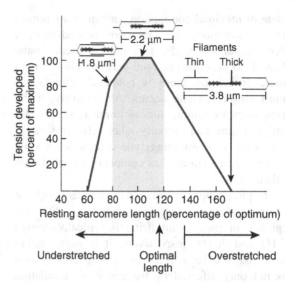

Figure 2.13 The length-tension relationship which dictates that the tension produced during contraction is dependent on the initial sarcomere length. (From Tortora and Derrickson, *Principles of Anatomy and Physiology, Twelfth Edition*, 2009, reproduced by permission of John Wiley & Sons Inc.)

formation. During the **contraction phase**, the sarcomere changes length to a point where peak tension occurs. Muscle tension then decreases in the **relaxation phase** (which usually occurs at a slower rate the contraction phase), when the sarcomere returns to its original length. In this phase, Ca^{2+} are pumped back into the SR so that they are available for contraction upon the delivery of the next action potential.

2.4.3 The length-tension relationship

The actual tension developed by a muscle fibre during contraction is a function of the sarcomere length at the *onset* of contraction, and thus the number of crossbridges formed between the thick and thin filaments. This relationship is known as the *length-tension relationship* and is shown in Figure 2.13. Here you can see that if the contraction were to begin at the initial resting sarcomere length shown in the green zone, then maximal tension would develop. This initial position is known as the optimal resting sarcomere length. If the contraction was to begin when there is very little overlap at the long sarcomere length, then not much force would develop at the beginning of contraction. Similarly, if the thick and thin filaments have too much overlap initially, where the thick filaments can only pull the thin filaments a short distance, then little force will be generated.

Furthermore, if there are no more binding sites available for myosin to form new crossbridges then no force will be generated.

2.4.4 Tetanus contractions

It is important to appreciate that the type of muscle contractions that occur in sport- and exercise-related activities are not the result of a single twitch contraction generated by the delivery of only one action potential. Rather, these types of contractions are due to multiple action potentials stimulating the muscle fibre within a short period of time. As a result of this increased **frequency** of action potentials, the muscle fibre does not have time to relax in between each twitch contraction and the actual force produced is additive, to create a much greater force than a single twitch. This process is known as *summation*.

If the frequency of stimulation (i.e. the number of action potentials per second) is high enough (usually around 60–100 Hz), relaxation between twitches is diminished until the fibre achieves a state of maximal contraction, known as a *tetanus*. In this situation, the contraction is said to be a *fused tetanus*, as the individual twitches have 'fused' to produce maximal tension. They remain there (providing there is continual stimulation) until muscle fatigue occurs. Alternatively, if the frequency of stimulation is lower (i.e. <30 Hz) and the fibre can partially relax between stimuli, the result is a wavering type contraction known as an *unfused tetanus*, as complete fusion has not taken place.

In physiological situations such as weak or strong voluntary muscle contractions, the frequency of motor unit firing is typically around 5 Hz and 70 Hz, respectively. It is important to note that the force produced during contractions is not only affected by frequency of stimulation but also by recruiting an increasing amount of motor units, as would be the case when we increase exercise intensity. An example myogram illustrating differences in tension produced during single, unfused and fused contractions is shown in Figure 2.14.

2.4.5　Force-velocity relationship

In most sporting situations, it is important to appreciate that the tension produced by a muscle fibre not only depends on fibre type, but also on the relationship between velocity of shortening and the load placed on the muscle. This relationship can be shown graphically by the force-velocity curve outlined in Figure 2.15. This relationship dictates that the absolute force produced during contraction is greatest at slow, concentric speeds. In other words, the speed of contraction (i.e. movement) is greatest at low workloads – a relationship which is true for both slow and fast twitch fibres. Indeed, it is easy to flex your biceps muscle quickly when no dumbbell is in your hand, compared to when you are holding a 20 kg dumbbell!

Given that most sporting events require the development of power (a product of force × velocity), it follows that there is a trade-off between training with the optimal load and velocity in order to develop the power-generating capacity of the muscle.

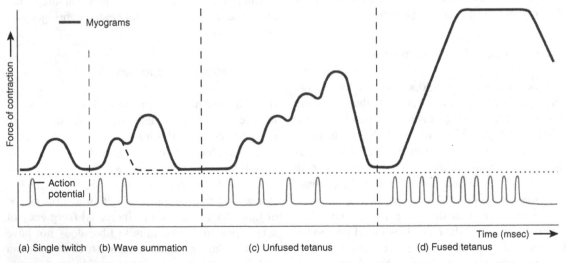

Figure 2.14 Differences in tension produced during single and multiple twitches. (From Tortora and Derrickson, *Principles of Anatomy and Physiology, Twelfth Edition*, 2009, reproduced by permission of John Wiley & Sons Inc.)

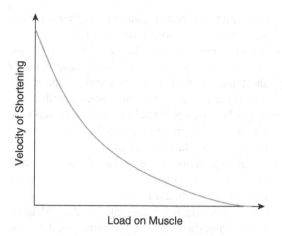

Figure 2.15 Force-velocity relationship during skeletal muscle contraction

2.4.6 Muscle fatigue

One of the most highly research areas within the sport and exercise sciences are the mechanisms by which muscles become fatigued during exercise. Fatigue can be most simply defined as *an inability to maintain a given force or power output during repeated muscle contractions*.

Though relatively straightforward in definition, actually undertaking research to ascertain the underlying physiology and biochemistry underpinning exercise-induced fatigue has proved a major challenge for exercise scientists (see Allen *et al.*, 2008 for an excellent review). Furthermore, much of this research has also been conducted in animal models using isolated single fibres. While such approaches have proved insightful in terms of elucidating potential detailed biochemical mechanisms of fatigue, it is likely that the findings produced are not entirely relevant to the exercising human performing whole-body exercise.

Despite the uncertainty surrounding this area, two general theories of fatigue have emerged. The first describes *central fatigue*, meaning that the processes underpinning the decline in force are due to disturbances at the level above the NMJ. Alternatively, the cause of fatigue could be peripheral in location (i.e. *peripheral fatigue*), due to metabolic disturbances below the NMJ and in the muscle itself (refer back to Figure 2.7 for an overview of the chain of events involved in force production).

Given that the focus of this text is on *skeletal muscle*, we are concerned with those events that are peripheral in nature which could lead to inability to produce force. Examination of Figure 2.8 suggests this could be due to a failure of propagation of the action potential along the sarcolemma, in EC coupling, in crossbridge formation and also reduced energy availability. Furthermore, the precise location(s) and cause(s) of fatigue within this chain of events is also likely to be highly dependent on the type of contraction, the predominant muscle fibre type involved, exercise mode, duration, intensity and environment, as well as the nutritional and training status of the individual, etc. For this reason, potential causes of muscle fatigue are discussed in Part 3 of this book, where we will examine specific exercise scenarios of high-intensity, endurance and intermittent exercise.

2.5 Key points

- Muscle fibres are long, cylindrical cells that are multinucleated and postmitotic.
- Myofibrils runs the entire length of the muscle fibre and contain the thin (actin) and thick (myosin) filaments.
- Myofibrils are composed of sarcomeres, the basic contractile units of muscle fibres.
- ACh release from the synaptic end bulbs activate ACh receptors on the motor end plate to generate an action potential.
- Action potentials travel to the T-tubules and signals the SR to release Ca^{2+} into the cytoplasm.
- Ca^{2+} binds to troponin C and exposes the myosin binding site on the actin filaments.

- ATP hydrolysis causes the myosin head to bind actin and form crossbridges.
- The power stroke causes the myosin heads to rotate, thereby generating force which pulls the actin filaments towards the M-line according to the sliding filament mechanism.
- During contraction, the I-band shortens, whereas the A-band does not change length.
- Muscle fibres can be categorized as type I (slow twitch), type IIa (fast oxidative glycolytic) or type IIx (fast glycolytic) fibres, according to their structural, biochemical and functional properties.
- Most muscles contain a mixture of fibre types, with approximately 50% slow and the remainder equally shared between the fast fibres.
- Elite athletes tend to have a higher proportion of fibre types that are most suited to the demands of the specific sport.
- Muscle fibres are recruited in an exercise-dependent fashion, with slow twitch being used during sub-maximal contractions and fast twitch becoming recruited during higher-intensity activities, when more force is required.
- Muscles can produce force through dynamic contractions, where the muscle lengthens or shortens, or during an isometric contraction, where the muscle does not change length.
- A single action potential produces a twitch contraction which can be separated into latent, contraction and relaxation phases.
- Increasing frequency of action potentials generated causes summation and induces a high-force contraction termed a tetanus.
- The contractile force generated is dependent on initial sarcomere length, as determined by the length-tension relationship.
- The force-velocity relationship dictates that the absolute contractile force produced is greater at slower speeds of shortening.
- Muscle fatigue (i.e. inability to maintain a desired force) may be either central or peripheral in location.

3

Biochemical concepts

Learning outcomes

After studying this chapter, you should be able to:

- identify the main chemical elements in the human body;
- describe and draw basic atomic structure;
- identify the differences between atoms, ions, molecules and compounds;
- distinguish the difference between ionic and covalent bonds;
- define a chemical reaction and identify the difference between an endergonic and exergonic reaction;
- define energy and the units of energy;
- describe the role of ATP within the cell;
- describe the common forms of chemical reactions including synthesis, decomposition, reversible, exchange, phosphorylation/dephosphorylation and oxidation/reduction reactions;
- outline the functions of water and the chemical property underpinning water's ability to act as a solvent;
- define the terms mole, molar and molarity;
- define the terms acid, base and salt;
- draw and define the pH scale and describe what is meant by the terms acidic and alkaline;

- describe basic cell structure with particular emphasis to the plasma membrane, nucleus, cytoplasm and mitochondria.

Key words

acid	chemical reaction
alkaline	cholesterol
amino	chromosomes
anabolic	compound
anion	concentration
atom	condensation
atomic mass	covalent bond
atomic mass unit	cytoplasm
atomic number	cytoskeleton
ATP	cytosol
Avogadro's number	dalton
base	decomposition
buffers	dehydrogenation
calorie	DNA
carbon	dephosphorylation
carbon skeleton	electrons
carbohydrates	electron acceptor
catabolic	electron shell
cation	elements
chemical bonding	endergonic
chemical energy	

Biochemistry for Sport and Exercise Metabolism, First Edition. Don MacLaren and James Morton.
© 2012 John Wiley & Sons, Ltd. Published 2012 by John Wiley & Sons, Ltd.

endoplasmic
   reticulum
energy
exercise metabolism
exchange
exergonic
extracellular fluid
fats
functional groups
glycolipids
golgi apparatus
genes
histones
hydrogen
hydrolysis
hydrophilic
hydrophobic
inorganic
   compounds
integral proteins
intracellular fluid
ion channels
ionic bond
ions
irreversible
isotopes
isomers
joules
kilocalorie
kilojules
lactate
lactic acid
lipid bilayer
macronutrients
mass number
matter
megajoule
metabolism
minerals
mitochondria
mitochondrial
   matrix
molarity
mole
molecular formula
molecule

neutral
neutrons
nitrogen
nonpolar
nuclear envelope
nucleolus
nucleus
organs
organelles
organic compound
oxidation
oxidative
   phosphorylation
oxygen
peripheral proteins
pH scale
phospholipids
phosphorylation
plasma membrane
polar
products
proteins
protons
proton acceptor
proton donor
redox
reversible
ribosomes
reactants
receptor proteins
reducing equivalents
reduction
salts
solute
solution
solvent
sport and exercise
   metabolism
synthesis
tissues
transmembrane
   proteins
transporter proteins
vitamins
water

3.1 Organization of matter

3.1.1 Matter and elements

All things, living and non-living, consist of *matter*, defined as anything that occupies space and has mass. Matter, in turn, is made up of chemical building blocks known as *elements* – substances which cannot be split into simpler substances by ordinary chemical means. There are 112 known chemical elements, 92 of which occur naturally on Earth. Of these 92 elements, there are 26 which occur normally in our bodies. Each element can be symbolized using a one- or two-letter abbreviation which, in the following paragraphs, we include in brackets after stating the name of the element in question.

The most abundant elements which make up our bodies (constituting approximately 96% of our body's mass) are **oxygen** (O), **carbon** (C), **hydrogen** (H) and **nitrogen** (N).

Eight other elements make up 3.8% of our body's mass. These include calcium (Ca), phosphorous (P), potassium (K), sulphur (S), sodium (Na), chlorine (Cl), magnesium (Mg) and iron (Fe).

The remaining 0.8% of the body's store of elements consists of 14 elements known as the *trace elements*. These include aluminium (Al), boron (B), chromium (Cr), cobalt (Co), copper (Cu), fluorine (F), iodine (I), manganese (Mn), molybdenum (Mo), selenium (Se), silicon (Si), tin (Sn), vanadium (V) and zinc (Zn).

Elements are important for human life. They are components of the **energy** sources of **carbohydrates**, **fats** and **proteins**, and they also provide us with **water** and important **vitamins** and **minerals** that are needed to sustain healthy living. An overview of the main chemical elements within the human body is shown in Table 3.1.

3.1.2 Atoms and atomic structure

Each element is made from *atoms*, which are the smallest units of matter. Atoms are extremely

Table 3.1   An overview of the body's main chemical elements and some of their known functions

Chemical element (symbol)	Percentage abundance in the human body	Function
Oxygen (O)	65	Used to generate energy using aerobic processes and also part of water and energy sources such as carbohydrates, fats and proteins.
Carbon (C)	18.5	Important component of organic (i.e. carbon-containing) molecules such as carbohydrates, fats, proteins and deoxyribonucleic acids (DNA – a cell's genetic material).
Hydrogen (H)	9.5	Component of water and most organic molecules.
Nitrogen (N)	3.2	Component of all proteins and DNA.
Calcium (Ca)	1.5	Important component for maintenance of bones and teeth; also involved in regulatory processes such as hormone release, muscle contraction and enzyme activation.
Phosphorous (P)	1	Component of ATP (the immediate energy supply for muscle contraction) and DNA.
Potassium (K)	0.35	Important component of intracellular fluid and needed to generate the action potential required for muscle contraction.
Sulphur (S)	0.25	Component of vitamins and many proteins.
Sodium (Na)	0.2	Component of extracellular fluid; essential for maintaining water balance and also needed to generate the action potential required for muscle contraction.
Chlorine (Cl)	0.2	Component of extracellular fluid and essential for maintaining water balance.
Magnesium (Mg)	0.1	Important component of many specialized proteins known as enzymes.
Iron (Fe)	0.005	Important component of red blood cells and many enzymes.

small and are impossible for us to see with the naked eye. In fact, approximately 200,000 atoms could fit on the end of a pencil! Atoms are made from the special arrangement of sub-atomic particles known as *protons, neutrons* and *electrons*. The basic structure of an **atom** consists of a central core known as the *nucleus* in which exist positively charged protons (p^+) and uncharged neutrons (n^0). Negatively charged electrons (e^-) orbit regions around the nucleus known as *electron shells*, the number of which depends on the specific element.

This basic structure of an atom is shown in Figure 3.1. For ease of understanding, electron shells are depicted diagrammatically as 'circles' around the nucleus, although it should be noted that, in reality, electrons do not follow a fixed path or spherical orbits but form negatively charged clouds which surround the nucleus in 'shells'. Each **electron shell** can only hold a specific number of electrons. For example, the first shell (closest to the nucleus) can only ever hold two electrons, while the second can hold eight, the third can hold a maximum of 18 and so on. It

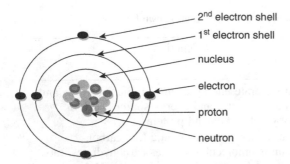

2nd electron shell
1st electron shell
nucleus
electron
proton
neutron

Figure 3.1 Basic diagrammatic representation of an atom. In this example, the atom's nucleus contains six protons and six neutrons, and there are also six electrons in the orbit. As always, the first electron shell holds two electrons and in this case the second shell holds four

is important to note that the number of electrons and protons in an atom of an element are always equal. For this reason, the overall charge of an atom is zero.

3.1.3 Atomic number and mass number

What makes the atoms of one element different from another is the number of protons present in the nucleus. This is called the *atomic number*. For example, atoms of hydrogen, oxygen, carbon, nitrogen and so on are primarily different because they each contain different numbers of protons.

The *mass number* of an atom is the sum of its protons and neutrons. Atoms of elements will always have the same atomic number (i.e. number of protons), but in some cases they may have different numbers of neutrons and hence different mass numbers (see Figure 3.2 for examples). Such atoms are referred to as *isotopes*. In most cases, these are *stable isotopes* because their nuclear structure does not change over time. Atoms of the common elements of carbon, nitrogen and oxygen, for example, can exist as stable isotopes. Although isotopes of an element have different numbers of neutrons, they each have identical chemical properties because they all contain the same number of electrons. Progressing from what you learned from Figure 3.1, Figure 3.2 shows how the atomic structure of specific atoms differ from one another on the basis of the number of protons they have.

3.1.4 Atomic mass

The *atomic mass* (often referred to as *atomic weight*) of an element is the average mass of all its naturally occurring isotopes. The standard unit for atomic mass (*atomic mass unit*, *abbreviated as 'amu'*) is the *dalton*, which is symbolized as Da. The mass of a neutron is 1.008 Da, the mass of a proton is 1.007 Da and the mass of an electron is 0.0005 Da. In its purest sense, the Da can be defined as one-twelfth of the mass of a carbon ^{12}C atom and therefore equates to the extremely small mass of 1.66×10^{-24} grams! When rounded to the nearest whole number, the atomic mass of an element typically coincides with the mass number of the predominant isotope of that element (see Figure 3.2).

3.1.5 Ions, molecules, compounds and macronutrients

As stated previously, the electrical charge of an atom is **neutral** because the number of positively charged protons is equal to the number of negatively charged electrons. However, atoms have a characteristic way of becoming charged by gaining or losing one or more electrons. When an atom undergoes this process (called *ionization*), it now becomes known as an *ion*. More specifically, it will be either an *anion* (a negatively charged ion because it has gained an electron) or a *cation* (a positively charged ion because it has lost an electron). We can symbolize the ion by writing the chemical symbol of the atom in question followed by the number of positive or negative charges in superscript. For example, Ca^{2+} designates a calcium ion with two positive charges because it has lost two electrons. Similarly, Cl^- designates a chlorine atom (now know as a chloride ion) with a negative charge because it has gained one electron.

Within our bodies, atoms not only exist in free form by themselves but can also join together with other atoms of the same element, or atoms of other elements, to form molecules. A *molecule* exists when two or more atoms join together. For example, when two oxygen atoms join

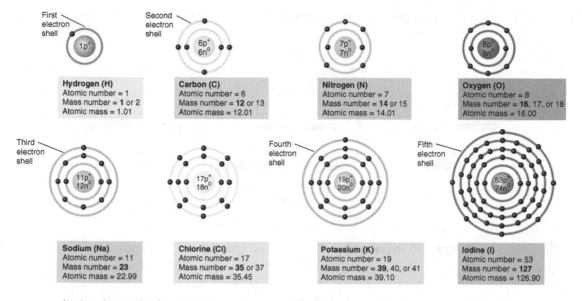

First electron shell

Second electron shell

Hydrogen (H)
Atomic number = 1
Mass number = **1** or 2
Atomic mass = 1.01

Carbon (C)
Atomic number = 6
Mass number = **12** or 13
Atomic mass = 12.01

Nitrogen (N)
Atomic number = 7
Mass number = **14** or 15
Atomic mass = 14.01

Oxygen (O)
Atomic number = 8
Mass number = **16**, 17, or 18
Atomic mass = 16.00

Third electron shell

Fourth electron shell

Fifth electron shell

Sodium (Na)
Atomic number = 11
Mass number = **23**
Atomic mass = 22.99

Chlorine (Cl)
Atomic number = 17
Mass number = **35** or 37
Atomic mass = 35.45

Potassium (K)
Atomic number = 19
Mass number = **39**, 40, or 41
Atomic mass = 39.10

Iodine (I)
Atomic number = 53
Mass number = **127**
Atomic mass = 126.90

Atomic number = number of protons in an atom
Mass number = number of protons and neutrons in an atom (boldface indicates most common isotope)
Atomic mass = average mass of all stable atoms of a given elements in daltons

Figure 3.2   Basic diagrammatic representation of the atomic structure of several stable atoms. Note the difference in atomic structures between atoms. You should also note that because these atoms exist as stable isotopes, the mass number can differ because they can differ in the number of neutrons present in the nucleus. (adapted from Tortora and Derrickson, *Principles of Anatomy and Physiology, Twelfth Edition*, 2009, reproduced by permission of John Wiley & Sons Inc.)

together they form an oxygen molecule which is symbolized as O_2.

A *compound* is a substance which has molecules comprised of atoms of two or more different elements. For example, water is a compound because it consists of two hydrogen atoms joined together with an oxygen atom, and it is thus symbolized as H_2O. It is important to note that while *all compounds are molecules, not all molecules are compounds*.

Most of the chemical elements in our bodies exist in the form of compounds which can be further classified as *inorganic compounds* (lacking carbon) or *organic compounds* (containing carbon). Some of the most important organic compounds that are relevant to **sport and exercise metabolism** include carbohydrates, fats and proteins. Collectively, these compounds are called the *macronutrients*, and it is through the action of specific biochemical processes (i.e. **chemical reactions**) that our bodies utilize these food sources to provide our muscles with the energy to exercise. Figure 3.3 shows the general flow of chemical organization from atom to macronutrient.

3.2   Chemical bonding

Atoms join together to make molecules or compounds through the process of **chemical bonding**. There are two main types of chemical bonds (*ionic and covalent*) by which atoms can join together, though both bonds involve the use of electrons in the outermost shell (i.e. the *valence shell*) to form the chemical bond. The valence shells of most atoms in elements are not typically stable with even numbers of electrons. However, if the conditions are appropriate, two or more atoms can interact by either sharing electrons or donating electrons to one another so that each atom can obtain a stable valance shell.

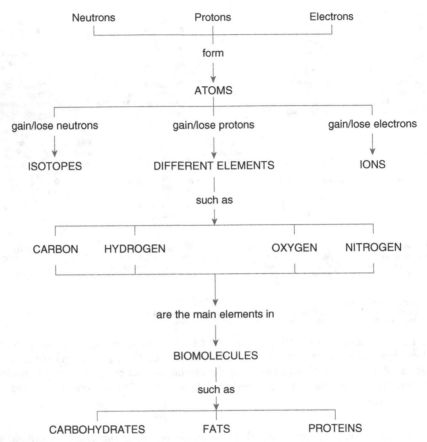

Figure 3.3   The basic flow of matter. Atoms of elements such as oxygen, carbon, hydrogen and nitrogen ultimately combine to make biomolecules, examples of which include the foodstuffs and fluids that we eat and drink in order to fuel our muscles during exercise and, more importantly, to sustain daily life

3.2.1   Ionic bonds

We have seen above how atoms can become **ions** by losing or gaining an electron, which ultimately results in a positively or negatively charged ion, respectively. If you have two atoms that can achieve a stable valence shell by either donating or gaining an electron, the result is a force of attraction which can bond the oppositely charged atoms together via an ***ionic bond***. This is most simply illustrated through the bonding of sodium (Na) and chlorine (Cl) atoms to make the compound sodium chloride (NaCl), which is the chemical name for common table salt (see Figure 3.4). It is important to remember that whenever atoms

bond via ionic bonds, the net charge of the newly formed compound is always zero.

3.2.2   Covalent bonds

In contrast to ionic bonds, ***covalent bonds*** (the strongest of all chemical bonds) work on the principle of atoms *sharing* electrons. Atoms can form covalent bonds by sharing one, two or three pairs of their valence electrons to make a *single, double* or *triple* covalent bond, respectively (see Figure 3.5). The larger the number of electron pairs shared, the stronger the covalent bond.

Covalent bonds can be further classified as ***nonpolar*** or ***polar***. In nonpolar covalent bonds,

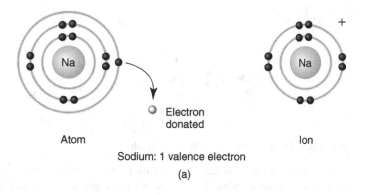

Electron
donated

Atom   Ion

Sodium: 1 valence electron

(a)

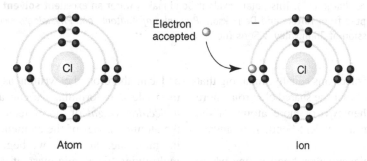

Electron
accepted

Atom   Ion

Chlorine: 7 valence electrons

(b)

Ionic bond in sodium chloride (NaCl)

(c)

Packing of ions in a crystal
of sodium chloride

(d)

Figure 3.4   Ionic bond formation. In this example, sodium forms an ionic bond with chlorine by donating an electron to the chlorine atom. The sodium atom now becomes positively charged and the chlorine atom now becomes negatively charged. (adapted from Tortora and Derrickson, *Principles of Anatomy and Physiology, Twelfth Edition*, 2009, reproduced by permission of John Wiley & Sons Inc.)

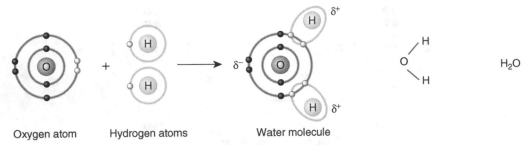

Oxygen atom   Hydrogen atoms   Water molecule

Figure 3.5 Covalent bond formation. In this example, electrons are shared equally between oxygen and hydrogen atoms. This bond is referred to as a polar covalent bond because the oxygen atoms attract the electrons more strongly. As such, the oxygen end of the water molecule has a partial negative charge (δ^-) and the hydrogen ends have a partial positive charge (δ^+). This polar covalent bond makes water an excellent **solvent**, as discussed later in this chapter. (adapted from Tortora and Derrickson, *Principles of Anatomy and Physiology, Twelfth Edition*, 2009, reproduced by permission of John Wiley & Sons Inc.)

the atoms share the electrons equally, meaning that one atom does not attract the shared electrons more than the other. When two or more atoms of the same element form a covalent bond, it is always nonpolar.

In contrast, a polar covalent bond is one where the sharing of electrons between atoms is unequal, so that one atom attracts the shared electrons more than the other. An important example of polar covalent bond is a water molecule (H_2O); here, it is the oxygen atom which has the greater power to attract electrons to itself (greater *electronegativity*) from the two hydrogen atoms.

3.2.3   Molecular formulae and structures

In briefly recapping what we have covered so far, you should now appreciate that atoms from elements can combine together, largely through the action of ionic or covalent bonds, to make molecules and compounds. In biochemistry, we can depict the atoms which form the molecule or compound through writing its **molecular formula**, which involves writing the chemical symbols of the atoms involved and moreover, the number of atoms of each element involved.

For example, one molecule of glucose (a vital energy source for exercise) contains six carbon atoms, 12 hydrogen atoms and six oxygen atoms

and can therefore be written as $C_6H_{12}O_6$. From the molecular formula, we can also calculate the *molecular weight* of the molecule, i.e. the sum of the atomic masses of the elements which make up the molecule. Note that we begin this process by multiplying the atomic mass of the element by the number of atoms present in the compound. For example, since glucose contains six carbon atoms, 12 hydrogen atoms and six oxygen atoms and the atomic masses of each element are 12, 1 and 16 respectively, the molecular weight can be calculated as follows:

$$C_6H_{12}O_6 = (12 \times 6) + (1 \times 12) + (16 \times 6) = 180$$

In addition to molecular formula, we are also interested in knowing the molecular structure (i.e. *constitutional formula*) of the compound – the structural arrangement by which the atoms have bonded to form the compound.

Figure 3.6a shows the molecular structure of a glucose molecule. A single line symbolizes a single covalent bond between atoms and a double line symbolizes a double covalent bond. Similarly, if there were a triple covalent bond between atoms present in this molecule, it would be symbolized by a triple line. In this example, the structure of glucose is shown in an open chain format which appears to exist as a two-dimensional structure. However, it is important to note

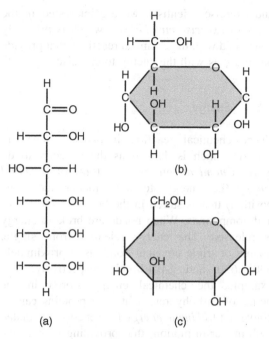

Figure 3.6 (a) Molecular structure of a glucose molecule. Note that the single and double lines represent a single or double covalent bond, respectively. (b) Molecular structure of glucose as shown as a ring like structure. (c) Molecular structure of glucose as written in shorthand method. In this example, carbon atoms are understood to be at locations where two bond lines interact and single hydrogen atoms are not shown

that in reality, molecules and compounds exist as three-dimensional structures. Furthermore, many compounds are also formed in special structural shapes. For example, the majority of glucose molecules in our bodies are stored in a ring-like structure comprising a ring-shaped 'carbon skeleton' with hydroxyl groups attached (hydroxyl groups consist of an oxygen and carbon atom joined by a single covalent bond) (see Figure 3.6b). Given that organic molecules and compounds are often relatively big, we sometimes draw their constitutional formula using shorthand methods (see Figure 3.6c).

In understanding molecular formulae and structures, it is important to note that some compounds can have the same molecular formula (i.e. the same number and type of atoms) but can differ in constitutional formula because the atoms have

bonded in a different structural arrangement. Such molecules are called *isomers*, and one example is that of glucose and fructose, which both have a formula of $C_6H_{12}O_6$. We will re-visit these compounds in Chapter 5.

3.2.4 Functional groups

Since we have now covered the basic processes of chemical bonding, it is also important to note that many atoms can bond repeatedly within compounds in certain combinations to yield specific *functional groups*. Indeed, during chemical reactions (see next section) the atoms contained within these functional groups tend to move between compounds as a *unit* rather than as individual atoms. Much of these functional groups can bond to a carbon atom (or to a chain of carbon atoms known as a carbon skeleton) via a single covalent bond to form ring-like structures or straight or branched chains. Some of the most important functional groups are shown in Table 3.2, where we also show the shorthand notation and bond structure.

Table 3.2 Common functional groups found within biological compounds. R denotes carbon skeleton to which the functional group is attached to

Name	Shorthand notation	Bond structure
Carboxyl	–COOH	O ‖ R–C–OH
Hydroxyl	–OH	R–O–H
Amino	–NH₂	H / R–N \ H
Phosphate	–PO₄	O ‖ R–O–P–O⁻ ‖ O⁻
Carbonyl	–CO	O ‖ R–C–R
Sulphydryl	–SH	R–S–H

3.3 Chemical reactions, ATP and energy

Within our bodies, there are thousands of *chemical reactions* occurring which underpin all of the body's essential processes. A **chemical reaction** occurs when the bonds between atoms are broken or when new bonds are formed between atoms. As outlined in the previous section, it is the interactions of electrons in the valence shell of atoms which form the basis of all chemical reactions. In simple terms, a chemical reaction consists of a substance or substances known as the *reactants*, which subsequently react to form the product or *products*. This is shown in Figure 3.7, which also uses the example of the reaction between hydrogen and oxygen molecules to produce water. The arrow in the equation represents the direction of the reaction, although, as will be explained later, some reactions are **reversible** – they can occur in both directions.

Notice that in this reaction, two molecules of hydrogen are required. This is due to the *Law of Conservation of Mass*, which states that the total mass of the reactants equals the total mass of the products (i.e. the number of atoms of each element is the same before and after the reaction). Although the total number of atoms is the same, the structural arrangements of the atoms have been changed, and it is for this reason that the newly formed products have different chemical properties.

The term *metabolism* refers to all of the chemical reactions which occur in our bodies. As sport and exercise scientists, we are interested in the study of *exercise metabolism*, which is primarily concerned with the chemical reactions that provide our muscles with the energy to exercise.

3.3.1 Energy

Every chemical reaction involves changes in *energy*, which is defined as the capacity to do work. ***Chemical energy*** is a form of *potential energy* (i.e. energy stored by matter due to its position) that is stored in the bonds of molecules and compounds. When bonds are broken, energy is released. The energy released from single, double or triple covalent bonds is approximately 330, 630 and 840 kJ/mol, respectively. For example, the chemical energy stored in the bonds of carbohydrates, fats and proteins can be converted to *kinetic energy* (i.e. energy associated with matter in motion) thus providing us with the *mechanical* energy needed to exercise.

According to the *Law of Conservation of Energy*, energy cannot be created or destroyed but it can be converted from one form to another. For instance, in the previous example, energy stored in the food we eat was converted to kinetic (mechanical) energy to provide us with the energy to exercise. Conversion of energy from one form to another also releases *heat* energy, which is why our bodies can get very hot during exercise. Both muscle and body (core) temperature can rise by 5°C and 3°C, respectively, during intense exercise (Drust *et al.*, 2005).

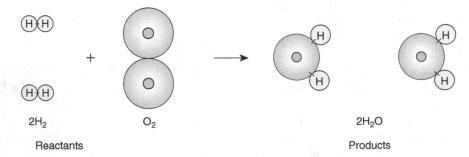

$2H_2$ O_2 $2H_2O$

Reactants   Products

Figure 3.7 Chemical reactions between two hydrogen molecules and one oxygen molecule to form two molecules of water, as formed by the breaking of old bonds and linking of new ones

The chemical reactions which take place in our bodies are of two main types:

1. **Exergonic reactions**: these are often referred to as *energy-producing* reactions as they release more energy than they absorb, i.e. the energy released when new bonds form is greater than the energy needed to break old bonds. Good examples of **exergonic** reactions are those that occur when we break down the bonds contained in carbohydrates, fats and proteins. In such circumstances, the energy produced can be subsequently stored inside the covalent bonds of a compound known as adenosine triphosphate (**ATP**).

2. **Endergonic reactions**: these are often referred to as *energy-consuming* reactions as they absorb more energy than they release, i.e. the energy released when new bonds form is less than the energy needed to break old bonds. A good example of an **endergonic** reaction is the process of muscle contraction, which requires the energy released from the breakdown of the covalent bonds of ATP to allow contraction to occur.

3.3.2 ATP

An important aspect of metabolism is the coupling between exergonic and endergonic reactions (see Figure 3.8). For example, the food we eat can be broken down to provide energy (an exergonic reaction), which can be subsequently used to make ATP (an endergonic reaction). In turn, the ATP can be broken down to provide energy (an exergonic reaction), which can be subsequently used for energy-consuming reactions such as allowing muscles to contract (an endergonic reaction).

ATP is often referred to as the *energy currency* of the cell, as it functions to transfer the energy produced in exergonic reactions to cellular activities that require energy (endergonic reactions) such as exercise, movement of substances within and between cells, synthesis of larger molecules from smaller ones, etc. Indeed, ATP is the only form of chemical energy which can be converted to other forms of energy used by living cells.

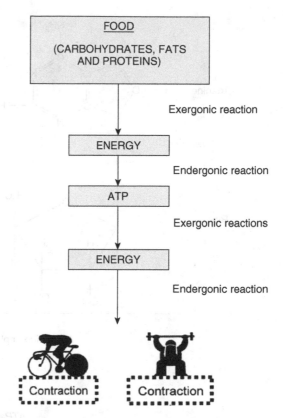

Figure 3.8 Schematic illustration of the coupling between exergonic (energy-liberating) and endergonic (energy-consuming) chemical reactions

The structure of an ATP molecule is shown in Figure 3.9a and essentially comprises of an adenosine molecule (adenine and ribose) with three phosphate groups attached. ATP can provide energy, as shown by the equation outlined in Figure 3.9b. Although we use the energy derived from ATP **hydrolysis** to fuel various cellular activities, a cell's ATP store is small (usually 20–30 mmol/kg dry muscle) and would be completely depleted within seconds of maximal exercise! However, we can regenerate ATP so as to sustain exercise for a longer period of time, so muscle ATP stores are never depleted by more than 20–40% even during exhaustive exercise (Spriet *et al.*, 1989).

The fundamental aim of this book, therefore, is to highlight how muscle cells can extract energy

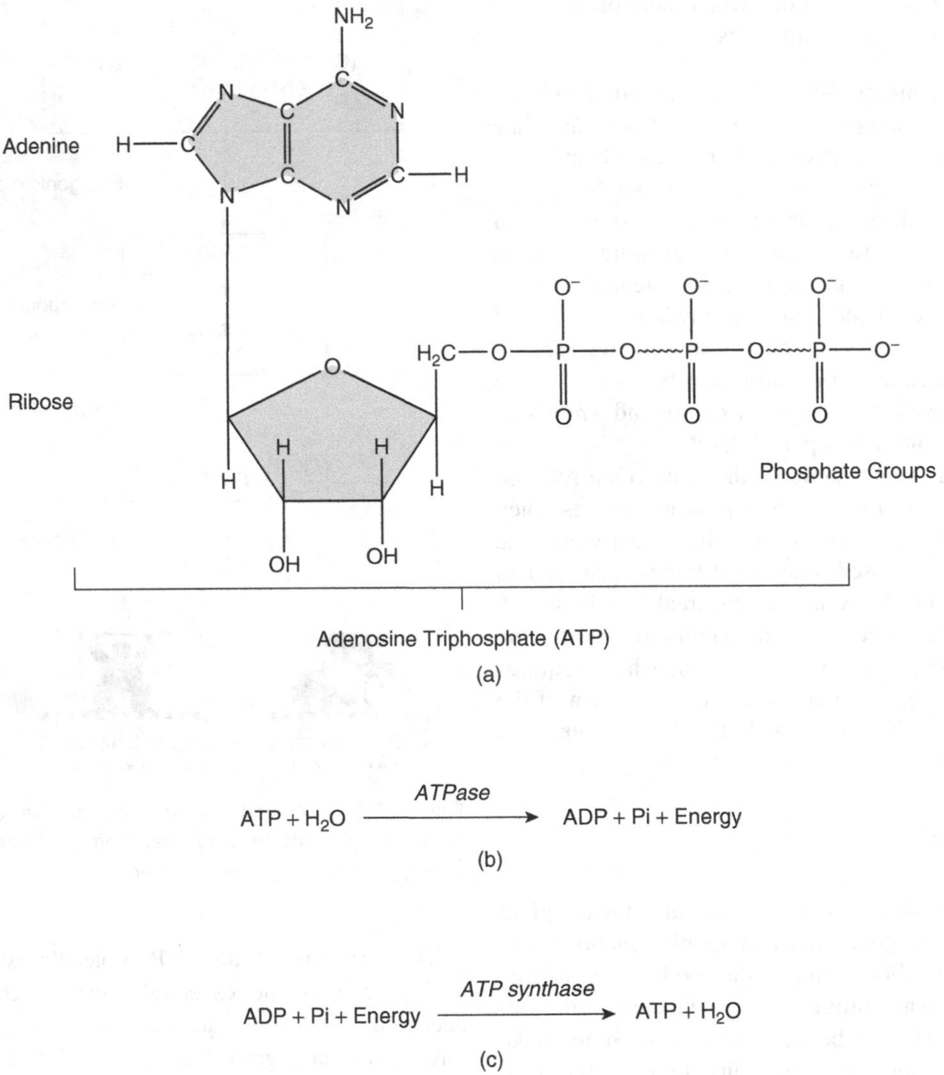

Adenine

Ribose

Phosphate Groups

Adenosine Triphosphate (ATP)

(a)

$$ATP + H_2O \xrightarrow{\text{ATPase}} ADP + Pi + Energy$$

(b)

$$ADP + Pi + Energy \xrightarrow{\text{ATP synthase}} ATP + H_2O$$

(c)

Figure 3.9   (a) The structure of ATP. (b) ATP hydrolysis to produce energy to fuel cellular activities, as catalysed by the enzyme ATPase. (c) The resynthesis of ATP, as catalysed by the enzyme ATP synthase. In this case, the energy is provided from breaking the bonds contained in compounds such as carbohydrates, fats and proteins. The importance of enzymes in facilitating chemical reactions is covered in Chapter 4

from compounds such as carbohydrates, fats and proteins, so as to replenish ATP stores and sustain exercise capacity and performance. Chapters 4, 5 and 6 will outline the biochemical pathways involved in these processes, while the chapters in Part 3 will specifically examine the regulation of the utilization of these pathways during different types of exercise.

3.3.3   Units of energy

Free energy changes are measured in units known as **calories**, one calorie being defined as the amount of heat required to raise the temperature of 1 gram of water by 1°C. We can measure the energy content of food using a 'bomb calorimeter', which is essentially a sealed chamber filled with oxygen that is enclosed in a water tank. By completely burning the food (*oxidation*), the chemical bonds in the structure are broken, thus releasing heat energy which subsequently heats the water. From measuring the rise in water temperature, the energy content of the food can then be calculated.

Given that the calorie is a relatively small unit, the terms *kilocalorie* (kcal) or *Calorie* (Cal, note the spelling with an upper case C) is more often used to measure energy. A kcal is equal to 1,000 calories and refers to the amount of heat required to raise 1 kg of water by 1°C. Thus, if we say that a slice of bread contains 80 Calories, we are actually referring to 80 kcal. In this situation, the 80 kcal in the slice of bread would therefore contain enough energy to raise the temperature of 80 kg of water by 1°C. From studies using the bomb calorimeter and after accounting for the process of digestion, the energy available from carbohydrate, protein and fat equates to 4, 9 and 4 kcal per 1 gram of substrate.

In addition to the kilocalorie, the standard international units for measuring energy are the *joule* (J) and the *kilojoule* (kJ). To convert from kilocalories to kilojoules, we must multiply the kcal value by 4.184. Thus in the above example, the energy value of a slice of bread is 80 kcal or 334.7 kJ. In order to avoid working with large numbers, we also use the term *megajoule* (MJ), which is equivalent to a 1,000 kJ.

Most healthy adults consume in the region of 2,000 to 3,000 kcal per day (or 8.4–12.6 MJ). Due to the intense energy demands of training and competition, elite athletes need to consume more; for example, Tour de France cyclists have been reported to consume up to 35 MJ per day during competition when they can be riding for eight hours daily (Saris *et al.*, 1989). For sports nutrition professionals, a thorough understanding of an athlete's energy expenditure is therefore crucial in order to optimize nutritional programmes for energy provision and recovery from training and competition.

Energy expenditure can be measured directly by having an athlete exercise in a specially designed bomb calorimeter and subsequently measuring the heat produced during exercise. However, because such methods are expensive and technically challenging, we can indirectly measure energy expenditure by measuring oxygen consumption (VO_2), owing to the fact that VO_2 increases with exercise intensity, thus providing an indirect measure of heat production. As a general rule of thumb, approximately 5 kcal of energy is produced for every 1 litre of oxygen consumed, although the precise amount of energy produced depends on the proportion of carbohydrate and fat oxidized.

3.3.4 Types of chemical reactions

When a chemical reaction occurs, the atoms in a newly formed product are arranged structurally different from how they were arranged when present as reactants. As a result, the newly formed product is likely to have different chemical properties. The chemical reactions which occur in our bodies can be classified as specific types of reaction, according to how the products have been formed. The common reactions which occur in our bodies are summarized below.

Synthesis reactions

When two or more atoms, ions, molecules or compounds combine to make larger molecules, the reaction is known as a *synthesis* reaction. This can be summarized as follows, where A and B join together to make a larger compound known as AB.

$$A + B \rightarrow AB$$

Synthesis reactions are also known as *anabolic* reactions and are usually endergonic, as energy is required in order for A and B to combine. In some cases, synthesis reactions can also be referred to as *condensation* reactions, as water is produced as a by-product of the reaction. A good example of a synthesis reaction which involves condensation is when **amino acids** join together through peptide bonds and a water molecule is produced. We will cover this issue in more detail in Chapter 4.

Decomposition reactions

When molecules or compounds split into smaller atoms, ions or molecules, the reaction is known as a *decomposition* reaction. For example, in the reaction below, molecule AB has been split into molecules A and B.

$$AB \rightarrow A + B$$

Decomposition reactions are also known as *catabolic* reactions and are usually exergonic, because they release more energy than they absorb. In some cases, decomposition reactions involve *hydrolysis* (i.e. splitting with water), as water reacts with the molecule or compound, causing the breakage of the bonds. For example, when our muscles break down ATP to provide energy for muscle contraction (as shown in Figure 3.9b), it does so via the addition of a water molecule.

Reversible reactions

In the above examples, you should notice that the direction of the arrow was from left to right only. This means that the reaction can only proceed in this direction and it is said to be *irreversible*. However, there are also many chemical reactions which are said to be *reversible*, meaning that the products from one reaction can also be converted to their original reactants. We can symbolize reversible reactions using an arrow which points in both directions:

$$AB \leftrightarrow A + B$$

Phosphorylation and dephosphorylation reactions

Many metabolic reactions occurring in the body, especially during exercise, involve the addition or removal of a phosphate group to or from a compound, respectively. For example, in the below reaction, molecule A has had a phosphate group attached (abbreviated as P_i for inorganic phosphate) and is now said to have been *phosphorylated*.

$$A + P_i \rightarrow A\,P_i$$

Removal of a phosphate group is known as *dephosphorylation* and can be written as follows:

$$A\,P_i \rightarrow A + P_i$$

As we will see in Chapter 4, many enzymes (proteins which assist in accelerating metabolic reactions to take place) exist in both dephosphorylated and phosphorylated forms. Usually (but not always), the enzymes are inactive when in their dephosphorylated form but, upon becoming phosphorylated, they become active and gain function. This switching between **phosphorylation** state has been likened to the turning on (phosphorylation) and off (dephosphorylation) of a light switch (Houston, 2006) in that it induces a rapid change in activation.

Exchange reactions

Many reactions occurring in our bodies are also known as *exchange* reactions and they consist of both synthesis and decomposition reactions. In exchange reactions, atoms or ions which exist in a larger molecule or compound can be transferred to another molecule or compound and vice versa. For example, in the following reaction, the bonds between A and B and between C and D have been broken (decomposition), thus allowing new bonds to form between A and C and B and D (synthesis).

$$AB + CD \rightarrow AC + BD$$

Oxidation-reduction reactions

Oxidation reactions involve the removal of electrons from an ion, molecule or compound, whereas *reduction* reactions involve the addition of electrons to the relevant molecular structure. A simple way to remember these reactions is through the use of the acronym OIL RIG (Oxidation Is Loss, Reduction is Gain). Where a molecule has undergone oxidation or reduction, it is said to have been *oxidized* or *reduced*, respectively.

Oxidation and reduction reactions are always coupled, meaning that every time a molecule has been oxidized, another molecule has simultaneously been reduced. Such reactions are also frequently referred to as *redox* reactions. Given that redox reactions involve the transfer of electrons from one molecule to another, they can also be considered as a form of exchange reaction as outlined below. For example, in this reaction, ion A has become reduced because it has gained an electron (thus lowering its positive charge), while molecule B has been oxidized as it has lost an electron to ion A (thus increasing its positive charge).

$$A^{3+} + B^{+} \rightarrow A^{2+} + B^{2+}$$

Although, strictly speaking, redox reactions involve the transfer of electrons, the most common form of redox reaction involves the exchange of hydrogen atoms between molecules (where the molecule has been oxidized, the reaction can therefore be further classified as a **dehydrogenation** reaction). In such cases, the reaction is still an example of a redox reaction because, every time a hydrogen atom leaves a molecule, it does so with an electron attached. For this reason, hydrogen atoms are often referred to as **reducing equivalents**, because they are equivalent to electrons (recall from Figure 3.1 that hydrogen atoms have a single proton and electron).

Redox reactions involving the transfer of hydrogen atoms are essentially the underpinning basis for exercise metabolism during endurance-type exercise, because it is the transfer of hydrogen atoms from the food we eat to oxygen molecules (to produce water) which produces the energy store (ATP) to fuel our muscles during exercise. In such circumstances, oxygen is said to be the final **electron acceptor**, as it undergoes a four-electron reduction (by accepting four hydrogen atoms) to produce water. Collectively, this process is known as **oxidative phosphorylation** and we will cover this in detail in Chapter 5.

Oxidation reactions are usually exergonic reactions as they involve the loss of hydrogen atoms from energy-rich reduced compounds (containing many hydrogen atoms) to lower-energy compounds. In the case of oxidation of food such as carbohydrates, some of the energy released through the breakage of bonds (i.e. removal of hydrogen atoms) is used to phosphorylate ADP to ATP (i.e. *substrate phosphorylation*). The energy has therefore been transferred and stored in ATP molecules so that it can later be used to drive energy-consuming processes such as exercise.

Misconception:

Because of the name of *oxidation* reactions, it is a common misconception that oxidation reactions always involve oxygen atoms. In reality, however, many biological compounds which do not contain oxygen can be oxidized, providing they have lost an electron (or a hydrogen atom).

3.4 Water

Water (H_2O) is the most important abundant inorganic (i.e. lacking carbon) compound in the body, and it is essential to the maintenance of life. Whereas we might be able to live for weeks without food, we can die without water in days. Indeed, athletes involved in weight-making sports such as wrestling and boxing often rely on dehydration to 'make the weight' and, in extremes cases of intended dehydration, this has led to death (Centers for Disease Control and Prevention, 1998). The adult human body is about 60% water by weight, and the water content also varies among different **tissues**. For example, blood is about 90% water, muscle 75%, bone 25% and adipose tissue 5%. Approximately two-thirds of body water is found inside our body cells and exists as **intracellular fluid**, and one-third exists outside our cells as **extracellular fluid**.

3.4.1 General functions of water

Water serves many important functions, such as *transportation* (via the blood) of nutrients and oxygen to different tissues (e.g. our muscles), and it also serves to remove waste products (e.g. carbon dioxide) from tissues. The transportation function of water is therefore very important to exercise. Water in urine removes other waste products such as urea, excess salt and ketones from the body. Water also has *protective* functions such as *cleansing* (e.g. tears can lubricate our eyes and wash away dirt), *lubrication* (e.g. saliva lubricates the mouth and helps us to chew and swallow our food) and *cushioning* (e.g. water inside the brain, eyes and spinal fluid can help cushion against shock). One other important function of water for exercise metabolism is related to chemical reactions, as water serves as the medium for most chemical reactions in the body (e.g. ATP hydrolysis) and also participates as a reactant or product in certain reactions (e.g. the formation of peptide bonds in protein synthesis).

As we saw in Section 3.3, the breakage of the bonds contained within our food during exercise also releases heat energy. In order, therefore, to prevent us from overheating during exercise, water can help to regulate body temperature via increased sweating. As the sweat evaporates, heat is then removed from the body surface. It is important to note, however, that unless body water is replaced at appropriate times and in appropriate amounts, we may become dehydrated, which can subsequently impair exercise performance. In fact, decrements in exercise performance are associated with dehydration equivalent to as little as 2% of body mass loss (Armstrong *et al.*, 1985).

3.4.2   Water as a solvent

Another important function of water is to act as a *solvent* which can dissolve another substance called the *solute* to make a *solution*. For example, in the common commercially available sports drinks, water acts as a solvent for glucose and electrolytes such as sodium.

It is water's property as a polar compound which makes it an excellent solvent. As seen in Section 3.3, a water molecule is formed through a polar covalent bond, where the oxygen atom is slightly negatively charged and the hydrogen atoms are slightly positively charged. This makes water an excellent solvent for other ionic or polar substances (solutes), as the slightly negatively charged oxygen atoms and the slightly positively charged hydrogen atoms are attracted to other charged substances.

Solutes that contain polar covalent bonds are referred to as **hydrophilic** (meaning they are 'water-loving') and they dissolve easily in water; examples include sugar and salt. Solutes that mainly contain nonpolar covalent bonds are referred to as **hydrophobic** ('water-fearing') and they are not soluble in water. A common hydrophobic compound is household vegetable oil, which, if placed in a saucepan of water, will not dissolve at all. It is water's ability to act as a solvent which makes it an excellent medium for many of the body's metabolic reactions and to also carry out its transportation roles.

3.5   Solutions and concentrations

When a solute is dissolved in a substance to make a solution, it is useful to know the ***concentration*** of the subsequent solution, i.e. just how much of the solute is actually present in the solvent. A common way to express concentration is in *moles per litre* (abbreviated as mol/L or $mol.L^{-1}$), which refers to the number of molecules in a litre solution.

An understanding of the '**mole**' is a must for all aspects of chemistry and biology. A *mole* of substance is always equal to the atomic mass in grams of the substance, and contains 6.023×10^{23} atoms of that substance. This latter number is known as ***Avogadro's number*** and it is used the same way we use the term a dozen. For example, if we put a dozen baked beans into a bath tub, there are 12 baked beans present. If we put one mole of baked beans in the bath tub, it means there are 6.023×10^{23} baked beans present in the tub. It is important to note that whereas a mole refers to the amount of a substance, the ***molarity*** of a substance refers to its concentration, i.e. the number of moles of a substance in a given volume. A *1 molar* (1 M) solution contains one mole of a substance in one litre of solution.

A simpler way to understand the mole (especially in relation to making solutions with specific concentrations) is to refer to the atomic mass of the substance. For example, as outlined earlier, one mole is equal to the atomic mass in grams of the substance. In other words, as the atomic mass of glucose is 180, then 1 mole of glucose is equal to 180 grams of glucose, which contains

6.023×10^{23} molecules of glucose. Similarly, the atomic mass of water is 18, meaning that 1 mole of water is the equivalent to 18 grams of water, which is the equivalent of 6.023×10^{23} molecules of water. We can now use our understanding of moles to solve problems and make specific concentrations of solutions (see box: Laboratory focus: making concentrated solutions).

Laboratory focus – making concentrated solutions

For a laboratory experiment, a researcher is required to make 10 ml of a 5 mM glucose solution.

Step 1: Calculate the atomic mass (i.e. molecular weight) of glucose as this provides the amount in grams of 1 mole of glucose:

Molecular formula of glucose $= C_6 H_{12} O_6$
Atomic mass of glucose $= (12 \times 6) + (1 \times 12) + (16 \times 6) = 180$
1 molar (M) glucose solution therefore $= 180 \, g/L$

Step 2: Convert units to mM and mg:
$$1 \text{ M } = 180 \, g/L$$
$$1 \text{ mM} = 180 \, mg/L$$

Step 3: Multiply up (in this case by a factor of 5) for required concentration:

$$5 \text{ mM} = 900 \text{ mg/L } or$$
$$900 \text{ mg in 1000 ml}$$

Step 4: Scale down from a 1 L solution to a 10 ml solution:

$$5 \, mM \text{ in 1 L } = 900 \, mg \text{ in 1000 ml}$$
$$5 \, mM \text{ in 10 ml} = (900/1000) \times 10 = 9 \, mg$$

Answer: to make a 5 mM 10 ml glucose solution, dissolve 9 mg of glucose in 10 ml of the required solvent.
A simple formula to use for making concentrations is as follows:
Molecular weight of substance $\times$ required volume (L) $\times$ required concentration (M) = required mass of substance (g)
In the above example, this would read as follows:
$180 \times 0.01 \, L \times 0.005 \, M = 0.009 \, g$, thus equating to 9 mg.

In addition to making solutions according to molarity, we can also make solutions according to a percentage concentration that is equivalent to mass per volume. For example, many of the common sports drinks are referred to as 6% solutions, meaning they contain 6 g of glucose per 100 ml of water.

3.6 Acid-base balance

3.6.1 Acids, bases and salts

An *acid* is a compound that, when dissolved in water, is able to donate a hydrogen ion (H^+). Given that H^+ is a single proton with one positive charge, acids are also commonly referred to as *proton donors*. Examples of acids in our bodies include hydrochloric acid (HCl), carbonic acid (H_2CO_3) and **lactic acid** ($C_3H_6O_3$), the latter of which we produce in our muscles during high-intensity exercise (Karlsson & Saltin, 1970).

In contrast, a *base* is a compound that is able to accept hydrogen ions. For this reason, a base is therefore commonly referred to as a ***proton acceptor***. Common bases include hydroxyl ions (OH^-) and bicarbonate ions (HCO_3^-).

Acids and bases can chemically react together via exchange reactions to form compounds known as *salts*. For example, in the below equation, hydrochloric acid reacts with the base potassium hydroxide (KOH) to form the salt potassium chloride (KCl) and water:

$$HCl + KOH \rightarrow H^+ + Cl^- + K^+ + OH^-$$
$$\rightarrow KCl + H_2O$$

Misconception: lactic acid and lactate are not the same thing!

The terms '**lactic acid**' and '**lactate**' are often used interchangeably. Consequently, many people assume they are the same thing. However, when lactic acid is produced, it is quickly ionized by releasing a hydrogen ion. It was traditionally assumed that the remaining lactate was a dead end waste product, but we now know that the carbon skeleton contained in this compound can be shuttled within and between other tissues to provide an additional source of energy! This concept is discussed in later chapters. The molecular structures of lactic acid and lactate are shown below:

Lactic Acid   Lactate

3.6.2   pH Scale

In order to maintain homeostasis of body fluids (i.e. maintain their volume and composition), there must be almost balanced quantities of acids and bases. When acids are dissolved in a solution, they dissociate into one or more H^+ ions and one or more anions. For example, in the case of hydrochloric acid, the acid dissociates into H^+ ions and chloride ions (Cl^-). Bases, in contrast, dissociate into one or more OH^- ions and one or more cations. The more H^+ ions that are dissolved in the solution, the more *acidic* the solution becomes; the more OH^- ions dissolved in the solution, the more **alkaline** the solution becomes.

We can quantify the acidity or alkalinity of the solution on the basis of the *pH scale*, which is essentially a logarithmic scale ranging from 0–14 that is based on the concentration of H^+ ions in moles per litre. The pH of a solution is defined as the negative decimal logarithm of the free H^+ concentration and can be expressed according to the following equation, where $[H^+]$ is the hydrogen ion concentration:

$$pH = \log\{1/[H^+]\} = -\log[H^+]$$

The midpoint of the pH scale is 7, and it is at this point that the concentration of H^+ and OH^- are equal. A solution with a pH of 7 is referred to as *neutral*, and the common example is pure water. If a solution has a neutral pH, this means that it contains 1×10^{-7} moles of hydrogen ions per litre. Where the solution has more H^+ ions than OH^- ions, the solution is referred to as an acidic solution and it therefore has a pH below 7. Conversely, where the solution has more OH^- ions than H^+ ions, the solution is referred to as an alkaline solution and has a pH greater than 7.

Because the pH scale is logarithmic, it is important to note that a change in one whole number on the scale represents a ten-fold difference in H^+ concentration. For example, a pH of 6 (1×10^{-6} moles of hydrogen ions per litre) denotes 10 times more H^+ ions than a pH of 7. Similarly, a pH of 8 (1×10^{-8} moles of hydrogen ions per litre) denotes 10 times fewer H^+ ions than a pH of 7. The pH scale is shown in Figure 3.10.

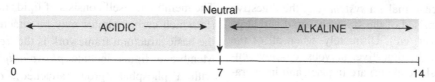

Figure 3.10   The pH scale. Note that a pH of 7.0 is referred to as neutral. The normal resting pH of arterial blood is 7.4 and that of muscle is 7.1. When the pH increases or decreases from these values, the cells are said to be alkaline or acidic respectively

As will be seen in subsequent chapters, the pH of the intracellular fluid in skeletal muscle cells can become reduced due to the H^+ ions which are produced in muscle as a result of the chemical reactions that occur to provide ATP during high-intensity exercise. In turn, these H^+ ions can diffuse into the blood thus lowering the pH of the blood also. This increased acidity can impair important biochemical processes required for exercise by lowering the activity (or causing complete inhibition) of enzymes involved in exercise metabolism or by directly interfering with the proteins involved in the process of muscle contraction itself.

3.6.3   Buffers

Most bodily fluids are reasonably well maintained around the neutral pH of 7. Indeed, even in the face of the severe metabolic acidosis caused by maximal intensity exercise (such as a 30-second maximal sprint), muscle pH does not fall below 6.5 (Bogdanis *et al.*, 1995). The body's ability to regulate pH is underpinned by *buffers*, defined as compounds that can convert strong acids or bases into weaker respective compounds. The carbonic acid-bicarbonate buffer system is one such system that can help regulate pH, especially in extracellular fluids. For example, in acidic conditions HCO_3^- ions can function as a weak base and remove H^+ ions, as shown below:

$$H^+ + HCO_3^- \rightarrow H_2CO_3 \rightarrow H_2O + CO_2$$

Similarly, in alkaline conditions, carbonic acid (H_2CO_3) can function as a weak acid and provide H^+ ions that are needed to reduce the pH towards the appropriate physiological range as follows:

$$H_2CO_3 \rightarrow H^+ + HCO_3^-$$

Important intracellular buffers in skeletal muscle include *carnosine, phosphocreatine* and *phosphates*, which collectively help to minimize the fall in muscle pH that can occur during high-intensity exercise as a result of increased lactic acid production and the associated increase in H^+ ion concentration. The increased H^+ ions subsequently diffuse into the blood, which also be buffered by bicarbonate in plasma and *haemoglobin* in red blood cells. We will cover the issue of metabolic acidosis further in subsequent chapters.

3.7   Cell structure

The previous parts of this chapter have focused on the chemical level of organization outlining how atoms of elements can bond to make molecules and compounds. Molecules, in turn, combine to make *cells*, the basic structural and functional unit of an organism. Humans are considered as *multicellular* organisms, as there are about 200 different types of cells in our bodies, such as muscle cells, blood cells, skin cells, brain cells and so on.

Cells then combine to make *tissues*, defined as groups of cells that work together to perform a particular function. There are four basic types of tissues in our bodies: *epithelial, connective, nervous* and *muscle* (further classified as skeletal, cardiac and smooth).

When two or more tissues combine, the result is an organ (e.g. the stomach) which, in turn, can also work together to make a *system* (e.g. the digestive system, comprised of the stomach, small and large intestines, liver, etc). Ultimately, when all of the systems (e.g. the digestive, nervous, cardiovascular, musculoskeletal etc) are in place and in operation together, the result is a living organism – for example, the person reading this book!

It is important to note that not all cells are the same. Nevertheless, the average human cell is $10–20\,\mu m$ in diameter and our bodies contain approximately 10^{14} cells. Most cells are 70–80% water and have many structural features in common. The basic structure of a cell is shown in Figure 3.11.

3.7.1 The plasma membrane

The boundary of cells is known as the ***plasma membrane***, which is essentially a sturdy but flexible barrier that encloses the cell (see Figure 3.12).

The membrane itself consists of lipids and proteins (to which carbohydrates may be attached), where the basic structural framework is the ***lipid bilayer***. Membrane lipids include ***phospholipids*** (lipids with a phosphate group attached), ***cholesterol*** (a steroid with a hydroxyl group attached) and ***glycolipids*** (lipids with carbohydrate groups attached).

Proteins in the plasma membrane are divided into two categories – ***integral proteins*** or ***peripheral proteins***. Most integral proteins are also referred to as ***transmembrane proteins***, meaning they span right across the lipid bilayer and are in contact with both the intracellular and extracellular fluid. In contrast, peripheral proteins tend to associate with membrane lipids or integral proteins at either the inner or outer surface of the membrane. Membrane proteins have a variety of functions which are essential for maintaining cell viability.

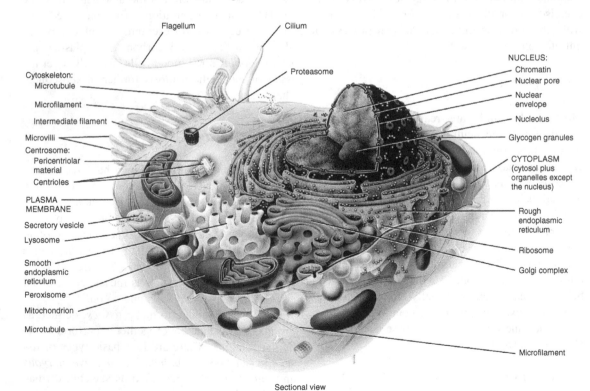

Sectional view

Figure 3.11   The basic structure of body cells. (From Tortora and Derrickson, *Principles of Anatomy and Physiology, Twelfth Edition*, 2009, reproduced by permission of John Wiley & Sons Inc.)

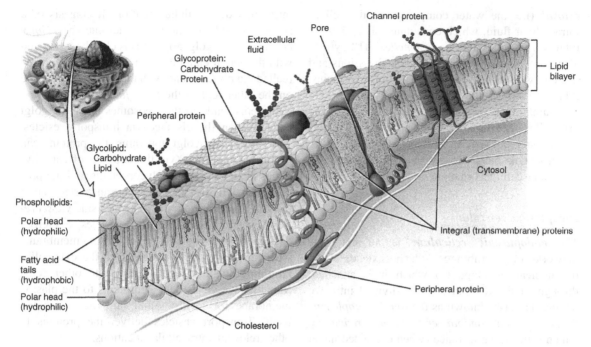

Figure 3.12   Basic structure of the plasma membrane. (From Tortora and Derrickson, *Principles of Anatomy and Physiology, Twelfth Edition*, 2009, reproduced by permission of John Wiley & Sons Inc.)

These include operating as ***ion channels*** (i.e. proteins with pores through which ions can pass into and out of the cell via the process of *diffusion*), ***transporter proteins*** (i.e. proteins which actively transport substances into and out of the cell via *facilitated transport*) and ***receptor proteins*** (i.e. proteins which recognize an extracellular signal, usually via the binding of hormones, which in turn then alters intracellular functions).

3.7.2   The nucleus

The ***nucleus*** is an oval-shaped structure which contains the genetic material within our ***genes***. Genes are arranged in single file along ***chromosomes***. Human cells contain 46 chromosomes, of which we inherit 23 from each of our parents. Each chromosome is a long molecule of deoxyribonucleic acid (abbreviated as ***DNA***) that is coiled together with proteins known as ***histones***. Encoded within the DNA is the essential genetic information that is required for making new proteins

(protein synthesis). We will cover DNA structure and the process of protein synthesis in Chapter 4.

Similar to the plasma membrane, a lipid bilayer membrane known as the ***nuclear envelope*** separates the nucleus from the rest of the cell. Embedded within the nuclear envelope are *nuclear pores* which allow selective movement of molecules between the nucleus and **cytoplasm**. Inside the nucleus is a structure known as the *nucleolus*, which is responsible for making **ribosomes** – organelles which function in making new proteins. It is important to note that, while most cell types contain a single nucleus, some (such as red blood cells) contain none. In contrast, skeletal muscle cells contain many nuclei and are thus referred to as *multinucleated cells*.

3.7.3   Cytoplasm and organelles

The *cytoplasm* is the term used to refer to everything inside the cell except the nucleus. The cytoplasm, in turn, can be further divided as the *cytosol* (i.e. the water component of the cell or intracellular fluid, which constitutes about 55% of total cell volume) and the *organelles*. The cytosol also contains many components such as ions and the energy sources of glycogen, lipids, proteins, ATP and all of the necessary enzymes needed to maintain important cellular processes. The organelles are structures made up of biomolecules which carry out specific cellular functions.

Let's look more closely at some of the most important cellular organelles.

Endoplasmic reticulum

The **endoplasmic reticulum** is an extensive network of membranes which extends from the nuclear envelope (to which it is attached) throughout the cytoplasm. It is divided into two distinctive forms known as the *rough endoplasmic reticulum* and *smooth endoplasmic reticulum*, which differ in appearance (when examined under a microscope) and function.

The rough endoplasmic reticulum is so called because of its granular-like appearance, which is due to organelles known as *ribosomes* that are attached to its external surface. Ribosomes are the cellular organelles responsible for protein synthesis and consist of proteins and ribosomal ribonucleic acid (abbreviated as rRNA).

In contrast, the smooth endoplasmic reticulum has no ribosomes attached to it and is considered to have a 'smooth' appearance. It extends from its rough counterpart and is responsible for the synthesis of lipids and various steroids. In certain cells, the smooth endoplasmic reticulum is specialized to perform a variety of functions. For example, as seen in Chapter 2, calcium ions responsible for muscle contraction are released from the *sarcoplasmic reticulum*, a form of smooth endoplasmic reticulum unique to skeletal muscle.

Golgi apparatus

Whereas the ribosomes are the sites responsible for protein synthesis, the **golgi apparatus** (or *golgi complex*) is the organelle responsible for transporting these newly made proteins to their correct intra- or extra- cellular location. It consists of a series of cuplike membranous sacs known as *Golgi cisternae*. The golgi apparatus is closely associated with the rough endoplasmic reticulum on one side (called the *cis face*) and with the plasma membrane on the other (called the *trans face*).

Proteins made in the ribosomes enter the golgi apparatus on the cis face via transport vesicles. Once inside the golgi apparatus, the proteins can be further modified (via the addition of carbohydrates or lipids to form glycoproteins and lipoproteins, respectively) and are then transported to exit the golgi apparatus on the trans face side via *secretory, membrane* or *transport* vesicles. Secretory vesicles deliver proteins to the plasma membrane, where they are then discharged to the extracellular fluid for subsequent transport to other cells. Membrane vesicles deliver proteins to the plasma membrane for incorporation into the membrane itself. Transport vesicles deliver the proteins to other relevant intracellular locations.

Mitochondria

Mitochondria are oval-shaped structures that are often referred to as the *aerobic powerhouse* of the cell, as they generate the most ATP. Cells which are highly active, such as muscle, kidney and liver cells, etc. contain many mitochondria. An increase in the number and size of mitochondria in skeletal muscle that occurs with endurance training is one of the most important adaptations to training which improves endurance performance (Holloszy & Coyle, 1984).

Mitochondria contain both an outer *mitochondrial membrane* and *inner mitochondrial membrane*, with a small fluid filled space between them. The inner membrane is folded into tubules called *cristae*, which substantially increase the surface area for the electron transport chain. The large, fluid-filled cavity enclosed by the inner membrane is known as the **mitochondrial matrix**. Similar to the nucleus, mitochondria also contain their own special DNA (which we inherit from our mothers), which can make 13 proteins that are needed to make other important proteins for the mitochondria. As mitochondria can also make their own proteins, ribosomes (i.e. the protein-making factories) are present in the mitochondrial matrix.

Cytoskeleton

The **cytoskeleton** is a flexible network of fibrous proteins (referred to as *filaments*) which gives the cell structure and support, similar to how the skeleton provides support within our bodies. However, the cytoskeleton is not a rigid, fixed structure but rather undergoes continual reorganization as it disassembles and reassembles when necessary. Three types of protein filaments constitute the cytoskeleton, and these are named according to their size (increasing diameter): *microfilaments, intermediate filaments* and *microtubules*.

Microfilaments have the smallest diameter and have two general functions of helping to generate movement and providing mechanical support. One important microfilament is the protein actin, which is involved in the process of muscle contraction.

Intermediate filaments are exceptionally strong proteins that have a diameter between that of microfilaments and microtubules. In skeletal muscle cells, an important intermediate filament is myosin, which works with actin to produce contraction. The intermediate filament desmin is also important as it helps to 'anchor' the contractile proteins, and organelles such as the mitochondria and the nucleus in position.

The largest cytoskeletal proteins are known as microtubules and are mainly composed of the protein tubulin. Microtubules help to determine cell shape and also assist in the movement of organelles and chromosomes during cell division.

3.8 Key points

- Matter is made up of elements, the most important of which to living organisms are oxygen (O), carbon (C), hydrogen (H) and nitrogen (N).
- Elements are made from atoms, which consist of a nucleus (containing protons and neutrons) and electrons (which orbit the nucleus in electron shells).
- Isotopes are atoms of the same element which have different numbers of neutrons.
- An atom that gains or loses an electron becomes an anion or a cation, respectively.
- When two or more atoms combine, they form a molecule.
- When different elements combine, they form compounds.
- Inorganic compounds lack carbon atoms, whereas organic compounds contain carbon.
- Atoms join via chemical bonds to make molecules.
- Chemical bonds form by sharing electrons or by losing or gaining electrons in the valence shell.
- Ionic bonds form when atoms lose or gain electrons.
- Covalent bonds form when atoms share pairs of electrons.
- Polar covalent bonds form when one atom attracts the shared electrons more than the other.
- Non-polar covalent bonds form when both atoms attract the shared electrons equally.
- Isomers are compounds with the same molecular formula which have different molecular structures.
- Chemical reactions occur when bonds break or new bonds form.
- Endergonic reactions consume energy and exergonic reactions release energy.
- Units of energy are the kilocalorie (kcal) and the kilojoule (kJ).
- ATP is the cell's main form of chemical energy which can be transferred to other forms of energy.
- Synthesis reactions occur when elements or compounds combine to make larger or more complex molecules.
- Decomposition reactions occur when large molecules are broken down into smaller molecules or individual atoms.
- Exchange reactions involve the exchange of atoms between reactant molecules to produce new products.
- In oxidation reactions, the reactant molecule loses at least one electron, whereas in reduction

reactions, the reactant molecules gain at least one electron.

- Some reactions are reversible, meaning they can proceed in either direction.
- Acids are compounds which are able to donate hydrogen ions.
- Bases are compounds that are able to accept hydrogen ions.
- Acids and bases can react together to form salts.
- The more hydrogen ions dissolved in a solution, the more acidic the solution.
- The more hydroxide ions dissolved in a solution, the more alkaline the solution.
- The acidity and alkalinity of a solution can be expressed on the logarithmic pH scale.
- A neutral solution has a pH of 7.0.
- Cells contain biochemical buffers to protect against a fall or rise in pH.

- Cells are the basic structural and functional units of an organism.
- The three common features to most cells include the plasma membrane, the nucleus and the cytoplasm.
- The plasma membrane is a bilayer of lipids and proteins which surrounds the cytoplasm of the cell.
- The cytoplasm is the cellular contents between the plasma membrane and the nucleus and is further divided into the cytosol (the watery portion of the cell) and the organelles (special structures which perform key cellular functions).
- The nucleus is an oval-shaped structure which contains all of the genetic material of the cell.

Part Two

Fundamentals of Sport and Exercise Biochemistry

4

Proteins

Learning outcomes

After studying this chapter, you should be able to:

- list the variety of functions which proteins carry out within the human body;
- define the terms essential and non-essential amino acid;
- draw the general structure of an amino acid;
- describe the primary, secondary, tertiary and quaternary structure of proteins;
- define the function of enzymes and explain the basic mechanisms of enzyme action;
- list and describe the cellular alterations in homeostasis that can modify enzyme activity;
- explain how the provision of co-factors and coenzymes modify enzyme activity;
- explain the process of covalent and allosteric regulation of enzyme activity;
- define the terms DNA, gene and codon;
- describe the general structure of a DNA molecule;
- describe the principles of the genetic code;
- outline the major steps involved in transcription and translation that are required to convert the genetic code into a fully functional protein;
- define the term free amino acid pool and anaplerosis;

- describe the principles of transamination and deamination reactions in the context of amino acid metabolism;
- outline the main stages and enzymes involved in the metabolism of branched-chain amino acids;
- outline the function and components of the glucose-alanine cycle;
- explain the function of the urea cycle.

Key words

actin	biological catalysts
anticodon	β pleated sheets
activation energy	branched chain amino
aspartate	acids (BCAAs)
active site	branched chain amino
atrophy	acid aminotrans-
adenine	ferase (BCAAAT)
alanine	branched chain keto
aminotransferase	acid dehydrogenase
allosteric regulation	(BCKAD)
alpha helix	carbon skeletons
amino acid	catalytic site
amino acid residue	chromosomes
aminotransferase	codons
anaplerosis	cofactors
antibodies	coenzymes
base pairs	C-terminus
binding site	cytosine

Biochemistry for Sport and Exercise Metabolism, First Edition. Don MacLaren and James Morton.
© 2012 John Wiley & Sons, Ltd. Published 2012 by John Wiley & Sons, Ltd.

deoxyribose
dephosphorylation
diabetes
disulfide bonds
DNA
dystrophin
endocrine system
enzymes
enzyme substrate
    complex
essential amino acids
free amino acid pool
genes
genetic code
glucogenic amino
    acids
gluconeogenesis
glucose-alanine cycle
glutamate
glutamate
    dehydrogenase
glutaminase
glutamine
glutamine synthetase
guanine
haemoglobin
hormones
hydrogen bonds
hydrophobic
    interactions
hyperglycaemia
hypertrophy
insulin
isoleucine
ketogenic amino acids
ketone bodies
kinases
leucine
lysine
messenger ribonucleic
    acid (mRNA)
Michaelis constant
mRNA
myoglobin
myosin
nicotinamide adenine

dinucleotide
    (NAD$^+$)
non-essential amino
    acids
N-terminus
oxidative deamination
pancreas
peptide bond
peptide chain
phosphorylation
promoter region
prosthetic groups
protein
protein degradation
protein kinases
protein phospharases
protein synthesis
protein turnover
proteome
polypeptide
ribonucleic acid
ribosomes
RNA polymerase II
sense strand
serine
substrate
subunit
template strand
threonine
thymine
transamination
transcription
transfer RNA
translation
transcription factors
tricarboxylic acid
  • cycle
tRNA
tyrosine
uracil
urea
urea cycle
urine
valine
V$_{MAX}$

4.1 Protein function

When we ask students what they think of when they hear the word *protein*, we are usually greeted with the same response. Typically, they respond with the classic textbook answer that proteins 'are needed for growth and repair' of tissues and that we can obtain them by eating protein-rich food such as chicken, fish, eggs and milk, etc. However, from this point forth, we would like you to extend your understanding of proteins beyond growth and repair and begin to appreciate that proteins are the macromolecules that are essential to life. In short, they could be referred as the *cellular action molecules*. Houston (2006) captures this point entirely by stating: '*Everything we do, everything we are and everything we become depend on the action of thousands of different proteins.*'

There are hundreds of thousands of proteins present in the human body and each is likely to perform a unique role within our cells. The average adult contains approximately 10–12 kg of protein, of which 60–75% is located within our muscles. The term *proteome* refers to all of the proteins present within the cell, and many scientists are devoted to characterizing the function of all proteins present in the proteome. To use a simple analogy, you could begin your study of proteins by thinking of them in the same way that you view friends and family in your own lives. For example, similar to how friends and family members play a particular role in you life, each of our cellular proteins also play important roles, without which our cells would not operate as efficiently and may become susceptible to disease.

For example, the skeletal muscle cells of patients with McArdle's syndrome lack the protein (in this case an *enzyme*) known as *glycogen phosphorylase*, and due to this they cannot break down muscle glycogen stores to provide energy. As a result, these patients fatigue within seconds of intense physical exertion and report extreme pain and stiffness. Consequently, their overall quality of life is severely hindered (Salter, 1967). This example alone clearly illustrates the importance of correctly functioning proteins. In the next section, we look more closely at some of the diverse roles that proteins can play in our bodies, many of which you will already be familiar with from Chapters 1–3.

4.1.1 General protein function

Proteins can perform an array of cellular functions, such as participating in biochemical reactions, transporting substances into and out of cells, maintaining cell structure, producing movement and transmitting important information. For this reason, proteins are often classified into a number of categories based on their cellular function, as shown in Figure 4.1. It is important to note, however, that not all proteins can be confined to a solitary function – many proteins perform diverse roles.

Catalytic

Many proteins function as *enzymes* (i.e. *biological catalysts*), which are defined as substances that can accelerate biochemical reactions without being altered themselves. For example, we briefly outlined earlier how the enzyme glycogen phosphorylase is involved in breaking down muscle glycogen stores to provide our muscles with ATP and, thus, the energy to exercise. An understanding of enzyme function and their regulation is therefore crucial for the study of sport and exercise metabolism. For this reason, we dedicate a whole section to this topic later in this chapter.

Transport and storage

There are many substances that are transported into and out of cells, into and out of intracellular organelles and also from one site of the body to another. The transportation of these substances is possible through the action of proteins. For example, the oxygen we breathe can be transported to our muscles via the protein *haemoglobin*, the major protein found in the

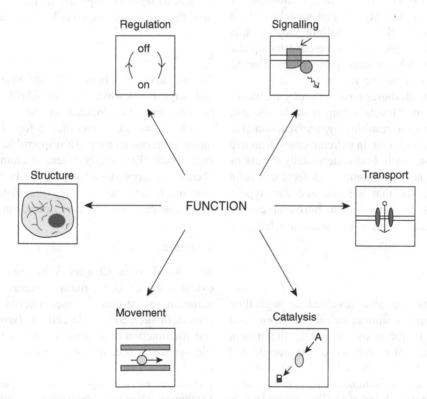

Figure 4.1 Schematic illustration of the diverse functions of proteins

blood. Similarly, the protein *myoglobin*, present in our muscles, can then receive this oxygen, store it and also transport it inside the muscle cell. Additionally, proteins can span across cell membranes and acts as channels or pumps, so as to regulate the flow of important molecules into and out of cells.

Hormones

Many proteins also function as *hormones*, defined as proteins secreted by cells of the *endocrine system*, which regulate activity of cells in other parts of the body. The importance of hormone action can be easily illustrated through the action of the hormone *insulin*, a hormone released from the **pancreas** following an increase in blood sugar (glucose) levels which occurs following the consumption of a meal, especially if it has a high carbohydrate content. Insulin regulates blood glucose concentration by binding to a receptor protein present in the plasma membrane of other cells (most notably skeletal muscle), which initiates an intracellular signalling cascade that ultimately causes the cell to increase its uptake of glucose, thereby returning the blood glucose concentration to baseline values.

Patients with **diabetes** have difficulty maintaining blood glucose levels within basal levels and, if left untreated, the resulting *hyperglycaemia* (i.e. high blood glucose) can, in extreme cases, lead to a coma and cause death. Fortunately, daily injections of insulin can help overcome the defects in insulin secretion or action that is associated with type 1 and 2 diabetes, respectively. The hormonal control of exercise metabolism is discussed in Chapter 7 of this book.

Signalling

Many proteins are also involved in signalling roles involving communication between and within cells. In the above example, the insulin receptor in the cell membrane of the muscle cell is bound by insulin released from the pancreas (i.e. cell-to-cell communication) which then initiates an intracellular signalling cascade (i.e.

intracellular communication), leading to increased glucose uptake.

Although the precise proteins involved in the insulin signalling cascade remains an active area of research, it is thought to work via series of phosphorylation reactions where proteins known as *kinases* phosphorylate a target protein, thereby rendering the latter active. This, in turn, may lead to phosphorylation of another protein (and so on) until the appropriate cellular response has been achieved. Similarly, when we perform repeated bouts of exercise (e.g. training) our muscle cells can respond to both extracellular and intracellular signals, which, in time, activate the relevant signalling cascade to help our muscles become more efficient to deal with the metabolic stress induced by exercise.

A simplistic way to think of proteins as signalling molecules is to imagine them in a game of dominoes. For example, when the signal has been initiated (i.e. the first domino has been toppled), it leads to repeated toppling of the domino chain until the necessary response has been achieved.

Contractile

As we saw in Chapter 2, the proteins **actin** and **myosin** (known as 'myofibrillar' proteins because they are located in the myofibrils of muscle cells) are sometimes referred to as the motor proteins, as they are responsible for muscle contraction. Essentially, these proteins turn the chemical energy stored within the bonds of ATP into mechanical work. They therefore form the molecular basis for muscle contraction.

Structural

As alluded to in Chapter 3 in reference to the cytoskeleton of cells, many proteins function to maintain cell structure. One important structural protein in skeletal muscle cells is *dystrophin*, the specific function of which is to anchor the contractile apparatus (i.e. the myofibrils) to the plasma membrane. The importance of the dystrophin protein is evident by examining patients with Duchenne muscular dystrophy (Kunkel, 1986).

The muscle cells of these patients do not contain dystrophin and as a result, their muscles become considerably weaker and smaller over time. Consequently, many patients are confined to a wheelchair by early childhood.

Other important examples of proteins with structural roles include *collagen*, which gives our skin and bones structure, and *keratin*, which forms the structural basis of hair and nails.

Immunological

Antibodies are proteins produced by cells of the immune system and they play an important role in fighting against infections. These proteins recognize and neutralize foreign substances (i.e. antigens) such as bacteria and viruses, etc. through the process of *phagocytosis*. Due to this important role of fighting infection, it is crucial that we

obtain enough protein in our diet so that we can consistently manufacture the appropriate supply of antibodies. When we are vaccinated for common diseases such as influenza and measles, etc. we are actually being injected with a small amount of the dead or inactive virus, which causes our bodies to make the corresponding proteins (antibodies) so that we can mount an effective immune response if we contract the disease at a later date.

Regulatory

Proteins known as **transcription factors** can bind to the relevant parts of the **DNA** within our **genes** which can ultimately lead to the formation of new proteins. The overall process of gene **transcription** and **translation** is known as **protein synthesis** and, because of its importance to sport and exercise metabolism, we outline the stages involved in this process later in this chapter.

Table 4.1 Amino acid names and their abbreviations

Amino acid name	Essential or non-essential	3-letter abbreviation	1-letter abbreviation
Alanine	non-essential	Ala	A
Arginine	non-essential	Arg	R
Asparagine	non-essential	Asn	N
Aspartate	non-essential	Asp	D
Cysteine	non-essential	Cys	C
Glutamate	non-essential	Glu	E
Glutamine	non-essential	Gln	Q
Glycine	non-essential	Gly	G
Histidine	non-essential	His	H
Isoleucine	essential	Ile	I
Leucine	essential	Leu	L
Lysine	essential	Lys	K
Methionine	essential	Met	M
Phenylalanine	essential	Phe	F
Proline	non-essential	Pro	P
Serine	non-essential	Ser	S
Threonine	essential	Thr	T
Tryptrophan	essential	Trp	W
Tyrosine	non-essential	Tyr	Y
Valine	essential	Val	V

4.2 Amino acids

In the same way that bricks build a house, *amino acids* are the building blocks of proteins. There are 20 amino acids that are needed to make proteins, eight of which are described as *essential amino acids* because the body cannot make them and they therefore have to be obtained from the food we eat. The remaining 12 amino acids are often considered as *non-essential amino acids*; the body can synthesize them from compounds already present in our cells. The specific names of each amino acid can also be abbreviated using three- or one-letter symbols as shown in Table 4.1.

4.2.1 Amino acid structure

Amino acids can all be depicted by the same general structure, as shown in Figure 4.2. Each amino acid consists of a central carbon atom to which an amino group, a carboxyl group, a hydrogen atom and a variable side chain group (referred to as R) are attached. The R group is different for each amino acid and, indeed, it is this variable side chain which gives each amino acid its unique characteristics and identity. At physiological pH, the amino and carboxyl group are ionized, with a positive and negative charge, respectively. This form is often referred to as the *zwitterion* form. The net charge of the amino acid is therefore neutral unless the side chain also carries a charge.

As discussed above, amino acids differ from one another on the basis of their side chain. The R group can vary in size, charge, polarity and reactivity. Figure 4.3 shows the structure of each amino acid and classifies them according to their polarity and charge.

4.3 Protein structure

Although proteins can be considered to function as little machines within our bodies, we also need to appreciate the huge, complex structure of proteins. Indeed, proteins are much larger molecules than carbohydrates and fats. The structure of proteins can be recognized by increasing levels of complexity beginning with the primary, secondary, tertiary and in some cases, a quaternary structure.

4.3.1 Primary structure

The primary structure of a protein refers to the linear sequence of amino acids which join together via *peptide bonds* (a form of covalent bond between the carbon atom of the carboxyl group of one amino acid and the nitrogen atom of the amino group of another) to make a *peptide chain*. When a peptide bond forms, a water molecule is produced, thus making the reaction a synthesis condensation reaction. In contrast, when a peptide bond is broken, it is an example of hydrolysis reaction, where the addition of a water molecule is needed.

An example of a peptide bond joining two amino acids is shown in Figure 4.4. When peptides are formed, there is a free amino group starting at the left hand side (referred to as the *N-terminus*) and a free carboxyl group at the right hand side (referred to as the *C-terminus*).

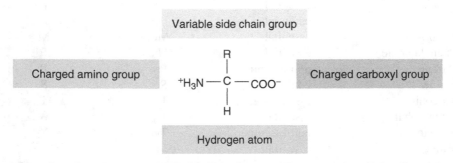

Figure 4.2   General structure of an amino acid

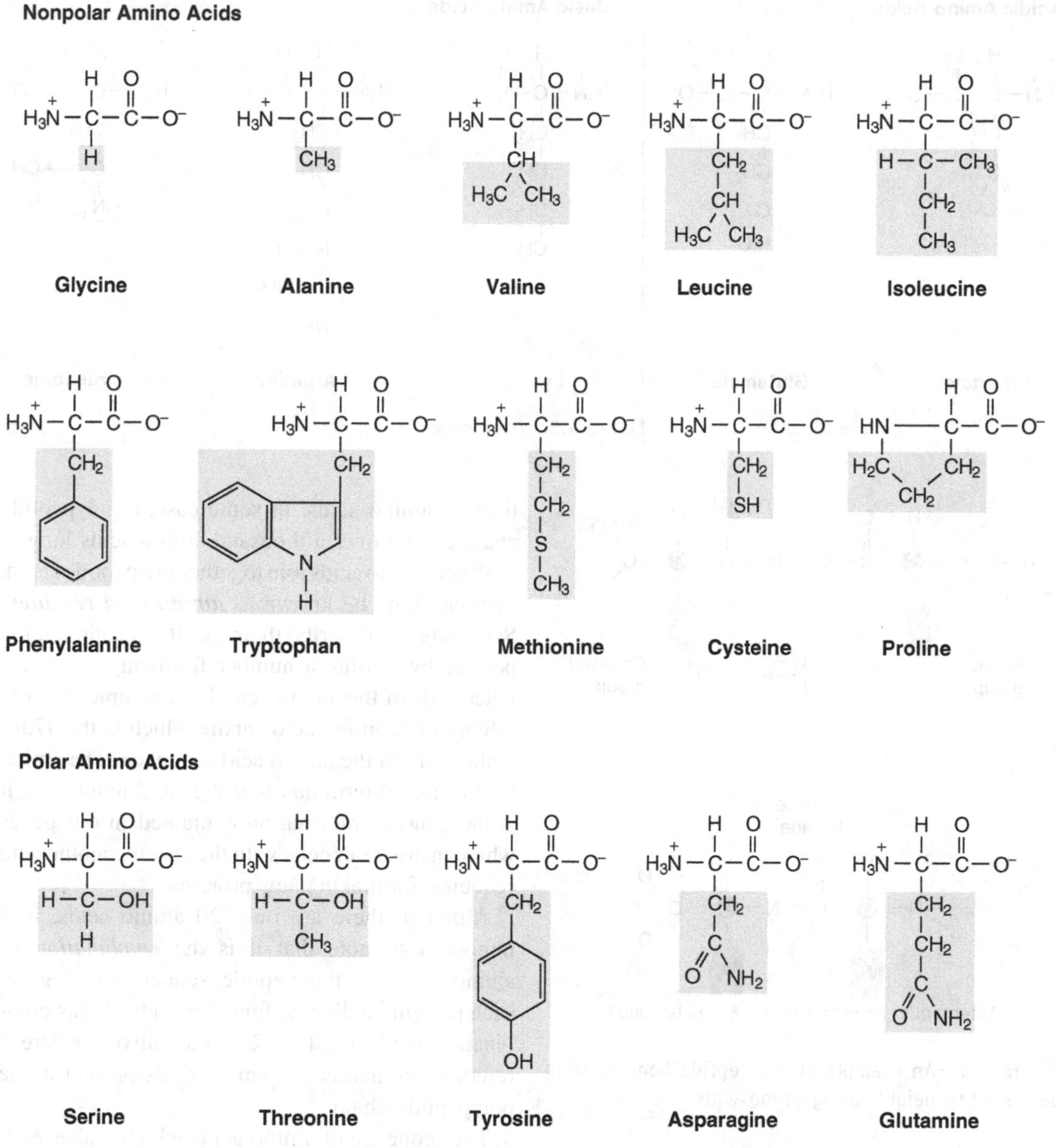

Nonpolar Amino Acids

Glycine	Alanine	Valine	Leucine	Isoleucine

Phenylalanine	Tryptophan	Methionine	Cysteine	Proline

Polar Amino Acids

Serine	Threonine	Tyrosine	Asparagine	Glutamine

Figure 4.3   The specific structure of each of the 20 amino acids

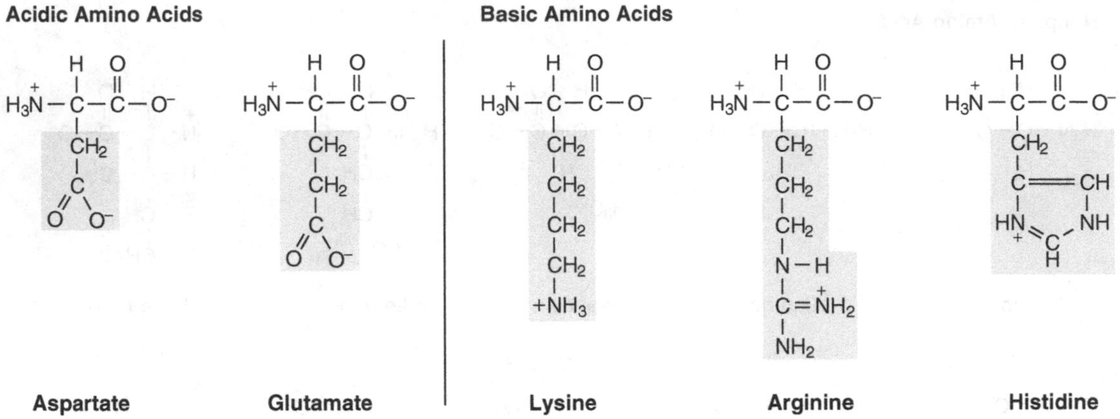

Acidic Amino Acids

Basic Amino Acids

Aspartate   **Glutamate**   **Lysine**   **Arginine**   **Histidine**

Figure 4.3   (*continued*)

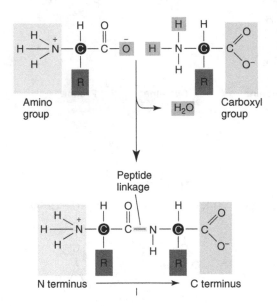

Figure 4.4   An example of the peptide bond forming between two neighbouring amino acids

Depending on the number of amino acids present in the peptide chain, we can use prefixes to characterize the number present. For example: *di* = two; *tri* = three; *tetra* = four; *penta* = five; *hexa* = six; *hepta* = seven; *octa* = eight; *nona* = nine and *deca* = ten. The term *oligopeptide* is used to refer to a peptide chain that consists of 10–20 amino acids. A *polypeptide* is the term used to describe a large peptide which contains more

than 20 amino acids. In some case, a polypeptide chain can be over a thousand amino acids long.

When amino acids join together in a peptide chain, they can now be known as **amino acid residues**. Scientists can describe their specific location in the peptide by writing a number following the three-letter code of the amino acid. For example, ser-473 refers to the amino acid **serine** which is the 473rd amino acid in the amino acid sequence. The amino acid at the N-terminus is designated number 1. It is the genetic information contained in our genes which instruct our cells with the specific amino acid sequence for making new proteins.

Although there are only 20 amino acids, it is important to note that it is the *combination* of amino acids in the peptide sequence that gives each protein its distinct function. Indeed, this combination could exist as 20^n alternatives, where n refers to the number of amino acids present in the polypeptide chain.

The sequence of amino acids which makes each specific protein can therefore be considered as similar to how letters of the alphabet can link together to form different words. There are only 26 letters in the standard alphabet, yet there are hundreds of thousands of words in the English language alone!

It is also important to consider that it only takes one amino acid to be out of its correct location for the protein to become potentially useless and dangerous. Indeed, the medical condition *sickle cell anaemia* (an abnormal red blood cell shape which results in restricted blood flow to organs) results from the replacement of **glutamate** with **valine** at the 6th position.

From an exercise science perspective, we are interested in knowing the specific locations of the amino acids **serine**, **tyrosine** and **threonine**, as these amino acids can be phosphorylated during exercise and this may therefore render the protein active or inactive. For example, the protein adenosine monophosphate kinase (AMPK) is phosphorylated at ser172 during exercise, and this protein is currently thought to be one of the regulatory proteins involved in increasing muscle glucose uptake during exercise, as well as signalling training adaptation (Richter & Ruderman, 2009).

4.3.2 Secondary structure

The backbone of the polypeptide chain does not extend in a straight line for its entire length. Instead, it repeatedly folds in a number of distinct forms, which ultimately gives rise to a three-dimensional structure. The secondary structure of a protein refers to the conformation of a short stretch of the polypeptide chain which can fold in two common forms known as the *alpha helix* or β *pleated sheets* (see Figure 4.5b).

In both forms of secondary structure, the protein is stabilized by *hydrogen bonds* which form at regular intervals along the polypeptide backbone between neighbouring elements such as oxygen. The hydrogen bond is a form of non-covalent bond between a hydrogen atom with a partial positive charge and an oxygen or nitrogen atom with a partial negative charge. Although hydrogen bonds are considerably weaker than covalent bonds, the considerable number of bonds between hydrogen and oxygen atoms in peptide units allows sufficient force for the secondary structure of proteins to be stabilized.

4.3.3 Tertiary structure

The tertiary structure of a protein refers to the three-dimensional shape of the entire polypeptide chain

(see Figure 4.5c). It is only when the protein has folded to its tertiary structure that it is able to function. Given the tertiary three-dimensional shape, it is possible for amino acids that are far apart in the primary structure to be now in close proximity.

Many types of chemical bonds are responsible for giving rise to the tertiary structure of proteins, the strongest of which is the covalent *disulphide bond*. Disulphide bonds are formed between the sulphydryl groups of two monomers of the amino acid cysteine and are symbolized chemically as S-S.

Other more frequent but less strong bonds include hydrogen bonds, ionic bonds and *hydrophobic interactions*. The latter also help to shape the tertiary structure of proteins, given that some amino acids are attracted to water (i.e. hydrophilic), whereas others are repelled from water (i.e. hydrophobic). Given that most proteins exist in water environments inside our cells, those amino acids which are hydrophobic therefore reside deep in the central region of the protein, away from the protein's surface, whereas the 'water-loving' hydrophilic amino acids reside nearer to the protein's surface in contact with the cytoplasm.

Cellular stresses such as heat, free radical production and changes in pH can all disrupt the tertiary structures of proteins. In such instances, the protein is said to have *denatured* and has therefore lost function. Fortunately, cells have a highly conserved family of proteins known as *heat shock proteins* (HSPs), which help to repair damaged and unfolded proteins in order to restore their function. The stress of even moderate-intensity exercise can up-regulate muscle HSP content in the days following the exercise protocol, and hence these proteins are thought to repair any damage to proteins induced by the exercise bout as well as protect the cell against future stresses (Morton *et al.*, 2006).

4.3.4 Quaternary structure

Some proteins are composed of more than one polypeptide chain and, in these instances, the protein is now considered to have a quaternary structure (see Figure 4.5d), defined as the structural arrangement of each polypeptide chain

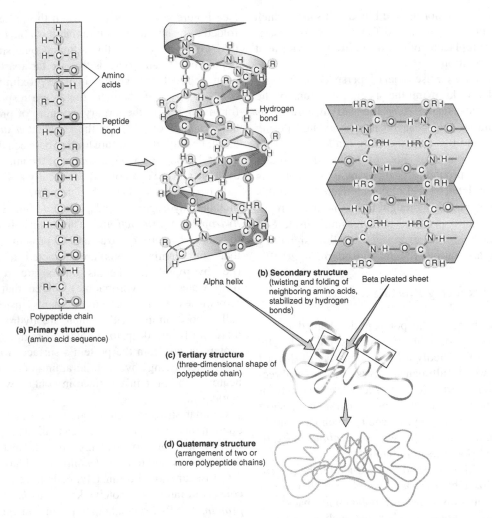

Figure 4.5 Overview of protein structure. (a) Primary structure refers to the linear sequence of amino acids in the polypeptide chain. (b) Secondary structure of proteins: the repeated twisting and folding of neighbouring amino acids that are bonded by hydrogen bonds in common conformations known as the alpha helix and the β pleated sheets. (c) Tertiary structure refers to the 3-dimensional structure of the protein that has arisen during the protein folding process. (d) Quaternary structure exists for those proteins with two subunits or more and refers to the arrangement of each subunit relative to another. (adapted from Tortora and Derrickson, *Principles of Anatomy and Physiology, Twelfth Edition*, 2009, reproduced by permission of John Wiley & Sons Inc.)

(or *subunit*) relative to one another. The bonds that hold each subunit together are similar to those in the tertiary structure. One example of a protein with a quaternary structure is haemoglobin, the protein that is responsible for transporting oxygen in our blood to cells and tissues. Haemoglobin is composed of four subunits, two α-globin units and two β-globin units. Myosin, the protein involved in the contractile apparatus of muscle cells, is composed of six subunits, two of which are known as *myosin heavy chains* and four of which are referred to as *myosin light chains*.

4.4 Proteins as enzymes

As discussed earlier, one of the most important functions of proteins is to act as enzymes – biological catalysts which speed up the rate of chemical reactions without being directly modified themselves. Without the action of **enzymes**, most cellular chemical reactions would go so slowly that the cell would die. Under the right conditions, enzymes can speed up chemical reactions at a rate that is 100 million to 10 billion times quicker!

The basic function of enzymes is shown schematically in Figure 4.6. In this example, the reactants A and B (i.e. the *substrates*) are converted to the products C and D through the action of the enzyme. In Figure 4.6a, the reaction is shown in the particular format to highlight that the enzyme is unchanged once the reaction has taken place. However, we usually write such reactions in a form of shorthand, where the enzyme is written above the reaction arrow (Figure 4.6b). Figure 4.6c shows an example of an enzymatic reaction where the enzyme *lactate dehydrogenase* (LDH) facilitates the production of lactate, a reaction which is highly active in our muscles during high-intensity exercise (Karlsson & Saltin, 1970). In the following sections, we discuss the basic processes of enzyme action and also outline some of the factors that can modify enzyme activity.

4.4.1 Mechanisms of enzyme action

All chemical reactions require an initial input of energy to initiate the reaction, known as the *activation energy*. You could think of this as analogous to pushing a boulder up a cliff top (i.e. the initial energy required to push the boulder to the correct position) and then rolling it over the edge. In a similar fashion, activation energy is the initial energy required to bring the reactants (the boulder) into the necessary position (top of the hill) to allow the reaction to proceed (the boulder rolling down the hill).

Enzymes can speed up the rate of chemical reactions by lowering the required activation energy, thus making it more likely that the

$$A + B + enzyme \longrightarrow C + D + enzyme$$

(a)

$$A + B \xrightarrow{\text{enzyme}} C + D$$

(b)

$$Pyruvate + NADH + H^+ \xleftrightarrow{\text{LDH}} Lactate + NAD^+$$

(c)

Figure 4.6 The basic processes of enzyme action. See text for accompanying information

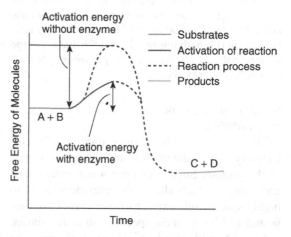

Figure 4.7 Enzymes lower the activation energy of chemical reactions

reaction will start (see Figure 4.7). Without enzyme action, the reaction would depend on *random* collisions between the reactants in order to bring them into the necessary alignment.

Enzymes lower the activation energy by reversibly binding to the to the reactant substrate(s) to form an *enzyme substrate complex*. Once binding has occurred, a specific part of the enzyme will carry out the necessary changes (e.g. bringing the substrates into close proximity or changing the shape of the substrate molecule to increase reaction susceptibility) in order for the reaction to take place. In this way, enzymes have specific amino acid residues which act as the

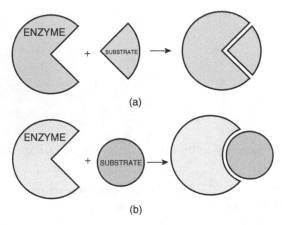

Figure 4.8 Enzyme and substrate binding to form the enzyme substrate complex. In example (a), the enzyme and substrate fit similar as to a how a key fits in a lock. In example (b), both the enzyme and substrate undergo a conformational change when they come into contact so that binding can occur

binding site and specific residues which act as the *catalytic site*.

The term *active site* is often used to refer collectively to both the binding and catalytic domains of the protein. Such sites have a particular shape and charge, which allows the enzyme to bind to highly specific substrates. Enzymes have been suggested to bind to their specific substrates similar to how a key fits in a lock. Alternatively, both the enzyme and substrate undergo a conformational change when their surfaces touch, such that they now fit each other accurately (see Figure 4.8).

4.4.2   Factors affecting rates of enzymatic reactions

The ability of the cell to increase or decrease the rate of enzymatic reactions is particularly important, so that the cell can tightly regulate the flow of biomolecules through energy-producing or energy-consuming pathways, according to the demands placed upon it (e.g. exercise). There are a number of important factors which can all affect the rate of an enzymatic reaction, and these are described below.

Substrate concentration

Increasing the substrate concentration while keeping enzyme concentration constant will accelerate the reaction rate, as more substrate molecules are now available to bind to the enzyme within a given time. This relationship is shown graphically in Figure 2.9. However, it is important to note that the relationship is only linear over the initial period of the reaction, after which point the curve becomes hyperbolic. Eventually, there comes a point at which increasing substrate concentration any further does not cause any further increase in reaction rate. At this substrate concentration, the enzyme is said to have *saturated* and has reached its *maximal velocity* (V_{MAX}). At such points, the enzyme is working as fast as it can in converting the substrate to the product.

Also shown in Figure 4.9 is the *Michaelis constant* (K_M), defined as the substrate concentration required to achieve half of the maximal velocity of an enzymatic concentration. The smaller the K_M value, the greater affinity the enzyme has for its substrate and, as such, the enzyme is active even when the substrate concentration is low. Within our cells, most substrates are generally present at concentrations equal to or less than the K_M value. This is beneficial, as it means that the enzyme can still respond to subtle

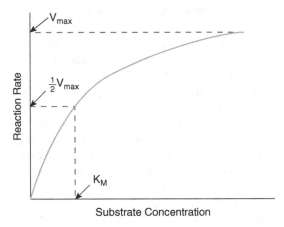

Figure 4.9   Effect of substrate concentration on reaction rate

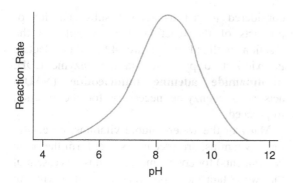

Figure 4.10 Effect of pH on reaction rate

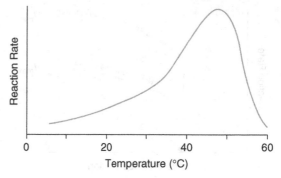

Figure 4.11 Effect of temperature on reaction rate

changes in substrate concentration, since it is still on the steep part of the curve.

pH

Cellular changes in pH can alter the affinity of an enzyme for its substrate, as the change in ionization state (i.e. addition or removal of protons) of the enzyme can alter the structure and charge of the binding site of the enzyme protein. Changes in pH can also alter the substrate directly, thus in turn influencing the rate of the reaction.

Enzymes usually function optimally over a narrow range of pH that is close to the physiological pH of the particular cell (see Figure 4.10). For example, enzymes in the stomach usually function optimally close to a pH of 2, given the acidic conditions present. In contrast, the enzymes in our muscles usually function optimally around 7.

While cellular changes in pH are usually small, skeletal muscle shows the largest change in pH, especially during high-intensity exercise conditions, where pH can fall from 7.1 to 6.6 (Bogdanis et al., 1995). For this reason, an acidosis-induced inhibition of metabolic enzymes involved in the glycolytic pathway is often associated with fatigue during high-intensity exercise (Hargreaves et al., 1998).

Temperature

One of the most profound factors influencing rates of enzymatic reactions is cell temperature, as this increases the kinetic energy of the reactants, thus

raising the chances of effective collisions. Rates of reaction show a linear increase up until approximately 50°C, after which point the enzyme protein denatures (i.e. loses its three-dimensional structure) and loses function (see Figure 4.11).

Such sensitivity to temperature underpins our need to actively warm-up prior to exercise, so as to increase muscle temperature and increase enzyme activity in our muscles. Indeed, muscle temperature can rise from around 35°C at rest to 41°C during intense exercise (Morton et al., 2006). To put this into a sporting performance context, professional soccer players typically cover less distance in the first five-minute period of the second half period, compared with the last five min of the first half, and this has been suggested to be due to a fall in muscle temperature to near resting values during the half-time period (Mohr et al., 2004). In such instances, the same researchers also observed that performing light exercise during half-time to keep muscle temperature (and enzymes active) high can offset such performance decrements.

Enzyme concentration

Once the enzyme is saturated with substrate and working at V_{MAX}, increasing the enzyme concentration itself will further augment reaction rate, as there are now more active sites available for substrate binding. Although increasing enzyme concentration will increase V_{MAX}, it is important to note that there is no concomitant increase in K_M. (see Figure 4.12).

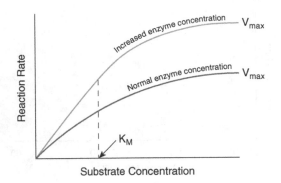

Figure 4.12 Effect of enzyme concentration on reaction rate

The ability of cells to adjust enzyme concentration in order to increase reaction rate is one of the underpinning mechanisms by which skeletal muscle adapts to endurance training. With repeated bouts of endurance training, our muscle cells respond by making new proteins through the process of protein synthesis (see later sections), thus increasing enzyme concentration so that metabolic reactions operate at a greater rate. As such, the stress of exercise is reduced for a given absolute intensity (Holloszy & Coyle, 1984).

4.4.3 Coenzymes and cofactors

Many enzymes require the presence of additional reactive groups known as *cofactors* in order to have full catalytic function. Cofactors may consist of inorganic molecules such as the metal ions of zinc, copper, manganese, magnesium, etc. In such instances, these cofactors directly alter the binding activity of the enzyme by changing the charge distribution and shape of the active site of the enzyme. Where cofactors are tightly bound to the enzyme at all times, they are referred to as *prosthetic groups*, e.g. copper, manganese, zinc, biotin, vitamin B6, etc.

Alternatively, cofactors may be organic molecules known as *coenzymes*. In contrast to inorganic cofactors, coenzymes do not alter the enzyme's binding activity but instead act as important compounds which directly participate in the reaction. Coenzymes can therefore be considered to act as second substrates for or products of the reaction. For example, in the reaction outlined in Figure 4.6, where lactate is oxidized to pyruvate via the enzyme LDH, **nicotinamide adenine dinucleotide (NAD$^+$)** acts as a coenzyme necessary for the reaction to proceed.

Many of the water-soluble vitamins, especially the B vitamins, are precursors (i.e. form the basic components) for coenzymes, and thus it is essential that we obtain the appropriate amount of vitamin B in our diets. Indeed, there are many diseases associated with vitamin B deficiency, given that certain enzymes cannot function optimally if they lack the necessary coenzyme. Members of the vitamin B family and the coenzymes they form are shown in Table 4.2, as are recommended dietary allowances (RDA) for 19–30 year old males (as recommended by the Food and Nutrition Board of the National Academy of Sciences). The coenzymes NAD$^+$ and FAD are especially important for *oxidation-reduction reactions*, as they form the basis for oxidative phosphorylation, the energy-producing pathway which is dominant during prolonged endurance-type exercise.

4.4.4 Classification of enzymes

As we saw in Chapter 3, there are many common types of chemical reaction. Similarly, the enzymes which facilitate many of these reactions can also be classified into six common classes and sub-classes (see Table 4.3), as designated by the International Union of Biochemistry. Most enzymes are recognizable by the suffix-*ase*, while the first part of the enzyme's name (everything that precedes the suffix) usually refers to the type of reaction and/or the substrate which they act upon. For example, the enzyme creatine kinase has phosphocreatine (PCr) as its substrate and, as a kinase, it transfers a phosphate group to ADP, thus making the products ATP and creatine (Cr). This reaction is highly active within the first 10 seconds of maximal exercise, providing a rapid source of ATP production to fuel muscle contraction (Parolin *et al*. 1999).

Table 4.2 The B vitamin family and the coenzymes they form

B vitamin	Coenzyme	Abbreviation	RDA
Thiamine (B1)	Thiamine pyrophosphate	TPP	1.2 mg/d
Riboflavin (B2)	Flavin adenine dinucleotide	FAD	1.3 mg/d
Niacin (B3)	Nicotinamide adenine dinucleotide	NAD$^+$	16 mg/d[a]
Vitamin B6	Pyridoxal phosphate	PLP	1.3 mg/d
Pantothenic acid	Coenzyme A	CoA	5 mg/d
Folate (folacin)	Tetrahydrofolic acid	THFA	400 μg/d[b]
Biotin	Biotin	n/a	30 μg/d
Vitamin B12	Methyl cobalamin	n/a	2.4 μg/d

[a]values expressed as Niacin equivalents;
[b]values expressed as dietary folate equivalents; d (day)

Table 4.3 Enzyme classes and sub-classes and descriptions of their general functions

Enzyme class	Sub-class	General function
Oxidoreductases	Dehydrogenases Oxidases Oxygenases Reductases Peroxidases Hydroxylases	Catalyze oxidation and reduction reactions
Transferases	Kinases Transcarboxylases Transaminases	Catalyze the transfer of elements from one molecule or compound to another
Hydrolases	Phosphatases Esterases Peptidases	Catalyze reactions where cleavage of bonds is achieved by adding water
Lyases	Synthases Deaminases Decarboxylases	Catalyze reactions in which groups of elements are removed to form a double bond or are added to an existing double bond
Isomerases	Mutases Isomerases Epimerases	Catalyze reactions that result in rearrangement of the structure of molecules
Ligases	Synthetases Carboxylases	Catalyze bond formation between two substrate molecules

4.4.5   Regulation of enzyme activity

We have seen thus far how the rates of enzymatic reaction can be altered by changing the cell temperature and pH as well as the substrate concentration and enzyme concentration itself. The provision of additional reactive groups in the form of cofactors and coenzymes can also modify reaction rates. However, there are two other major cellular mechanisms by which enzyme activity can be further modified.

Covalent modification

The most rapid way to modify enzyme activity is through the addition or removal of a phosphate group (which is provided from ATP) to the hydroxyl part of the amino acid side chains of serine, threonine or tyrosine residues (see Figure 4.13). Such processes alter the conformation of the enzyme and are known as **phosphorylation** (addition of phosphate) or **dephosphorylation** (removal of phosphate). This form of covalent modification of enzymes is in turn regulated by enzymes known as *protein kinases* (responsible for phosphorylation) or *protein phosphatases* (responsible for dephosphorylation).

Phosphorylation-dephosphorylation has been likened to turning on and off a light switch, as it rapidly alters enzyme activity and it also has an 'all or none' effect – the enzyme is either active or inactive (Houston, 2006). Usually the enzyme is active when in the phosphorylated state, though there are many examples when enzymes are actually active in the dephosphorylated state. For example, glycogen synthase, the enzyme responsible for glycogen synthesis, is inactive when phosphorylated and requires dephosphorylation by protein phosphatase 1 to become active.

The overall mechanism of controlling enzyme activity by phosphorylation or dephosphorylation is critical to sport and exercise metabolism, and there will be many examples of this type of regulation in subsequent chapters.

Allosteric modification

Whereas phosphorylation-dephosphorylation generally renders the enzyme as active or inactive, enzymes can also gradually grade their activity via *allosteric regulation*. In this process, small molecules known as *allosteric effectors* bind to regulatory domains other than the active site. This, in turn, alters the shape and/or charge of the active site (see Figure 4.14). In this way, the enzyme can therefore increase or decrease its affinity for binding of substrates, depending on whether positive or negative allosteric effectors have bound, respectively. If phosphorylation-dephosphorylation can be likened to turning on and off a light switch, allosteric regulation can be thought of as a dimmer switch, where the enzyme's activity can be fine tuned along a continuum of activity (Houston, 2006).

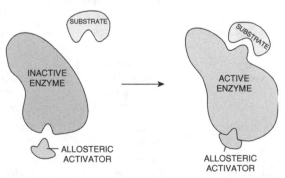

Figure 4.14 Regulation of enzyme activity through allosteric modification. Binding of the allosteric effector to the non-binding site alters the shape and/or charge of the binding site, thus increasing the enzyme's affinity for binding to its substrate

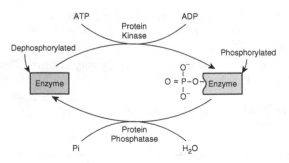

Figure 4.13 Regulation of enzyme activity through phosphorylation and dephosphorylation

Similar to covalent regulation, allosteric regulation of enzymes is highly important for sport and exercise metabolism, in order to regulate the rate of energy provision according to the intensity and duration of the exercise. In such circumstances, products of energy-producing reactions such as ADP, AMP, P_i and H^+, etc. can all act as a feedback loop mechanism to fine tune the rate of enzymatic reactions during exercise (Parolin et al., 1999). This will be highlighted in much more detail in future chapters, where we will examine the regulation of metabolism during different types of exercise.

4.5 Protein turnover

4.5.1 Overview of protein turnover

Although we have examined the basic structure and functions of proteins, it is also important to appreciate the dynamics of *protein turnover*. The proteins within our bodies are in a continual state of turnover, in that new ones are being made (*protein synthesis*) and old ones are being broken down to their constituent amino acids (*protein degradation*). The process of protein turnover is also energy-dependent, and can account for as much as 20% of daily basal energy expenditure.

The half-life of a protein can vary from minutes (e.g. enzymes in the liver) to days and weeks (e.g. enzymes in the muscle) and is usually dependent on the function of the specific protein. For example, in the case of the liver, the rapid ability to up-regulate enzyme protein content is a carefully regulated process involved in controlling the metabolic reactions that occur during feeding and fasting.

In skeletal muscle cells, the training-induced increase in mitochondrial proteins that occur over weeks and months can improve the muscle cell's ability to generate ATP through oxidative metabolism, thus giving rise to improved endurance performance (Gollnick et al., 1973; Holloszy & Coyle, 1984). Similarly, it is the accumulation of the myofibrillar proteins in response to resistance training that eventually results in

muscle *hypertrophy* (i.e. muscle growth) and allows us to become stronger (Wackerhage & Ratkevicius, 2008). In contrast, when the rate of protein degradation exceeds the rate of protein synthesis, such as during times of fasting or disuse, our muscles undergo *atrophy* and become smaller (Philips et al., 2009).

Understanding the basic processes of protein synthesis is therefore highly important for the exercise scientist and this is now one of the most active areas of research within the literature (Kumar et al., 2009).

The information required for our cells to make new proteins is stored within the nuclei and specifically within the *genes* in our *chromosomes*. All nuclei (with the exception of those in human egg and sperm cells) contain 46 chromosomes. Males contain two copies of chromosome 1 through to 22 plus an X and Y chromosome. Females also have two copies of chromosomes 1–22 but differ in that they possess two X chromosomes and no Y chromosome.

Each chromosome is essentially a single but extremely long strand of DNA, and it is the information contained within specific segments of our DNA (i.e. genes) which dictates which amino acids (and, moreover, the specific linear sequence of amino acids) are used to make the protein of interest. In order to make new proteins, our cells must make a copy of the relevant segment of DNA through a process known as *transcription*, which yields a newly formed compound known as *messenger ribonucleic acid* (**mRNA**). The process of transcription occurs in the nucleus. The information contained within the newly formed mRNA molecule subsequently determines the exact nature of amino acid binding to make a protein. This process is referred to as *translation* and occurs in the **ribosomes**. A simplified overview of the pathway from DNA to protein is shown in Figure 4.15.

4.5.2 DNA structure

Our chromosomes largely consist of long strands of DNA that are coiled together in a double helix format. Our DNA, in turn, is composed

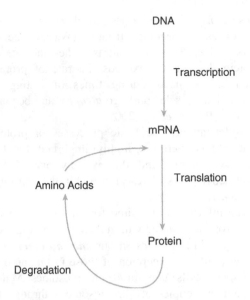

Figure 4.15 The pathway from DNA to protein

of a sugar (*deoxyribose*), a phosphate and four organic bases, two of which are pyrimidine bases (*cytosine* and *thymine*) and two of which are purine bases (*adenine* and *guanine*). The bases are often abbreviated using the capital of the first letter in their name i.e. C, T, A and G, respectively. A chain of sugar and phosphate essentially provides the backbone for which the bases to attach, as shown in Figure 4.16. In this example, the bases are ordered as A, G, T and C, although it is important to note that the precise ordering of bases will vary throughout the stretch of the DNA molecule. Indeed, a DNA molecule is typically millions of these units long, and if extended (as opposed to existing in its double helix format) would be around 2 m long!

We have already alluded to the double helix structure of DNA in that DNA is essentially structured as a double-stranded molecule which is held together by hydrogen bonds between bases. The bases therefore exist as *base pairs*, where the adenine in one strand is always joined to thymine in the other strand. Similarly, the guanine in one strand is always bonded to cytosine in the other strand. Each strand differs in polarity from one another, as one begins with a free phosphate

group attached to deoxyribose (known as the 5' end) and one strand ends with a free OH group attached to deoxyribose (known as the 3' end). In essence, the two strands are therefore *antiparallel*, as one runs from 5' to 3' and the other runs from 3' to 5' (see Figure 4.17).

4.5.3 Transcription

During the process of transcription, a specific segment of DNA (i.e. a gene) is copied to make a newly formed molecule known as **messenger ribonucleic acid (mRNA)**. The order of bases in the DNA therefore serves as a template for which to produce mRNA. The bases in the newly formed mRNA have the same base pairing as they do in DNA, with the exception that thymine in mRNA is actually replaced by *uracil* (U). Transcription begins when an enzyme known as *RNA polymerase II* binds to the *promoter region* of a gene, which is an approximate 100-base pair DNA sequence. RNA polymerase II is, in turn, first attracted to the promoter region of the gene following the binding of a regulatory protein known as a *transcription factor* (TF) to the promoter. In this way, effective binding of the transcription factor protein subsequently recruits RNA polymerase II to the promoter region. RNA polymerase then 'scans' the entire length of the gene, transcribing the base sequence in one strand of DNA into its complementary strand of mRNA (see Figure 4.18).

4.5.4 The genetic code

The sequence of the bases in the mRNA molecule can now determine the exact sequence of the amino acids in the primary structure of the protein to be made. For this to occur, the bases in the mRNA molecule are read in groups of three known as *codons*. It is the specific sequence of bases within the codons which underpins the *genetic code*, a code which is used to translate the three-base sequence into a corresponding amino acid. The genetic code is shown in Table 4.4,

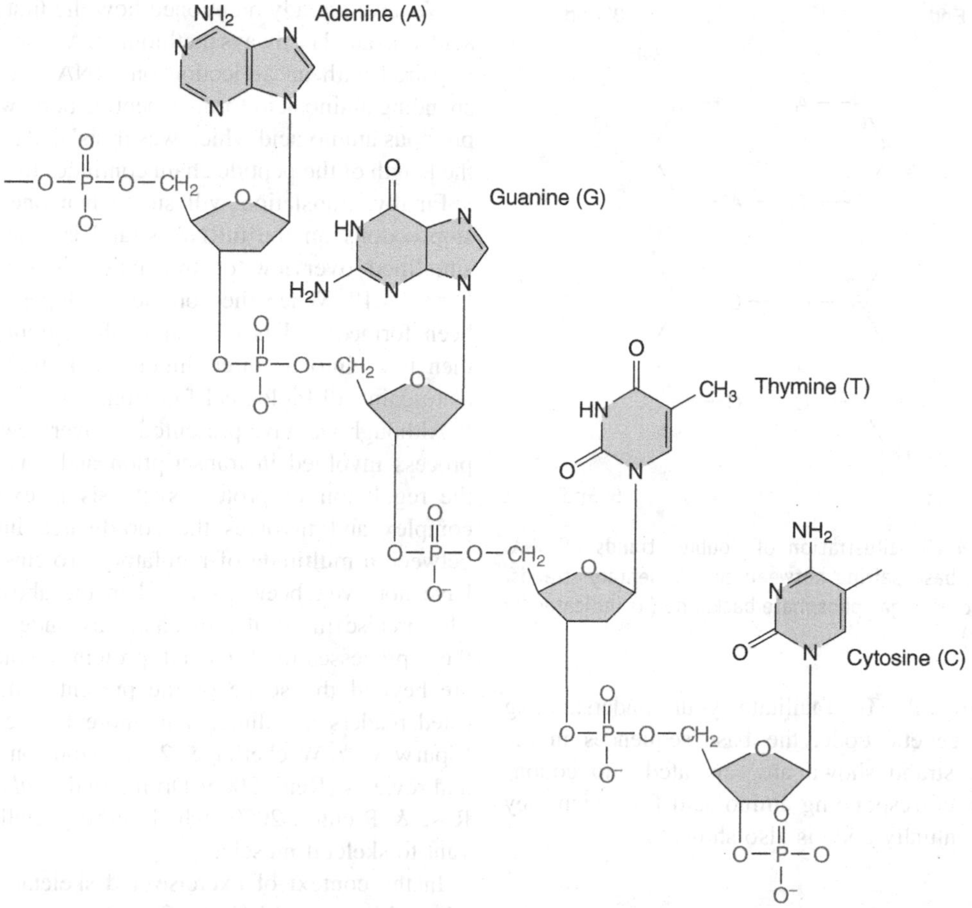

Figure 4.16 Example of a strand from a DNA molecule, showing the attachment of the bases (indicated by black text) to the sugar-phosphate backbone (indicated by red text)

where the amino acid (symbolized by its three-letter abbreviation) corresponding to a particular codon is written adjacent to the base sequence.

Given that there are four bases present in mRNA and that they are read in combinations of three, theoretically this gives rise to 4^3 codons (i.e. 64) and hence 64 amino acids. However, there are, of course, only 20 amino acids used to make proteins, so multiple codons can therefore code for the same amino acid. (see Table 4.4). Of the 64 codons, 61 code for amino acids and three are 'stop' or 'termination' signals (UAA, UGA and UAG). The latter codons signal the end of translation of the information contained in mRNA into a polypeptide chain. The start codon or initiation codon is always

AUG, which also corresponds to the amino acid methionine. For this reason, methionine is always the first amino acid used for protein synthesis.

Returning to Figure 4.18, we can see that only one strand of DNA is used for transcription, and this is known as the *template strand*. The template strand is read in the 3' to 5' direction. The DNA strand which is not copied is known as the *sense strand* and has the same base sequence as the mRNA, with the exception that U now replaces T. In this way, the polarity of the sense strand and mRNA are the same, but are opposite to that of the template strand. The mRNA strand is therefore read in the 5' to 3' direction, which is often referred to as from 'upstream to

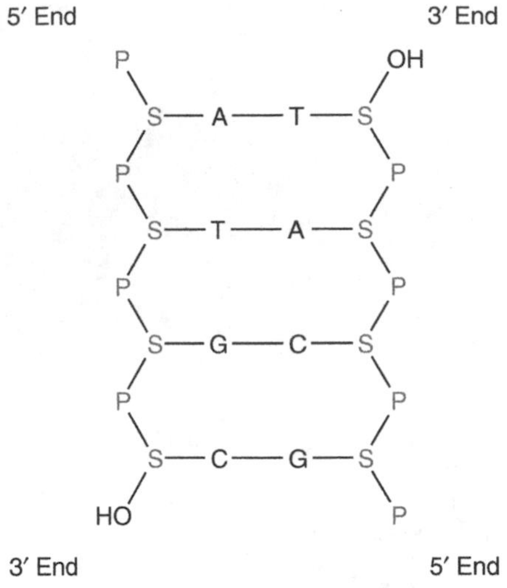

5′ End   3′ End

```
        P                          OH
         \                         /
          S — A — T — S
         /                         \
        P                          P
         \                         /
          S — T — A — S
         /                         \
        P                          P
         \                         /
          S — G — C — S
         /                         \
        P                          P
         \                         /
          S — C — G — S
         /                         \
       HO                          P
```

3′ End   5′ End

Figure 4.17 Illustration of double strands of DNA, showing base pairing between complementary strands. S-P denotes sugar-phosphate backbone (as indicated by red text)

downstream'. To facilitate your understanding of the genetic code, the base sequences in the mRNA strand shown are separated into codons and the corresponding amino acid for which they will eventually code is also shown.

4.5.5   Translation

Having formed the mRNA molecule in the cell nucleus, the next stage in the process of protein synthesis is to translate the base sequence in mRNA into its corresponding amino acid. As discussed above, the process of translation is underpinned by the genetic code. However, for translation to occur, the mRNA has first to exit the pores in the nuclear membrane and travel to the *ribosomes* (the 'factories' where proteins are made) – the cellular location where translation occurs.

As the strand of mRNA emerges along the ribosome, each codon is recognized by an **anticodon** which is bound to a **transfer RNA (tRNA)** molecule. The other binding site on tRNA molecules is that which binds the corresponding amino acid.

We have already mentioned how the first amino acid translated is always methionine. As each codon is paired with an anticodon on tRNA, the corresponding amino acid forms a peptide bond with the previous amino acid which was translated and thus the length of the peptide chain continues to grow.

Finally, translation will stop when one of the stop codons on the mRNA strand is reached. A simplified overview of translation is shown in Figure 4.19. When the complete polypeptide has been formed and is present in the cytoplasm, it then folds into its three-dimensional structure so as to gain full biological function.

Although we have presented an overview of the process involved in transcription and translation, the regulation of protein synthesis is extremely complex and involves the coordinated interplay between a multitude of regulatory proteins which have not even been discussed in the above text. The precise molecular mechanisms underpinning these processes (and, indeed, protein degradation) are beyond the scope of the present text; interested readers are directed to more focused texts (Spurway & Wackerhage, 2006; Houston, 2006) and reviews (Reid, 2005; Drummond *et al.*, 2009; Rose & Richter, 2009) which are especially relevant to skeletal muscle.

In the context of exercise and skeletal muscle adaptation, transcription of genes is thought to occur during and/or in the hours following an exercise session, such that changes in mRNA content for a specific gene can be detected within this timescale. However, up-regulation of the actual protein content is usually only detected within hours to days after the exercise bout. More often, it usually takes weeks of repetitive exercise sessions (i.e. training) before changes in protein content are observed.

It is this repetitive and transient change in gene expression which is thought to form the molecular basis for training adaptation (Coffey & Hawley, 2007). Understanding how differences in exercise intensity, duration and mode can affect the transcriptional responses to exercise is therefore one of the major challenges facing the exercise scientist in the coming decades. Such research is not only important for helping to optimize athletic

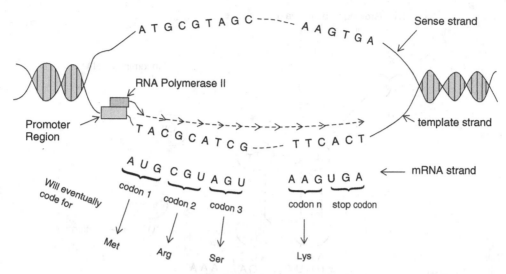

Figure 4.18 Schematic illustration of the process of transcription. Note that in order for transcription to occur, the DNA strands first have to be unravelled from the double helix structure. The sequence of bases in the mRNA strand is identical to those in the sense strand, with the exception that U replaces T

Table 4.4 The genetic code, detailing how the combinations of bases in the 1st, 2nd and 3rd position code for different amino acids

First position (5' end)	Second position				Third position (3' end)
	U	C	A	G	
U	UUU Phe	UCU Ser	UAU Tyr	UGU Cys	U
	UUC Phe	UCC Ser	UAC Tyr	UGC Cys	C
	UUA Leu	UCA Ser	UAA Stop*	UGA Stop*	A
	UUG Leu	UCG Ser	UAG Stop*	UGG Trp	G
C	CUU Leu	CCU Pro	CAU His	CGU Arg	U
	CUC Leu	CCC Pro	CAC His	CGC Arg	C
	CUA Leu	CCA Pro	CAA Gln	CGA Arg	A
	CUG Leu	CCG Pro	CAG Gln	CGG Arg	G
A	AUU Ile	ACU Thr	AAU Asn	AGU Ser	U
	AUC Ile	ACC Thr	AAC Asn	AGC Ser	C
	AUA Ile	ACA Thr	AAA Lys	AGA Arg	A
	AUG Met**	ACG Thr	AAG Lys	AGG Arg	G
G	GUU Val	GCU Ala	GAU Asp	GGU Gly	U
	GUC Val	GCC Ala	GAC Asp	GGC Gly	C
	GUA Val	GCA Ala	GAA Glu	GGA Gly	A
	GUG Val	GCG Ala	GAG Glu	GGG Gly	G

*Stop codons do not have an amino acid assigned to them.
**Codes for the amino acid methionine but also is the start or initiation codon.

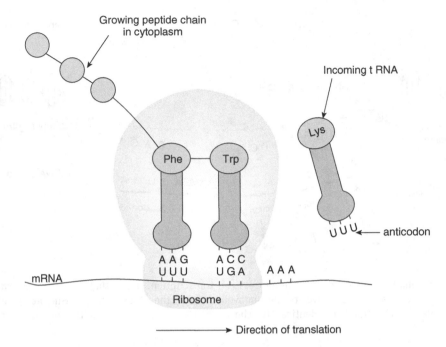

Figure 4.19 Schematic illustration of the process of translation. tRNA molecules originating from the cytoplasm enter the ribosome. Codons on the mRNA strand are recognized by specific anticodons on tRNA and hence by the corresponding amino acid. With continuing codon-anticodon binding, amino acids are joined by peptide bonding and are later folded into their three-dimensional structure in the cytoplasm

performance, but also in optimizing exercise training protocols which may improve health and well-being and offer protection against metabolic related diseases such as diabetes and obesity, etc. (Booth & Laye, 2009).

4.6 Amino acid metabolism

So far in this chapter, we have covered the basic functions and structures of proteins, where we paid particular attention to the role of proteins as enzymes. We then explored the dynamics of protein turnover and outlined the basic cellular processes of protein synthesis in terms of transcription and translation. Given the rapid turnover rates of proteins and, moreover, the importance of proteins to maintenance of life, it is therefore essential that we eat protein-rich foods in order to provide our cells with the essential amino acids needed to make specific proteins. Indeed, the average person will consume 10–15% of their daily calorie intake in the form of protein. Many athletes often consume extra protein, especially during times of intense training.

In addition to providing amino acids for protein synthesis, proteins can also be used as a source of energy, where 1 g of protein provides 4 kcal of energy. It is important to note, however, that protein is not considered as a primary energy source, given the important structural, functional and regulatory roles which proteins play within our bodies.

Nevertheless, during times of fasting or starvation, when energy availability is low, we can metabolize our body's protein stores to provide an additional source of energy. As skeletal muscle comprises our largest store of protein, in such instances we are essentially eating our own muscles! Although it is not advised, many athletes involved in weight-making sports such as boxing and wrestling often have to metabolize muscle protein (i.e. lose muscle mass) in order to make their competitive weight (Morton *et al*., 2010).

In this section, we outline the basic biochemistry of amino acid metabolism, with specific emphasis on skeletal muscle, in order to provide a platform for Part 3, where we will examine how exercise affects the regulation of these pathways.

4.6.1 Free amino acid pool

When dietary protein is consumed, it is broken down to its constituent amino acids in the gut and the small intestine through the enzymatic action of a variety of proteases. Following absorption, the blood then provides the medium for which to transport the amino acids to appropriate tissues, namely that of the liver and skeletal muscle. Although skeletal muscle possesses the largest store of free and protein-bound amino acids (approximately 40% of adult body weight is composed of skeletal muscle, of which 20% is comprised from protein), it is the liver which is the most metabolically active in terms of amino acid metabolism. The liver is also the organ responsible for synthesizing the non-essential amino acids previously outlined in Table 4.1 and, as such, it can therefore be considered as a key player in regulating amino acid delivery for incorporation into other tissues – not just that of skeletal muscle.

The amino acids present in the blood and extra-cellular fluid of tissues (i.e. amino acids that have not yet been taken up by cells for intracellular protein synthesis) represent the *free amino acid pool*. This free amino acid pool can also be complemented by the delivery of amino acids catabolized from the degradation of intracellular proteins. In this way, the amino acid pool therefore collectively consists of those amino acids arising from dietary intake and from the degradation of existing cellular protein (from a variety of tissues) and also those that were synthesized in and released from the liver (see Figure 4.20).

Given that, unlike carbohydrates and fats, we have no storage capacity for amino acids, the free amino acid pool is relatively small and is in a continual state of exchange. Essentially, those amino

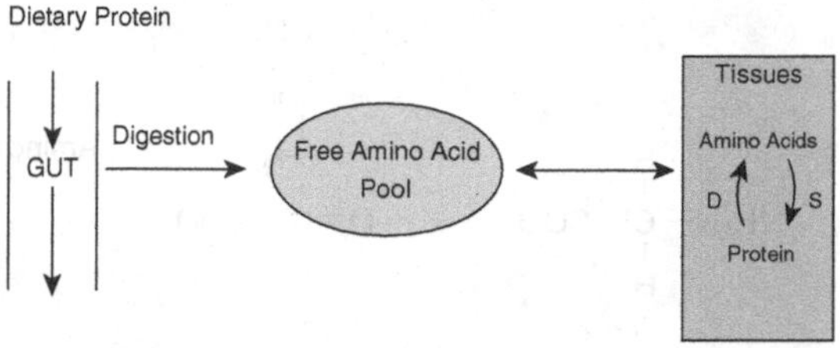

Figure 4.20 A basic overview of amino acid metabolism, showing the continual exchange of amino acids between the amino acid pool and tissues. S = synthesis, D = degradation

acids that are not used for immediate protein synthesis are largely metabolized to provide a source of chemical energy, in the form of intermediate compounds for the *tricarboxylic acid cycle* (abbreviated as TCA, and also known as the *citric acid* or *Krebs cycle*). Alternatively, they can be used to provide substrates for the process of *gluconeogenesis* – the formation of glucose from non-carbohydrate sources. We have not yet covered the reactions or, indeed, the importance of the TCA cycle or gluconeogenesis, but this will be covered in detail in Chapter 5.

4.6.2 Transamination

The initial stage of degradation of amino acids is the removal of nitrogen by removing the α-amino group. We need to remove nitrogen because we cannot use the nitrogen-containing portion of an amino acid in energy production. The majority of amino acids will remove their α-amino group by transferring it to α-*ketoglutarate* (often referred to as 2-oxoglutarate) to make the newly formed amino acid *glutamate*. This reaction is known as *transamination*, and it is catalyzed by a variety of enzymes collectively known as *aminotransferases*.

Recalling what we discussed in Section 4.4 when discussing the classification of enzymes, you should now appreciate that this class of enzymes is so called because they use amino groups as their substrates and they operate by transferring the substrate to another compound. Most of these

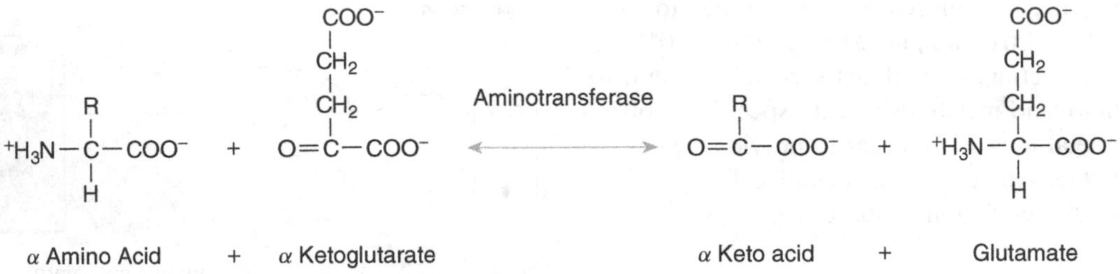

Figure 4.21   The process of transamination

enzymes require vitamin B6 as a prosthetic group (i.e. pyridoxal phosphate, abbreviated as PLP) and the enzymes are also specific to the particular amino acid, e.g. **alanine aminotransferase**, etc.

An example of a transamination is shown in Figure 4.21. The α-amino acid transfers its amino group to α-ketoglutarate (an intermediate of the TCA cycle), thus forming glutamate. The resulting carbon skeleton that is left, following removal of the α-amino group, then forms a variety of α-keto acids, which can be used in energy production. An α-keto acid is an organic acid containing a ketone functional group and a carboxylic acid group.

The α-keto acids produced are (or can later be) converted to intermediates of the TCA cycle, as shown in Figure 4.22, thus providing important energy-containing compounds which contribute to TCA cycle flux. The process of forming TCA cycle intermediates through transamination of amino acids is known as **anaplerosis**.

In addition to providing TCA cycle intermediates, the **carbon skeletons** produced from transamination can also provide important substrates for gluconeogenesis (the full biochemical pathway of this process is shown in Chapter 5). Indeed, many amino acids form *pyruvate* and *oxaloacetate*, which are two of the major precursors for gluconeogenesis. Additionally, the other α-keto acids produced, such as α-ketoglutarate, succinyl-CoA and fumarate, will eventually convert to oxaloacetate via the TCA cycle.

In this way, 18 of the 20 amino acids are a source of glucose and are therefore known as **glucogenic amino acids**. In contrast, the amino acids of **leucine** and **lysine** are considered as

ketogenic amino acids, as the acetyl-CoA or acetoacetyl-CoA which form from their degradation are **ketone bodies** which cannot be later converted to glucose (the formation of ketone bodies is discussed in more detail in Chapter 6).

4.6.3   Deamination

In recapping transamination, amino acids can transfer their amino group to α-ketoglutarate, thus forming glutamate and an α-keto acid, where the precise α-keto acid formed depends on the initial amino acid (it is important to note that this reaction is reversible, in that glutamate itself can form a new amino acid). The amino group that has been transferred to the newly formed glutamate can now be removed as ammonia via a process known as *oxidative deamination*. This reversible reaction is catalyzed by the enzyme **glutamate dehydrogenase**, which is located in the mitochondrial matrix (Figure 4.23).

The reaction is considered an **oxidative deamination**, as not only has glutamate lost its amino group, but it has also been oxidized by NAD^+ or $NADP^+$. The ammonia produced from the reaction (in the form of the ammonium ion, NH_4^+) is subsequently fed into the **urea cycle** (in the liver) to make **urea**, which is then excreted from the kidneys when **urine** is formed. It is important to dispose of ammonia because, in high concentrations, it is toxic to the cell. The α-ketoglutarate produced in the deamination reaction is beneficial, as it can then also participate in transamination reactions again (as outlined in Figure 4.21) or, alternatively, it can enter the TCA cycle directly.

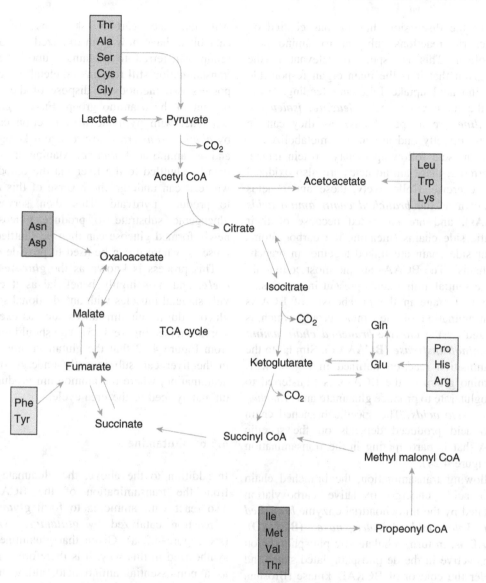

Figure 4.22 Entry of carbon skeletons of amino acids into the TCA cycle as important intermediates

Glutamate dehydrogenase

$$\text{Glutamate} + \text{NAD (P)}^+ + H_2O \longleftrightarrow \alpha\text{-ketoglutarate} + NH_4^+ + NAD(P)H + H^+$$

Figure 4.23 The process of oxidative deamination

4.6.4 Branched chain amino acids

Most of the discussion thus far has centred on the generic reactions inherent to amino acid metabolism. This is especially relevant to the liver, given that it is the main organ responsible for amino acid uptake following feeding. However, the three amino acids *leucine*, *isoleucine* and *valine* are a special case, as they can be taken up directly and are mainly metabolized in skeletal muscle following dietary protein intake. Furthermore, these amino acids are also oxidized during exercise. Collectively, these amino acids are known as the *branched chain amino acids* (**BCAAs**), and are so called because of their aliphatic side chains (meaning the carbon atoms in their side chain are linked together in branch-like chains). The BCAAs are the most commonly found essential amino acids present in proteins.

The first stage in the metabolism of BCAAs is transamination of the amino group, which is catalyzed by the enzyme *branched chain amino acid aminotransferase* (**BCAAAT**). Similar to the transamination reaction outlined in Figure 4.21, the amino group of the BCAAs is transferred to α-ketoglutarate to produce glutamate and *branched chain α-keto acids*. The specific branched chain α-keto acid produced depends on the specific BCAA that is participating in the transamination (see Figure 4.24).

Following transamination, the branched chain α-keto acids undergo oxidative carboxylation facilitated by the mitochondrial enzyme *branched chain keto acid dehydrogenase* (**BCKAD**). BCKAD is, in turn, regulated by phosphorylation (and is active in the de-phosphorylated state) and is under the control of BCKAD kinase (Brosnan & Brosnan, 2006). The products of this reaction are then further oxidized in a reaction catalyzed by the enzyme *acyl-CoA dehydrogenase* (ACDH). Ultimately, the carbon skeletons produced from the metabolism of the BCAAs eventually find their way to the TCA cycle to be oxidized to CO_2 and H_2O.

4.6.5 Glucose-alanine cycle

Although the carbon skeletons of BCAA catabolism have now been oxidized, the α-amino group transferred to glutamate upon the initial transamination still remains. Skeletal muscle cells possess two methods to dispose of the nitrogen present in the α-amino group. Firstly, glutamate can react with pyruvate in a reaction catalyzed by *alanine transferase* to produce α-ketoglutarate and the amino acid *alanine*. Alanine, in turn, can then be shuttled to the liver via the bloodstream, where it can undergo the reverse of this reaction to produce pyruvate. This then serves as a glucogenic substrate to produce glucose. The newly formed glucose can then be shuttled to the muscles, where it can be used to provide energy.

This process is known as the *glucose-alanine cycle*, and it is highly beneficial as it can provide skeletal muscles with an additional source of glucose during circumstances such as exercise or starvation (see Figure 4.25). You should remember from Figure 4.23 that the glutamate now formed in the liver can subsequently undergo oxidative deamination, where the ammonium produced will ultimately feed to the urea cycle.

4.6.6 Glutamine

In addition to the above, the glutamate formed from the transamination of the BCAAs can also react with ammonia to form *glutamine* in a reaction catalyzed by *glutamine synthetase* (see Figure 4.26a). Given that glutamine can be synthesized in this way, it is therefore considered as a non-essential amino acid, although during times of muscle atrophy (i.e. loss of muscle mass) associated with fasting or disease, it is often beneficial to consume extra glutamine in our diets. Similar to alanine, the newly formed glutamine can then be shuttled to the liver, where it can be re-converted to glutamate via the enzyme *glutaminase* (Figure 4.26b). Finally, the

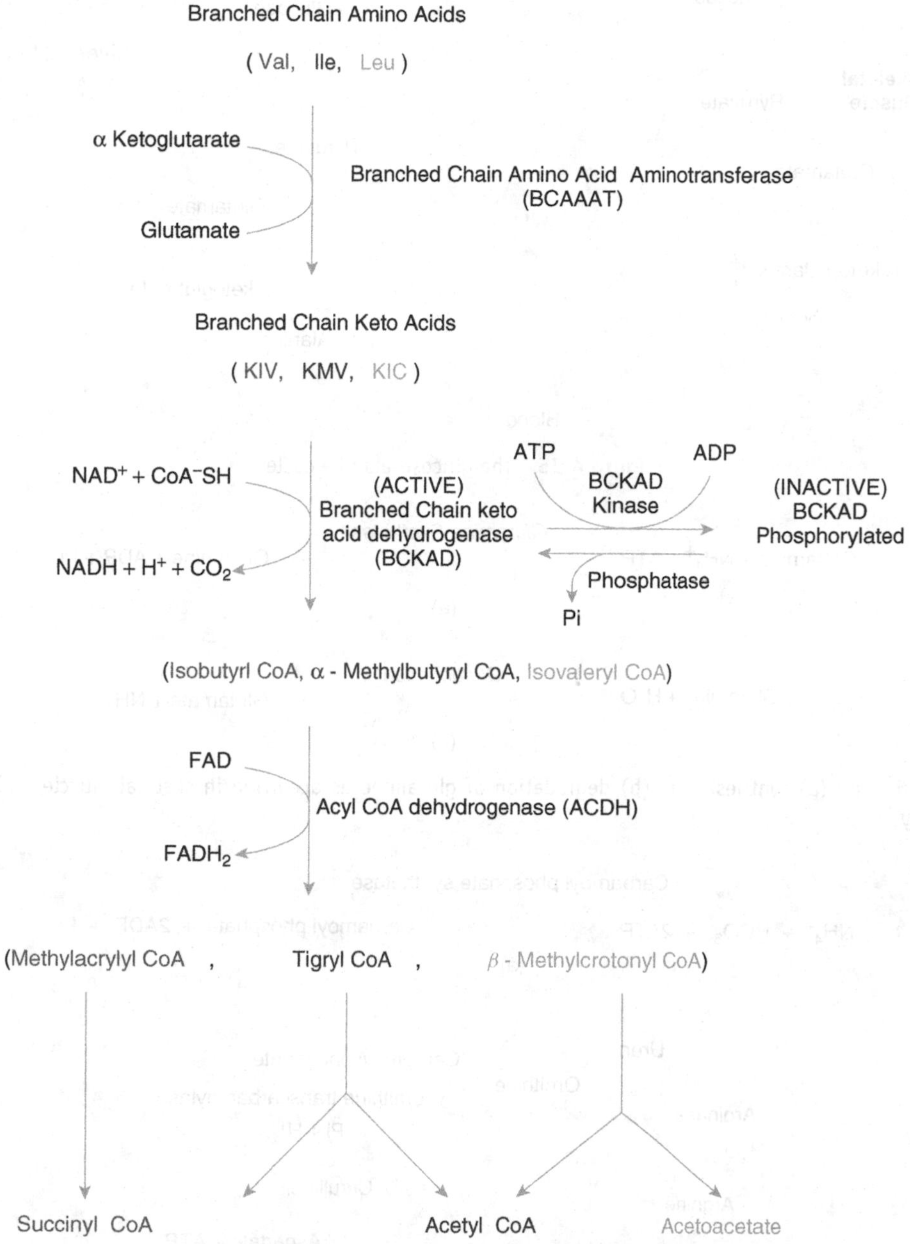

Branched Chain Amino Acids

(Val, Ile, Leu)

α Ketoglutarate

Branched Chain Amino Acid Aminotransferase
(BCAAAT)

Glutamate

Branched Chain Keto Acids

(KIV, KMV, KIC)

NAD$^+$ + CoA$^-$SH

ATP   ADP

(ACTIVE)
Branched Chain keto
acid dehydrogenase
(BCKAD)

BCKAD
Kinase

(INACTIVE)
BCKAD
Phosphorylated

NADH + H$^+$ + CO$_2$

Phosphatase

Pi

(Isobutyrl CoA, α - Methylbutyryl CoA, Isovaleryl CoA)

FAD

Acyl CoA dehydrogenase (ACDH)

FADH$_2$

(Methylacrylyl CoA   ,   Tigryl CoA   ,   β - Methylcrotonyl CoA)

Succinyl CoA   Acetyl CoA   Acetoacetate

Figure 4.24 Degradation of the BCAAs. KIV = α-ketoisovalerate, KMV = α-keto-β-methylvalerate, KIC = α-ketoisocaproate

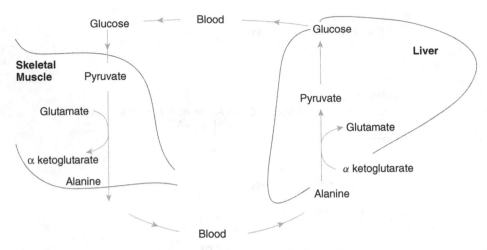

Figure 4.25   The glucose-alanine cycle

$$\text{Glutamate} + NH_4^+ + ATP \xrightarrow{\textit{Glutamine Synthetase}} \text{Glutamine} + ADP + Pi$$

(a)

$$\text{Glutamine} + H_2O \xrightarrow{\textit{Glutaminase}} \text{Glutamate} + NH_4^+$$

(b)

Figure 4.26   The (a) synthesis and (b) degradation of glutamine as occurring in skeletal muscle and the liver, respectively

Carbamoyl phosphate synthetase

$$NH_4^+ + HCO_3^- + 2ATP \xrightarrow{\hspace{2cm}} \text{Carbamoyl phosphate} + 2ADP + Pi$$

(a)

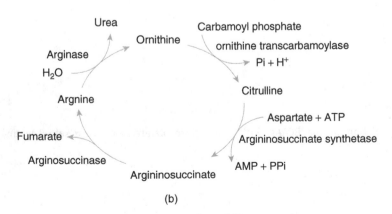

(b)

Figure 4.27   Overview of the urea cycle

glutamate can then dispose of its amino group through oxidative deamination to feed NH_4^+ to the urea cycle.

4.6.7 The urea cycle

As we bring our study of amino acid metabolism to a close, you should now appreciate that virtually all of the nitrogen degraded from the amino groups of α-amino acids is ultimately converted to ammonia in the liver. This accumulation of ammonia essentially arises from that provided from glutamine via the glutaminase reaction, from the oxidative deamination of glutamate and from any ammonia also taken up from the blood. Given that ammonia is toxic in high concentrations, and also because we cannot use the nitrogen present in ammonia, the liver subsequently converts the ammonia to *urea* in a series of reactions known as the *urea cycle*.

The four reactions that comprise this cycle are shown in Figure 4.27. The initial substrate of the cycle, carbamoyl phosphate, is formed in the mitochondrial matrix from the linking of ammonia and bicarbonate. The remaining reactions take place in the cytosol. The non-essential amino acid **aspartate** also contributes to the cycle by incorporating its amino group in reaction 2. The aspartate is formed from a transamination reaction, where glutamate transfers its amino group to oxaloacetate to produce aspartate and α-ketoglutarate in a reaction catalyzed by *aspartate aminotransferase*.

It is important to note that aspartate is the only amino acid to directly dispose of its amino group in the urea cycle. Urea is eventually formed after reaction 4 and, because it is water soluble, it leaves the liver via the bloodstream before being taken up and excreted by the kidneys as urine. Given urea's obvious link to amino acid metabolism, it is no surprise that urea excretion can increase 2–3 fold if a high protein diet is consumed!

4.7 Key points

- Proteins are the cellular 'action molecules' as they perform important functions essential to the maintenance of life.

- The diverse functions of proteins include operating in catalytic, transport, storage, signalling, contractile, structural, immunological and regulatory roles.
- Amino acids are the building blocks of proteins.
- Twenty amino acids are needed to make proteins, eight of which are considered essential (i.e. we have to obtain them from our food) and 12 of which are non-essential (i.e. we make these from compounds already stored within our bodies).
- The general structure of an amino acid consists of a central carbon atom, a charged amino group, a charged carboxyl group and a variable side chain symbolized as R.
- It is this R group which gives each amino acid its unique characteristics.
- Protein structure consists of a primary, secondary, tertiary and in some cases a quaternary structure.
- The primary structure refers to the linear sequence of amino acids in the polypeptide chain.
- The secondary structure refers to the repeated twisting and folding of neighbouring amino acids in conformations such as alpha helix and the β pleated sheets.
- The tertiary structure arises when the protein folds into a three-dimensional structure. It is only when the protein has tertiary structure that it has function.
- The quaternary structure refers to those proteins that consist of two or more subunits joined together.
- Enzymes are biological catalysts which speed up the rates of chemical reactions without being altered themselves.
- Enzyme activity can be altered by changing the substrate/enzyme concentration and cell temperature/pH.
- Many enzymes require the provision of additional groups known as co-factors or coenzymes in order to gain full function.
- Enzyme activity can also be altered through covalent or allosteric modification.
- Cells make proteins from the information contained within our DNA.

- Strands of DNA exist as a double helix structure in which the bases of adenine/thymine and cytosine/guanine exist as base pairs attached to a sugar-phosphate backbone.
- Transcription occurs in the nucleus, where the base sequence in the DNA template strand is copied to make mRNA.
- The base sequence in mRNA is read as codons and translated in the ribosome according to the genetic code, which determines the sequence of amino acids in the newly formed protein.
- The free amino acid pool represents those amino acids present in the blood and extracellular fluid of tissues. It is composed of amino acids arising from dietary intake, the degradation of existing cellular proteins and those that were synthesized in, and released from, the liver.
- Amino acids can be used to provide energy by providing intermediate compounds for the TCA cycle or by acting as substrates for gluconeogenesis.

- Transamination reactions involve the transfer of the α-amino group from the specific amino acid to α-ketoglutarate (catalyzed by aminotransferase enzymes) to produce glutamate and a corresponding α-keto acid.
- Deamination involves the removal of the α-amino group from glutamate (catalyzed by glutamate dehydrogenase) to produce ammonia, which is then removed via the urea cycle.
- Branched amino acids (BCAAs) are unique as they can be metabolized in skeletal muscle cells.
- Glutamate formed from transamination of BCAAs is converted to alanine or glutamine. Alanine can be shuttled to the liver from the muscle, where it can be converted to glucose, which in turn can be shuttled back to the muscle to provide energy. This process is known as the glucose-alanine cycle.

5

Carbohydrates

Learning outcomes

After studying this chapter, you should be able to:

- elucidate the role of carbohydrates in sport and exercise;
- draw the general structure of a glucose molecule and its isomers;
- draw the general structure of a fructose molecule;
- describe the formation of a disaccharide, illustrating how and where the glycoside bond is present;
- outline the variations in polysaccharides;
- describe the processes of glycogenolysis, glycolysis, gluconeogenesis, and glycogenesis;
- describe the formation and fates of lactic acid;
- outline the key reactions in the link reaction and the TCA cycle;
- explain the concepts of electron transfer and of oxidative phosphorylation;
- calculate the number of ATP molecules produced during breakdown of a glucose molecule via either the anaerobic and aerobic systems;
- describe the formation of fructose.

Key words

acetyl CoA	electron transfer
adenylate cyclase	ETC (electron transfer chain)
adrenaline	
aerobic	FADH
allosteric effector	free radicals
AMP	fructokinase
amylopectin	fructose
amylose	furanose ring
anaerobic	galactose
antioxidants	glucokinase
ATP	gluconeogenesis
carbon	glucose
catecholamines	glyceraldehyde
cellobiose	3-phosphate
CPT1	glycogenesis
Chemiosmotic theory	glycogen
c-AMP	glycogen synthase
cytochrome	glycogenolysis
dephosphorylation	glycolysis
dihydroxyacetone	glycoside bond
phosphate (DHAP)	hexokinase
1,3-diphos-	hexose
phoglycerate	hydrogen
disaccharide	

Biochemistry for Sport and Exercise Metabolism, First Edition. Don MacLaren and James Morton.
© 2012 John Wiley & Sons, Ltd. Published 2012 by John Wiley & Sons, Ltd.

hypoglycaemia	phosphorylation
insulin	PDH
isoform	PEP carboxykinase
isoenzyme	PFK (phosphofructoki-
Krebs cycle	nase)
lactic acid/ lactate	PKA
lactate dehydrogenase	polysaccharide
lactose	pyranose ring
LDH	pyruvate carboxylase
link reaction	pyruvate
malonyl CoA	dehydrogenase
maltose	pyruvic acid/pyruvate
monosaccharide	reactive oxygen
NAD/NADH	species (ROS)
oxidative	starch
phosphorylation	sucrose
oxygen	TCA cycle
3-phosphoglycerate	tetrose
phosphoenolpyruvate	triose
(PEP)	pentose
phosphorylase	UDP/UTP

5.1 Relevance of carbohydrates for sport and exercise

This chapter deals with the biochemistry of carbohydrates. An examination of the effects of carbohydrates on performance is followed by a perusal of the types and structure of carbohydrates before exploring some key biochemical processes in which carbohydrates are important. These include **glycogenolysis, glycolysis, glycogenesis** and **gluconeogenesis**. In addition, the reactions in the **TCA cycle, electron transfer** and **oxidative phosphorylation** will be examined. The regulation of carbohydrate metabolism is dealt with in Chapter 7.

Why are carbohydrates important from a sports science perspective? The answer lies in the fact that carbohydrates are an important fuel and energy supply for muscles, particularly during intense bouts of activity. The evidence for the importance of carbohydrates and performance can be seen in Figure 5.1, where the relationship between exercise intensity and muscle **glycogen** depletion is highlighted.

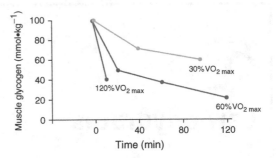

Figure 5.1 Muscle glycogen use during exercise of different intensities (adapted from Gollnick *et al.*, 1974)

Observe that after two hours of exercise at 60% VO_{2max} (i.e. relatively steady state exercise), there is a significant, if not total, depletion of muscle glycogen, whereas at 120% VO_{2max} (i.e. very intense exercise), muscle glycogen is significantly depleted although it doesn't appear to be totally depleted. This is because the data is from mixed muscle fibres, i.e. all muscle fibre types. If the type IIx (or fast glycolytic) fibres are examined after 120% VO_{2max}, a more likely scenario is that these fibres will be almost totally depleted, while the type I fibres (slow oxidative) are still quite full. Therefore, if an athlete wishes to engage in intense (single or repeated) bouts of activity, this appears to be possible only if the muscle glycogen stores (especially in the type IIx fibres) are not completely depleted. At 30% VO_{2max}, the muscle fibres hardly use muscle glycogen, and that is because fats are employed to a greater extent.

In Figure 5.2, another aspect of carbohydrate and its effect on performance can be observed, namely the likelihood of **hypoglycaemia** (low blood **glucose**, i.e. below a concentration of 4 mM) and fatigue. In this instance, the individual becomes hypoglycaemic at the first point of fatigue. In other words, the blood glucose concentration is below 4 mM. The normal level of blood glucose is around 5 mM, and after a meal this could increase to 9–10 mM. The reason why hypoglycaemia results in fatigue is due to the fact that the brain normally uses only blood glucose as a fuel; therefore, when this concentration drops below 4 mM, brain function is affected and results in poor decision-making, slower reactions and also a sensation that exertion requires more effort.

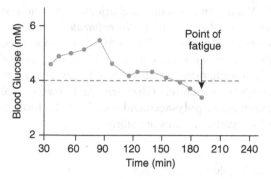

Figure 5.2 Evidence of hypoglycaemia during prolonged exercise (adapted from Christensen and Hansen, 1936)

A more recent concept concerning fatigue proposes that the brain is the 'governor' and that it senses diminished supplies of carbohydrate to bring about a reduction in performance as a protective mechanism. So we should be wary that the brain may play a part in the development of fatigue, and that inadequate carbohydrate content could be involved in this process.

In Figure 5.3, the results of a classical study carried out in the late 1960s in Scandinavia can be observed, whereby the relationship between muscle glycogen, diet over three days and exercise capacity were explored. When the muscle glycogen levels were low (60 mM glycosyl units) because of an inadequate daily carbohydrate intake, the average exercise duration was 60 minutes, whereas when the muscle glycogen content was elevated to 120 mM due to a greater dietary

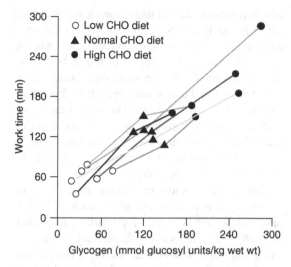

Figure 5.3 Relationship between muscle glycogen content, exercise capacity and diet (adapted from Bergstrom et al., 1967)

intake of carbohydrate, the duration of exercise was 120 minutes. In fact, when levels of muscle glycogen were raised even further (180 mM) by a high carbohydrate diet over the three days, the time to fatigue increased to about 180 minutes. The exercise was cycling at 70% VO_{2max} to fatigue.

Clearly there appears to be a relationship between diet and muscle glycogen content, and also between muscle glycogen content and the ability to exercise for a prolonged period of time.

Further evidence on the relationship between pre-exercise muscle glycogen and the capability for prolonged exercise can be seen in Table 5.1,

Table 5.1 Changes in muscle glycogen and distance covered during a football match (adapted from Saltin, 1973)

	Normal carbohydrate	Low carbohydrate
Number of players	5	4
Muscle glycogen before the game	100%	50%
Muscle glycogen at half time	40%	7%
Muscle glycogen at end of match	10%	0%
Distance covered 1st half	6,100 m	5,600 m
Distance covered 2nd half	5,900 m	4,100 m
Per cent walking	27	50
Per cent sprinting	24	15

which represent the findings from a study carried out in the early 1970s examining muscle glycogen utilization in a competitive football match. Muscle glycogen was significantly depleted at half time, and almost totally by the end of the match, indicating substantial use of muscle carbohydrate. Furthermore, those participants who started the match with a low muscle carbohydrate covered less distance both in the first half and (notably) in the second half, compared to those who started the game with normal carbohydrate stores.

These findings show two things: first, that muscle glycogen is used during sports such as football (and this would hold true for similar games such as rugby, netball, hockey, basketball, volleyball, and so on); and second, that starting a competitive match with a low muscle carbohydrate is likely to impair performance.

You should now appreciate that carbohydrates are important for sport performance, and consequently there is a need for a greater understanding of the biochemistry of carbohydrates.

5.2 Types and structure of carbohydrates

Carbohydrates consist of **carbon**, **hydrogen** and **oxygen** only, with a general formula of $C_n(H_2O)_n$. For a 6-carbon **monosaccharide** this would mean a formula of $C_6H_{12}O_6$ (where n = 6). The simplest of the carbohydrates are the *monosaccharides*, which contain between three and seven carbon atoms:

- Three-carbon monosaccharides are known as *trioses*, and an example is dihydroxyacetone ($C_3H_6O_3$).
- The four-carbon monosaccharides are *tetroses* ($C_4H_8O_4$).
- The five-carbon monosaccharides are the *pentoses*, of which ribose ($C_5H_{10}O_5$) is an important example (see nucleic acids e.g. deoxyribose nucleic acid (DNA) and ribonucleic acid (RNA) in Chapter 4).
- The 6-carbon monosaccharides are known as *hexoses* ($C_6H_{12}O_6$), of which *glucose* and *fructose* are examples.

When two monosaccharides are joined together, they form a **disaccharide**, of which **sucrose, maltose**, and **cellobiose** are examples. *Polysaccharides* consist of multiple numbers of monosaccharides attached in a larger and more complex structure. **Glycogen** and **starch** are examples of **polysaccharides** and are the form in which carbohydrates are stored.

5.2.1 Monosaccharides

Figure 5.4 shows how the structure of glucose can be represented either as an open chain or, if folded, into a ring known as a *pyranose ring*. The ring structure more adequately represents the biochemical properties of glucose and the other monosaccharides than does the open chain structure. Note that the ring only contains five carbon atoms; the sixth carbon is outside the ring. As you look at the structure of glucose, you should note the positions of the carbon atoms from 1 to 5 from right to left, and also that to each of the carbon atoms is attached a hydrogen (H) and a hydroxyl (OH) group.

Monosaccharides, as with many other biochemical compounds such as amino acids, have *isomers*, which are chemical compounds which have the same molecular or chemical formula but possess different structural formulae. Isomers can act differently, both physiologically and biochemically. Glucose, for example, exists as an alpha (α-) and a beta (β-) form (Figure 5.5). The difference between the two is in the carbon-1,

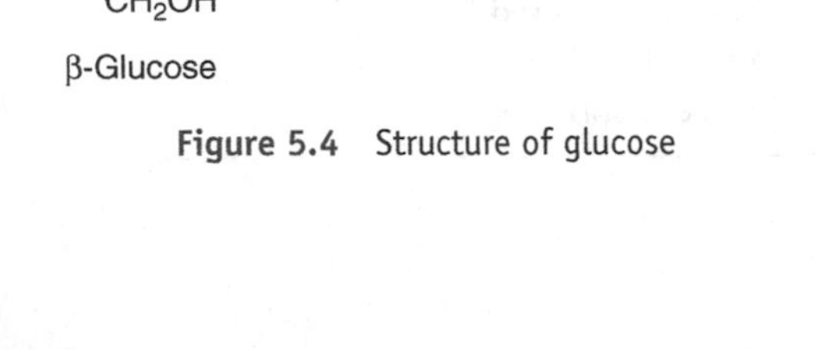

β-Glucose

Figure 5.4   Structure of glucose

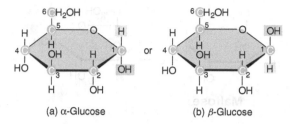

(a) α-Glucose   (b) β-Glucose

Figure 5.5 Isomers of glucose

position where the hydrogen (H) and hydroxyl (OH) lie in different planes.

Glucose also exists in two forms – dextro- (D-) and laevo (L-). Here the difference is that the two forms, when in solution, rotate polarized light to the left (L-form) or to the right (D-form). The D- and L- forms are also different in so much as the human body is only capable of dealing with the D-form of carbohydrates (unlike the amino acids, where the L-form is physiologically active).

The structure of fructose, although it is a monosaccharide, is different from that of glucose. Fructose is formed as a five-membered ring known as a *furanose ring*, in which there are four carbon atoms, whereas glucose is formed of a six-membered ring (Figure 5.6). This makes fructose and glucose physiologically different in the human body, and you will see later that fructose is metabolized by the liver but not by muscle, while glucose can be metabolized by both. Furthermore, fructose fails to stimulate **insulin** secretion, whereas glucose does.

5.2.2 Disaccharides and polysaccharides

When two monosaccharides are attached together, they do so by means of a *glycosidic bond* and

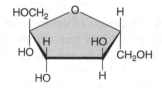

Figure 5.6 Structure of fructose

this results in the formation of a disaccharide. Figure 5.7 offers four examples of disaccharides, namely:

- **maltose**, which is a combination of 2 α-glucose units;
- **lactose**, which is a combination of glucose and **galactose** and is found in milk;
- **sucrose**, which is table sugar and is a combination of glucose and fructose; and
- **cellobiose**, a combination of two β- glucose units which is found in plant material.

Disaccharides

The **glycoside bond** is the essential bond that provides the backbone of larger carbohydrate molecules, in much the same way as a peptide bond does for protein structure. The *1,4 α-glycoside bond* is the most frequent form of glycoside bond and occurs between the carbon-1 of one monosaccharide and the carbon-4 of another monosaccharide. Figure 5.8 shows how the disaccharide maltose is formed from two glucose molecules and highlights the formation of a 1,4 α-glycoside bond. This is a condensation reaction and it results in the formation of water.

Cellobiose, on the other hand, is formed from two β-glucose molecules which are linked by a *1,4 β-glycoside bond* (Figure 5.9). Structurally, the 1,4 α and the 1,4 β bonds are different and, what is more, the enzymes necessary for breaking down 1,4 α links are present in our digestive system, whereas the enzymes needed to break down the 1,4 β links are not. The 1,4 β bonds are present in plant material and are often referred to as roughage or fibre in our diet. These foods pass through our digestive system undigested.

Examples of the glycoside bonds for the disaccharides maltose and sucrose can be seen in Figure 5.10.

Not all glycoside bonds are 1,4-bonds. There are also *1,6-glycoside bonds*, which you can see illustrated in figure 5.11. This bond takes place between the carbon-1 of one glucose molecule and carbon-6 of another glucose molecule, resulting in branching of the carbohydrate. The 1,6-glycoside

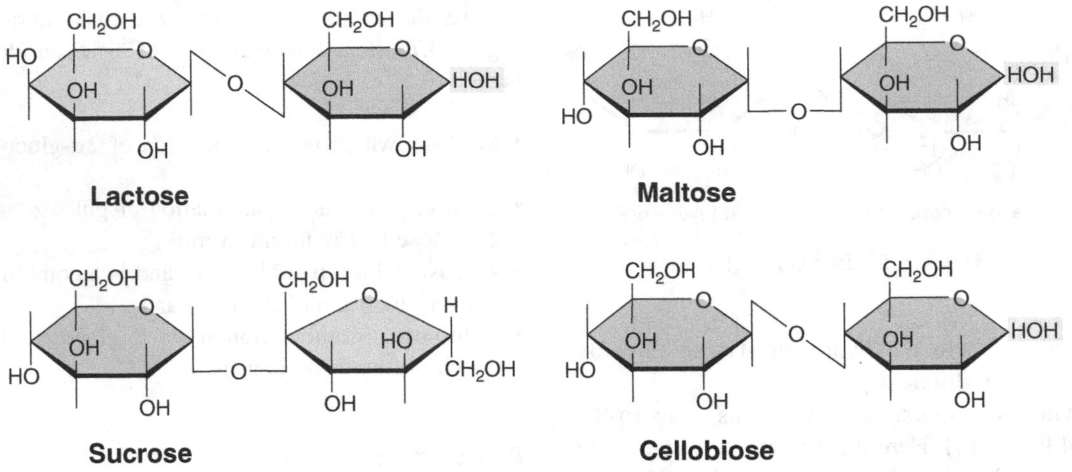

Lactose

Maltose

Sucrose

Cellobiose

Figure 5.7   Disaccharides

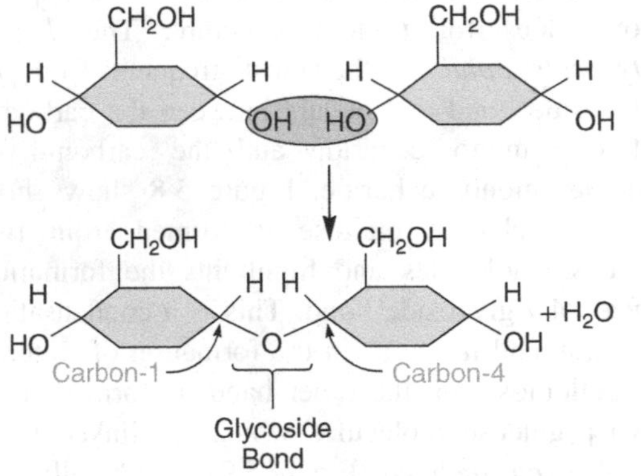

Figure 5.8   Formation of a disaccharide with a 1,4 α-glycoside bond

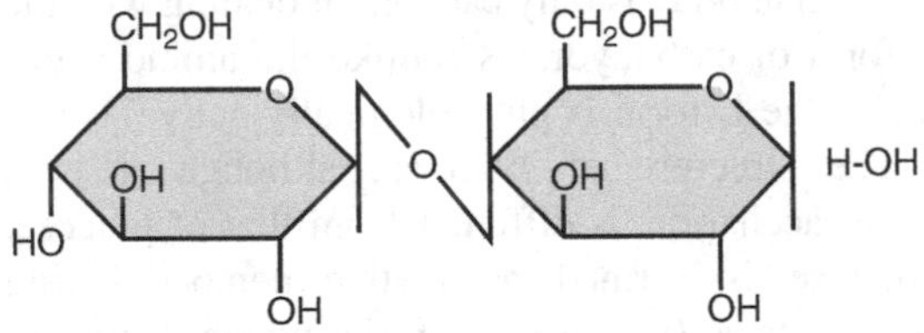

Figure 5.9   Formation of a disaccharide with a 1,4 β-glycoside bond

bonds are only found in polysaccharides, where chains of monosaccharides are linked in a larger more complex (and compact) structure. These bonds enable branching to occur, rather than the formation of long chains, and so help to make the structure more compact.

Polysaccharides

Polysaccharides are the storage forms of carbohydrates, of which the two major examples are starch (found in plants) and glycogen (found in animals). *Amylose* is a small polysaccharide consisting of

a straight chain of glucose units attached together with 1,4 α-glycoside bonds, whereas *amylopectin* contains 1,4 α-glycoside and 1,6-glycoside bonds. Since amylopectin is more highly branched than amylose, it is the major storage form of carbohydrate in some of the types of food we eat, such as potato, rice, wheat, and maize (Figure 5.12a and Table 5.2). Glycogen, which is the storage form of carbohydrate in animal muscle and liver, is much more branched than amylopectin (Figure 5.12b).

5.3   Metabolism of carbohydrates

Having explored aspects of the structure of carbohydrates, we should now turn our attention to the processes whereby energy may be generated from carbohydrates and also (briefly) how to synthesize the storage forms, that is, polysaccharides. We will see how polysaccharides are broken down

Maltose

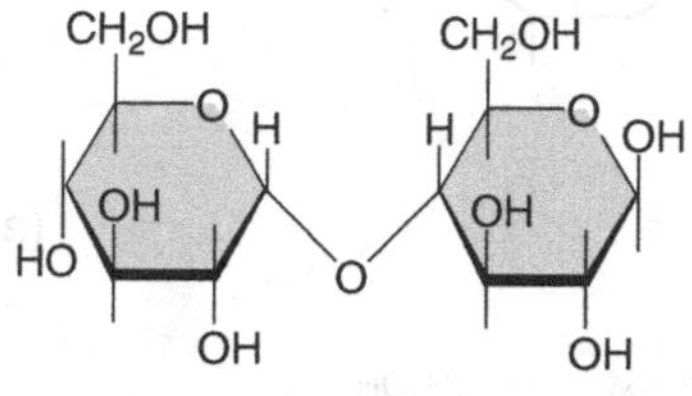

1-4 glycosidic linkage

Sucrose

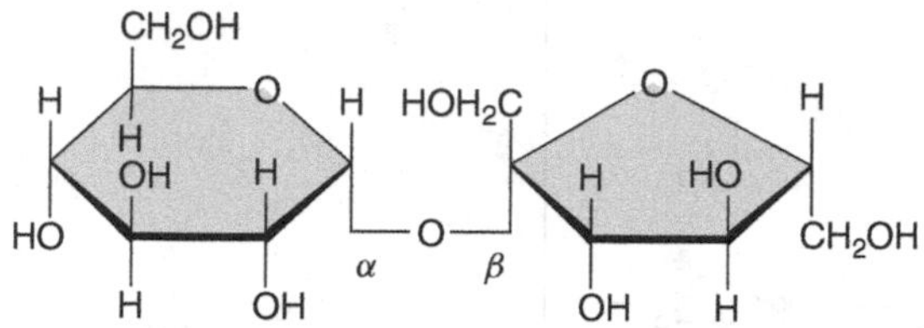

Figure 5.10 Glycoside bond in the formation of the disaccharides, maltose and sucrose

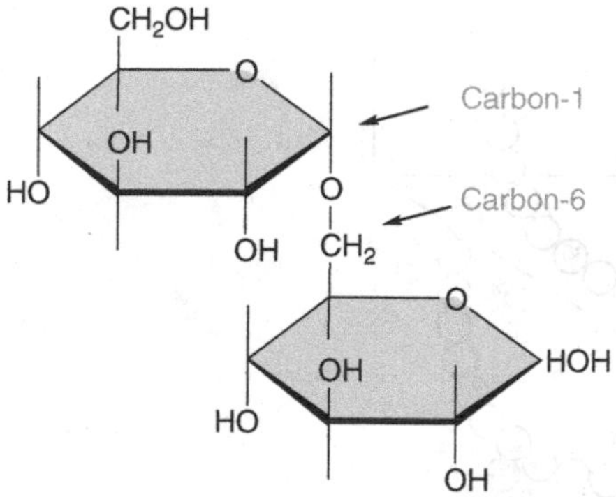

Isomaltose (glucose-β-1,6-glucose)

Figure 5.11 Formation of a 1,6 glycoside bond

to release monosaccharides, which are then further broken down to carbon dioxide and water (remember that carbohydrates contain carbon, hydrogen, and oxygen only), and the generation of useable energy in the form of **ATP**. The equations below highlight the basic principles of glucose breakdown In the cytoplasm, where oxygen is not necessary, as well as the complete oxidation in

Table 5.2 Polysaccharide composition of selected foods

	Amylose (%)	Amylopectin (%)
Maize	24	76
Potato	20	80
Rice	19	81
Tapioca	17	83
Wheat	25	75

the mitochondria:

$$\text{Glucose} \rightarrow 2\text{ Pyruvate} + 2\text{ ATP}$$

$$\text{Glucose} + 6\text{ Oxygen} \rightarrow 6\text{ Carbon Dioxide}$$

$$+ 6\text{ Water} + 38\text{ ATP}$$

In addition, it is necessary to understand how a polysaccharide, such as glycogen, is synthesized in muscle or liver.

Figure 5.13 is a schematic providing an overview of how carbohydrates, and in particular glucose, provide energy for muscles. Glucose is transported across the muscle membrane from blood using a transport protein (*GLUT4*), although muscle also has its own storage form of carbohydrate, namely glycogen. Glucose from blood and from glycogen can be used to furnish energy in the form of ATP at the muscle crossbridge. Note that the processes start in the cytoplasm (so they are called *anaerobic*, because oxygen is not required) and then completed in the mitochondria (a so called *aerobic* process).

In the cytoplasm, glucose molecules are converted to **pyruvic acid** (often referred to simply as **pyruvate**) via a process known as *glycolysis*. Energy is derived in this series of ten enzyme controlled reactions in the form of ATP. However, the glucose from muscle stores of glycogen must first be released in a process known as *glycogenolysis*.

5.3.1 Glycogenolysis

Glycogenolysis is the breakdown of glycogen into glucose molecules, specifically glucose-

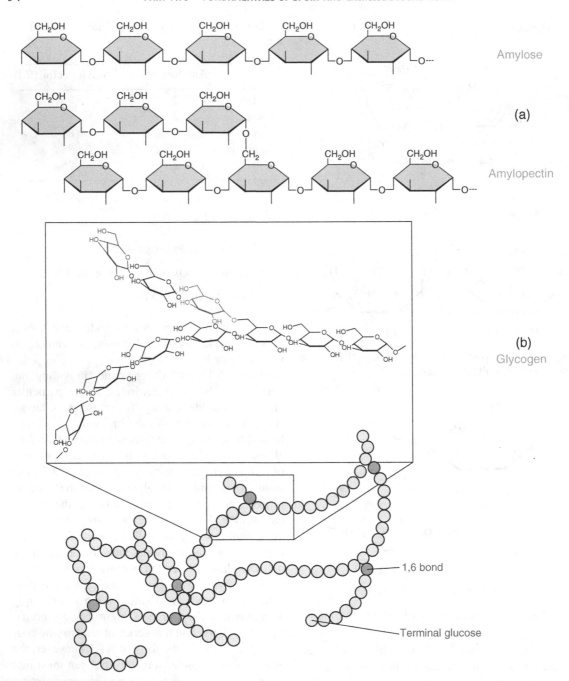

Figure 5.12   Basic structure of polysaccharides: (a) plant polysaccharides, amylose and amylopectin (b) glycogen (green circles denote locations of 1.6 glycoside bonds)

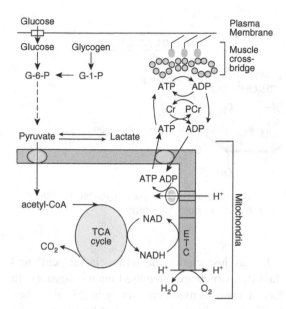

Figure 5.13 Schematic of energy production from carbohydrate in a muscle cell (adapted from Spriet, 2007)

1-phosphate (G-1-P), which is then converted to glucose-6-phosphate (G-6-P) before going through glycolysis (strictly speaking, the breakdown of glucose through a series of reactions to form pyruvic acid). Note that glycogenolysis feeds into glycolysis with the formation of glucose-6-phosphate. Figure 5.14 illustrates this interrelationship.

An important consideration for the process of glycogenolysis is that it is controlled by the enzyme **phosphorylase**. This enzyme (as with most enzymes regulating reactions in metabolism) exists in two forms; a relatively active form, phosphorylase$_a$ and a relatively inactive form, phosphorylase$_b$. We shall see more detail about this regulation in Chapter 7.

The glucose formed when removed from a glycogen molecule is glucose-1-phosphate, which means that the glucose has a phosphate group attached at the carbon-1 position. This is achieved because ATP is involved:

$$\text{Glycogen}_{(n)} + \text{ATP} \rightarrow \text{Glycogen}_{(n-1)}$$
$$+ \text{G-1-P} + \text{ADP}$$

The G-1-P is then converted to G-6-P, whereby the phosphate group is moved from carbon-1 to carbon-6 before undergoing glycolysis. Glycogenolysis is a process that must be capable of happening rapidly, since it provides an important and major source of energy during prolonged sprinting. This implies that glycogenolysis needs to be 'switched on' almost instantaneously. The regulation of this is explored in more detail in Chapter 7.

5.3.2 Glycolysis

Glycolysis is, in essence, a process where a six-carbon compound, glucose, is converted to two three-carbon compounds (i.e. two pyruvates), which are then converted to two two-carbon compounds (**acetyl-CoA**) with the liberation of carbon dioxide, and then into the *TCA cycle*, where it is completely oxidized to carbon dioxide and water. The conversion of glucose to pyruvate is through a series of ten reactions (Figure 5.15). Note that glucose is first phosphorylated to G-6-P by the enzyme *hexokinase* (although the liver uses *glucokinase*). This happens immediately as glucose enters the cell and utilizes an ATP molecule. Hexokinase is more specific than glucokinase. The G-6-P is then converted to fructose-6-phosphate and then, in the third reaction, the F-6-P is converted to fructose-1,6 diphosphate. This reaction involves the enzyme *phosphofructokinase* (**PFK**). PFK is the regulatory enzyme for glycolysis, and we shall see in Chapter 7 how PFK is activated and inactivated.

The next phase of glycolysis involves splitting the F-1,6 diphosphate (which, remember is a six-carbon compound) into two three-carbon compounds, **dihydroxyacetone phosphate (DHAP)** and **glyceraldehyde 3-phosphate**. The DHAP is then converted to **glyceraldehyde 3-phosphate** – so in effect there are now two glyceraldehyde 3-phosphates, which are in turn converted to **1,3-diphosphoglycerate**. In the latter process, an **NADH** is formed from **NAD**, NADH being the reduced form of **NAD**. The 1,3 di-phosphoglycerate is then converted to **3-phosphoglycerate** in a process that engenders ATP, before being converted

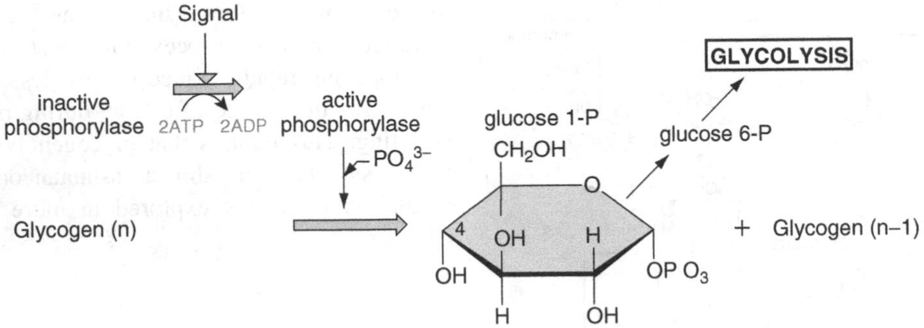

Figure 5.14 Glycogenolysis; removal of one glucose molecule to form glucose-1-P and a glycogen residue with one less glucose. The glucose 1-P is then converted to glucose 6-P and so enters glycolysis

to 2-phosphoglycerate and then to **phospho-enolpyruvate (PEP)**. The final stage sees the formation of pyruvate and another ATP from PEP.

Examination of glycolysis shows that after an initial use of two ATPs (reactions 1 and 3), a further four ATPs are produced (remember that in reactions 5 and 9 there are two reactants from the initial glucose molecule). So there is a net yield of two ATP. In addition, two NADH are formed from two NAD, and these can either be re-oxidized from aerobic events in the mitochondria (each producing three ATP – see Section 5.3.7) or from the conversion of pyruvic acid to **lactic acid** (Figure 5.16). The production of lactic acid ensures that glycolysis continues if aerobic re-oxidation of NAD from NADH is not possible. The latter tends to occur during very high intensity bouts of exercise. Regeneration of NAD is essential if glycolysis is to continue.

The formation of lactic acid occurs when significant amounts of pyruvate are formed in glycolysis. This happens mainly in the type II fibres which are recruited during intense exercise, but it can also take place in the type I fibres. The formation of lactic acid is a means whereby NAD can be regenerated from NADH and therefore allow reaction 5 in glycolysis to continue. If the exercise is low in intensity, then NAD can be regenerated from the NADH by oxidative processes taking place in the mitochondria, so the 'need' for lactic acid production is not required.

Let us just clarify the terms 'lactic acid' and 'lactate', which are often used interchangeably. In fact, 'lactate' is used consistently in this text when 'lactic acid' should be used – but be aware of the differences. Lactic acid is produced from pyruvic acid, but in normal physiological systems (such as in a cell), the lactic acid dissociates into a lactate ion and a hydrogen ion:

$$HLa \longleftrightarrow La^- + H^+$$

$$Lactic\ acid \longleftrightarrow Lactate^- - Hydrogen^+$$

Strictly speaking, therefore, lactate is the anion formed when lactic acid dissociates. In fact, 99% of lactic acid is normally in its dissociated forms.

The enzyme responsible for converting pyruvate to lactate is *lactate dehydrogenase* (**LDH**). This enzyme exists in five **isoforms**: LDH 1, LDH2, LDH3, LDH4, and LDH5. LDH 1 is also known as H-LDH (or heart-specific LDH), while LDH 5 is known as M-LDH (or muscle specific LDH).

The M-LDH (LDH5) is found in type IIx fibres, whereas H-LDH (LDH1) predominates in type I fibres. The essential difference is that LDH5 favours the formation of lactate from pyruvate, while LDH1 favours the formation of pyruvate from lactate. Formation of lactate therefore occurs more readily in type IIx (fast glycolytic) than type I fibres, whereas lactate formed during exercise can be taken up by the type I fibres and converted to pyruvate and then oxidized.

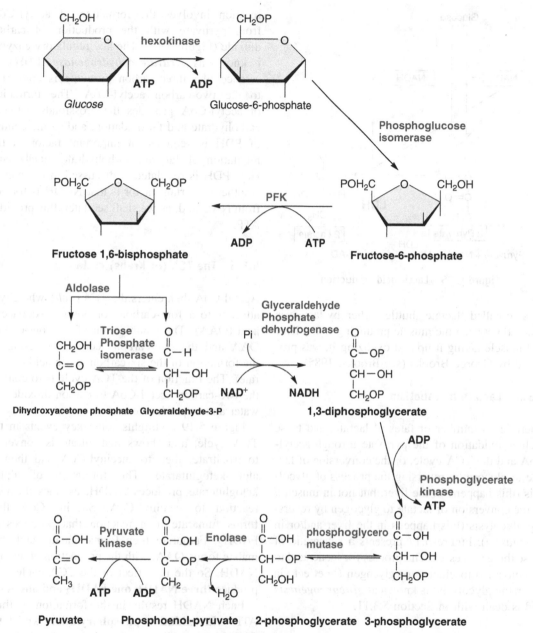

Figure 5.15   Glycolysis (the enzymes can be seen as red words)

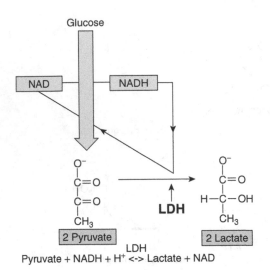

Figure 5.16   Lactic acid production

This so-called 'lactate shuttle', whereby lactate is shuttled between the muscle producing it and liver and muscle taking it up and oxidizing it, was proposed by George Brooks (see Brooks, 1985).

5.3.3   Lactate metabolism

There are a number of fates of lactate, and these include oxidation of the pyruvate through acetyl-CoA and the TCA cycle, or the conversion of lactate to glucose by reversing the process of glycolysis (this happens in the liver, but not in muscle), or the conversion of lactate to glycogen by reversing glycolysis (this happens in the liver and/or in the muscle). Figure 5.17 presents a schematic of these three processes. The process for lactic acid to be converted to glucose or glycogen (in effect via reversing glycolysis) is known as *gluconeogenesis* and is dealt with in Section 5.3.11.

5.3.4   The 'link' reaction; production of acetyl-CoA

Now let us go back to the fate of pyruvate. Remember that pyruvate was formed as the end result of glycolysis. Once it has been formed, it passes into the mitochondria and is converted to *acetyl-CoA* in the so-called 'link' reaction. This

reaction involves the formation of acetyl-CoA from pyruvate with the production of carbon dioxide (Figure 5.18). The key regulatory enzyme is known as **pyruvate dehydrogenase** (**PDH**). In essence, the three-carbon pyruvate is converted to the two-carbon acetyl-CoA. The formation of acetyl-CoA provides the crossroads between carbohydrate and fat oxidation, and so the control of PDH is seen as an important factor in the regulation of fat and carbohydrate metabolism. How PDH is regulated is discussed in Chapter 7. Another important factor is that NADH is formed from NAD and, as we shall see later, this provides ATP.

5.3.5   The TCA (or Krebs) cycle

Acetyl-CoA then enters the *TCA cycle*, whereby it attaches to a four-carbon compound, oxaloacetic acid (OAA). The combination of the four-carbon OAA and the two-carbon acetyl-CoA results in the formation of the six-carbon, citric acid (or citrate). The function of the TCA cycle is to convert the two-carbon acetyl-CoA to carbon dioxide and water and to produce energy.

Figure 5.19 highlights some key events in the TCA cycle, and shows that citrate is converted to isocitrate, then to succinyl-CoA and then to alpha-ketoglutarate. The formation of alpha-ketogluterate produces NADH, as does the next reaction to succinyl-CoA. Succinyl-CoA then forms fumarate in a reaction that produces an $FADH_2$. Fumarate then forms malate, and then malate forms OAA, with the production of another NADH. So the net effect of the TCA cycle is to produce **three NADH, one $FADH_2$** and **one ATP**.

Each NADH results in the formation of three ATPs via **oxidative phosphorylation** whilst the FADH is re-oxidized to form two ATPs via oxidative phosphorylation. How this occurs is explained in Section 5.3.7.

5.3.6   Electron transport chain

The basics of electron transfer can be realized in reduction-oxidation (*redox*) reactions in which a

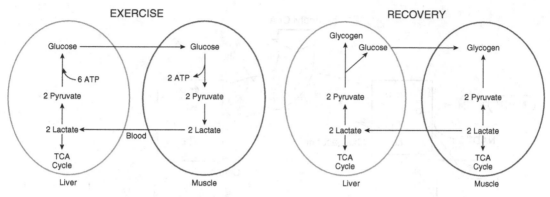

Figure 5.17 Fates of lactic acid

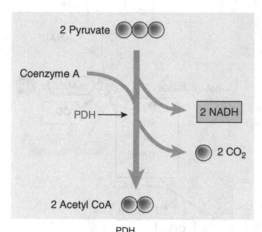

PDH

2 Pyruvate + 2 CoA + 2NAD -> 2 Acetyl CoA + 2CO$_2$ + 2NADH

Figure 5.18 The 'link' reaction (red dots denote carbon atoms)

molecule, when reduced, gains an electron. Once in its reduced form, a compound needs to become oxidized again to get rid of this electron. Thus, the reduced form gains an electron and an oxidized form loses an electron. When NADH is formed from NAD, NADH is the reduced form and the NAD is the oxidized form. For NADH to become NAD, it needs to donate an electron to another compound. If it does so, this other compound then becomes reduced.

The inner mitochondrial membrane contains a series of hydrogen carriers. These are the *cytochromes* or the *cytochrome chain*, and they are involved in what is termed the ***electron transfer chain*** (**ETC**). The purpose of the ETC (containing the cytochromes) is to take up and pass on electrons in a series of redox reactions. Figure 5.20 shows that there are four major components of the ETC, and these are complexes 1, 2, 3 and 4 (although there is some suggestion that there may be 5 components – see Figure 5.21). After complex 4 there is an *ATP-synthetase*, and this is where ATP is synthesized from an ADP.

Once NADH is formed from the TCA cycle in the matrix of the mitochondria, it donates its electron onto complex 1, which in turn becomes reduced. Complex 1 then donates its electron onto complex 2, and in doing so then becomes oxidized while complex 2 becomes reduced. Complex 2 donates its electron to complex 3, which then becomes reduced, while complex 2 becomes re-oxidized, and so on until the final electron acceptor is reached. Oxygen is the final electron acceptor and is reduced to water. For completeness, Figure 5.21 names the complexes as NADH-Q reductase (Complex 1), coenzyme-Q (Complex 2), cytochrome reductase (Complex 3), cytochrome-C, and cytochrome oxidase (Complex 4).

Note that FADH2 donates its electron to complex 2, not complex 1. The series of complexes, which are in effect large protein molecules on the inner mitochondrial membrane, exist in the sequence shown in Figure 5.20. These complexes contain cytochromes, which are iron-containing molecules, and hence iron deficiency in the human body may impair aerobic energy production.

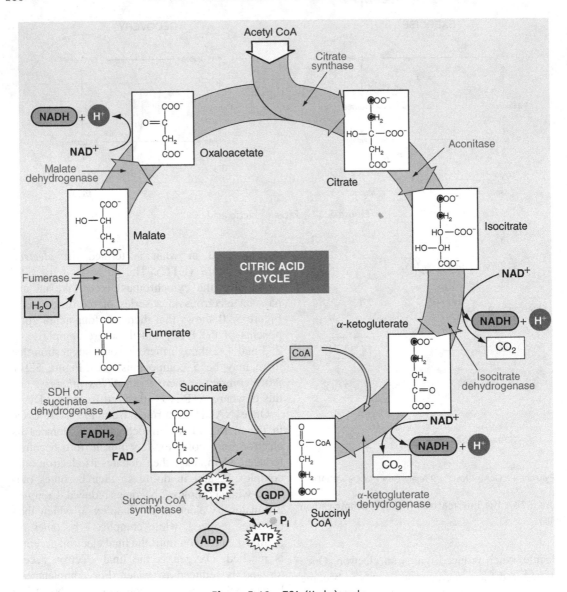

Figure 5.19 TCA (Krebs) cycle

5.3.7 Oxidative phosphorylation

To date we have noted that an NADH, when re-oxidized to NAD, produces three ATP molecules, and that an FADH, when re-oxidized to FAD, produces two ATP molecules. How does this happen? The **Chemiosmotic Theory** according to Peter Mitchell provides the answer. In his theory,

Mitchell (1961) stated that, as the electrons are donated from NADH or FADH to the complexes, H^+ ions are extruded into the inter-mitochondrial membrane space. The net effect is a series of H^+ making this area more positive with respect to the interior of the mitochondria (Figure 5.21). As a result of this ion charge difference, the H^+ ions then diffuse through an ATP synthetase molecule

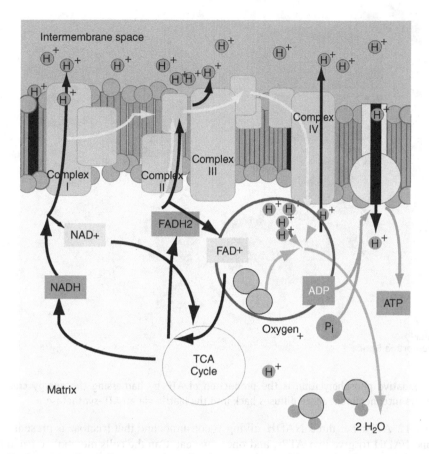

Figure 5.20 Electron transfer chain occurs when electrons are donated from molecule to molecule along a chain in the inner mitochondrial membrane. These are in effect a series of reduction-oxidation reactions. NADH and FAD, arising from the TCA cycle, instigate electron transfer

in the mitochondrial membrane. This process results in the conversion of ADP to ATP and is known as oxidative phosphorylation.

An issue arising from oxidative phosphorylation is the production of *free radicals* or **reactive oxygen species (ROS)**. These short-lived, but damaging, molecules can affect membrane integrity and DNA structure. Some scientists believe the greater the aerobic oxidation undertaken (such as in exercise), the more free radicals are produced, and therefore the more risk of damage to muscle membranes. The body produces *antioxidants*, whose function is to quench the free radicals and so limit the damage caused. Exercise results in the body producing more of its own antioxidants in order to compensate for the likely increase in

free radical production. From a nutrition perspective, antioxidants can be eaten in various fruit and vegetables.

5.3.8 Calculation of ATP generated in glucose oxidation

In order to calculate the number of ATP molecules produced from a glucose molecule, we need to appreciate that in glycolysis there is a net production of two ATPs and two NADH molecules, which then are re-oxidized to provide three ATPs each. This provides a total of eight ATP molecules. In addition, the so-called 'link' reaction produces a further two NADH, which, when re-oxidized gives six ATPs. Finally, one complete cycle of the TCA

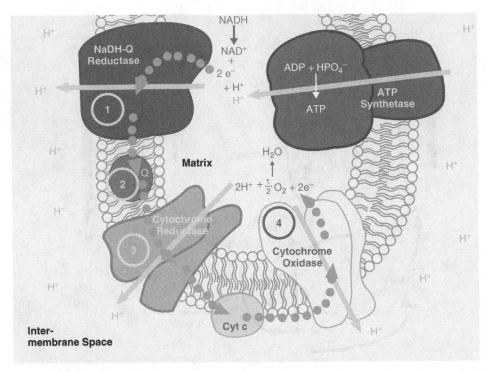

Figure 5.21 Oxidative phosphorylation is the production of ATP by harnessing the energy created when the extruded H^+ in the intermembrane space diffuses back into the matrix via an ATP-synthetase

cycle provides 12 ATPs i.e. three NADH giving nine ATPs, one FADH to give two ATPs, and one ATP. Bearing in mind that two acetyl-CoA are derived from one glucose molecule, a total of 24 ATPs are thereby generated via the TCA cycle (i.e. two cycles of the TCA cycle; see Figure 5.22).

5.3.9   Overview of glucose oxidation

Figure 5.23 is a schematic that provides an overview of carbohydrate oxidation in the cell from either glycogen or glucose to pyruvate via glycolysis, then the pyruvate entering the mitochondria, where it is converted to acetyl-CoA in the 'link' reaction, and then into the TCA cycle before electron transfer and the resultant generation of ATP from oxidative phosphorylation.

5.3.10   Fructose metabolism

It should be remembered that glucose is not the only monosaccharide available in the foods we

consume, and that fructose is present in most fruits we eat. Can the cells metabolize fructose, and if so does this happen in the same manner as glucose? Figure 5.24 highlights some key differences in the ability of the cells to handle fructose. You will note that muscle cells are incapable of oxidizing fructose, due to the fact that:

- they do not have the ability to transport fructose into the cell; and
- the enzyme **fructokinase** is *not* present in muscle.

On the other hand, liver cells *can* transport and metabolize fructose.

5.3.11   Gluconeogenesis

There are substrates other than lactate for gluco-neogenesis, and these include glycerol, alanine, and glutamine. Gluconeogenesis takes place in the liver and, to a certain extent, in the kidney, but not

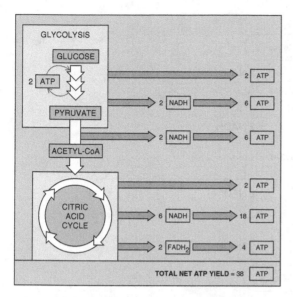

Figure 5.22 Number of ATP from glucose oxidation

fully in muscle. Figure 5.25 highlights the reactions involved in gluconeogenesis. In essence, the process initially requires pyruvate to be converted to PEP. During glycolysis, the conversion of PEP to pyruvate produces a great amount of energy, and the reverse process is physiologically difficult to achieve.

What happens, therefore, is that the liver produces PEP by a two-stage reaction, of which the first stage involves the conversion of pyruvate to oxaloacetic acid (OAA) using the enzyme **pyruvate carboxylase**. The OAA is then converted to PEP using the enzyme **PEP carboxykinase**. Both of these enzymes are found in the liver and in muscle, and they are regulated by the hormone glucagon.

Having formed PEP, the next stages of glycolysis can be reversed back to fructose 1,6-bisphosphate. The conversion of Fructose-1, 6-bisphosphate (F-1,6-bisP) to Fructose-6-phosphate (F-6-P) cannot use the enzyme PFK, which favours F-6-P to F-1,6-bisP. However, another enzyme, F1,6-bisphosphatase, can enable this to happen. This enzyme is present in both liver and muscle, so glycolysis can continue to be reversed until Glucose-6-phosphate (G-6-P) is reached.

The conversion of G-6-P to glucose cannot use glucokinase or hexokinase, so the enzyme glucose-6-phosphatase is required. This enzyme is present in liver but is not present in muscle, which is why muscle is not capable of forming glucose. Therefore, strictly speaking, gluconeogenesis cannot take place in the muscle, since glucose cannot be formed. Note, however, that the glucose-6-phosphate can be converted to glycogen, and so both the liver and muscle can form glycogen from lactic acid, whereas only the liver can form glucose. The glucose produced by the liver is then released into the blood and taken up by other tissues, including muscle.

Lactic acid is not the only substrate for gluconeogenesis, since pyruvate, alanine and glycerol can also undergo gluconeogenesis. Figure 5.26 highlights the positions wherein these substrates 'feed into' the process. Gluconeogenesis becomes an important blood glucose-producing process during prolonged exercise, and is promoted when insulin concentrations are low and glucagon levels are high. This happens during steady state exercise after about 30–45 minutes, so long as carbohydrate drinks or food are not ingested.

Remember, liver glycogen stores are limited and can easily run out. The capability of converting other 'energy' sources to maintain blood glucose levels, so preventing hypoglycaemia, is due to the liver taking up circulating alanine and glutamine (amino acids from protein breakdown) and glycerol (from fat breakdown) to produce glucose. Elevated levels of glucagon are essential for this to happen.

5.3.12 Glycogenesis

So far, the focus has been on catabolic reactions involving carbohydrate breakdown and oxidation. However, we should bear in mind that carbohydrates are stored within liver and muscle in the form of the polysaccharide glycogen. The process of glycogen formation is known as *glycogenesis*. For glycogenesis to occur, glucose must be made available inside the cell and insulin (a hormone which helps regulate blood glucose levels) elevated in the blood.

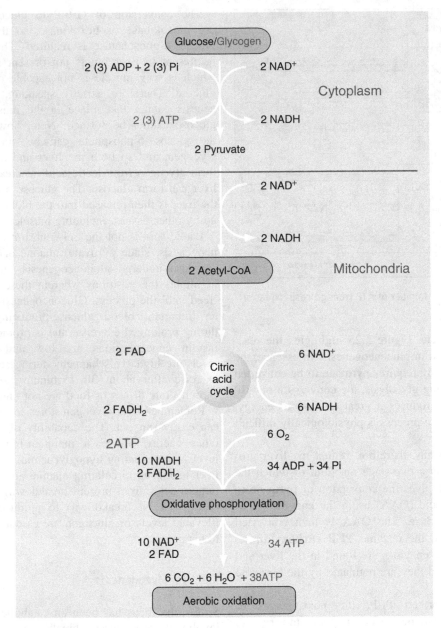

Figure 5.23   Overview of carbohydrate oxidation

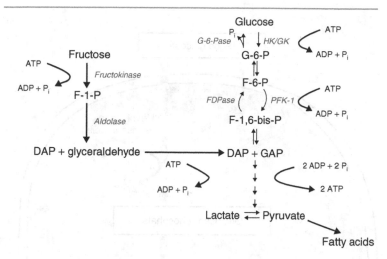

Figure 5.24 Fructose metabolism

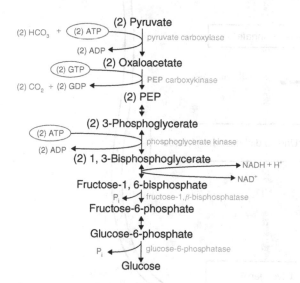

Figure 5.25 Gluconeogenesis of lactic acid (the enzymes can be seen in green)

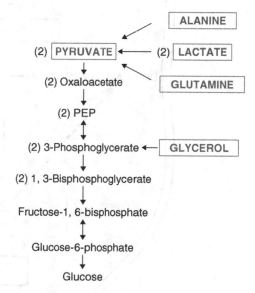

Figure 5.26 The four major substrates for gluconeogenesis can be seen in red

This typically occurs after a carbohydrate meal. Once glucose enters the cell, it is attached to **uridine di-phosphate** (**UDP**) to form *uridine di-phosphate glucose* (UDP-glucose). The UDP-glucose is then attached to the glycogen molecule by the enzyme **glycogen synthase**. Figure 5.27 highlights this process.

In effect, this means that the glycogen molecule becomes larger by the addition of one or more

glucose molecules. The central core of the glycogen molecule is never completely broken down, or it would not be possible for a glucose molecule to attach.

Being a synthesis reaction, glycogenesis requires energy. One ATP is used up when the glucose molecule enters the cell and is immediately phosphorylated to G-6-P; the other is

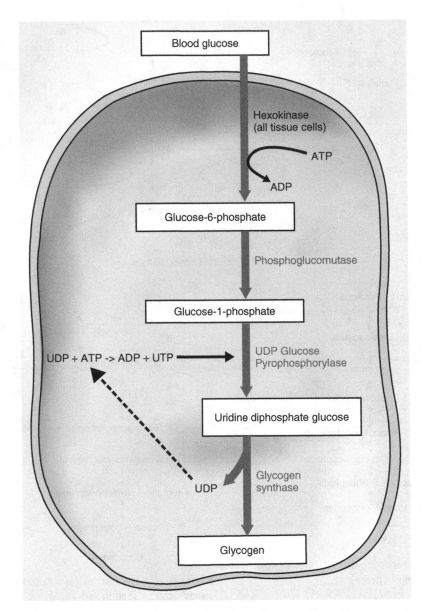

Figure 5.27 Glycogenesis is the formation of glycogen from glucose and involves the key enzyme, glycogen synthase

used in the form of *uridine triphosphate* (**UTP**), to which the G-1-P is attached to produce UDP-glucose. In order to restore UTP, the UDP is phosphorylated by ATP:

G-1-P + UTP ↔ UDP-glucose

UDP-glucose + glycogen(n) ↔ UDP

   + glycogen(n + 1)

UDP + ATP ↔ UTP + ADP

So the key regulatory enzyme for glycogenesis is glycogen synthase. In Chapter 7, we will explore how glycogen synthase is regulated in relation to phosphorylase, the enzyme which breaks down glycogen.

5.4 Key points

- Carbohydrates are an important source of energy for intense, and also prolonged, bouts of exercise.
- Muscle glycogen depletion and liver glycogen depletion leading to hypoglycaemia are potential factors for fatigue.
- Carbohydrates consist of carbon, hydrogen and oxygen only.
- Monosaccharides are the simplest form of carbohydrate.
- Disaccharides are made from two monosaccharides joined together by a glycoside bond.
- Polysaccharides are the storage form of carbohydrates.
- Glucose is the major useable form of carbohydrate for energy.
- Glycolysis results in the breakdown of glucose to form pyruvic acid; it takes place in the cytoplasm via a series of reactions in which the enzyme PFK is rate limiting.
- Glycogenolysis results in the formation of a number of glucose-1-phosphates, with phosphorylase as the key enzyme.

- Pyruvic acid is converted to lactic acid via LDH when muscles work intensely, and it thereby enables glycolysis to continue.
- During aerobic, steady state exercise, pyruvic acid passes into the mitochondria, where it is converted to acetyl-CoA via PDH.
- Acetyl-CoA enters the TCA cycle, where it is completely oxidized to carbon dioxide and water and produces 12 ATP molecules.
- The electron transfer chain involves a series of redox reactions using a sequence of mainly cytochrome containing complexes in the membrane of the mitochondria and thereby enables NADH and $FADH_2$ to be re-oxidized.
- Oxidative phosphorylation produces ATP from the resultant electron transfer.
- There is a net production of two ATP from 'anaerobic' breakdown of glucose to pyruvic acid and 38 ATP from complete oxidation.
- Fructose can only be metabolized by liver, since that organ possesses fructokinase whereas muscle does not possess this enzyme.
- Gluconeogenesis, using lactic acid as the substrate, in effect involves reversing glycolysis and producing glucose. All the necessary enzymes for this process can be found in liver (i.e. pyruvate carboxylase, PEP carboxykinase, fructose-6-phosphatase, and glucose-6-phosphatase), whereas muscle lacks glucose-6-phosphatase and so is unable to form glucose.
- Muscle can however synthesize glycogen from lactic acid.
- Alanine, glutamine, and glycerol are also gluconeogenic precursors.
- The hormone, glucagon, promotes gluconeogenesis.
- Glycogenesis is promoted by insulin (and the presence of glucose) and involves the enzyme glycogen synthase.

6

Lipids

Learning outcomes

After studying this chapter, you should be able to:

- list the variety of functions which lipids carry out within the human body;
- elucidate the role of lipids in sport and exercise;
- draw the general structure of a triacylglycerol molecule;
- draw the structure of a saturated and an unsaturated fatty acid molecule;
- outline differences in the types of lipoproteins;
- describe the structure of a cholesterol molecule and its similarity to steroid hormones;
- describe the processes of lipolysis, β-oxidation, and lipogenesis;
- list the key enzymes regulating the above processes;
- explain how fatty acids are transported in the blood and across both the plasma membrane and the mitochondrial membrane;
- calculate the number of ATP molecules produced from the oxidation of a fatty acid molecule;
- describe the formation of a ketone body;
- describe how excess carbohydrates can be converted to fatty acids.

Key words

acetyl CoA
acetyl-CoA carboxylase (ACC)
acyl carnitine
albumin
arachidonic acid
ATP-citrate lyase
β-oxidation
carnitine
cholesterol
chylomicron
CPT1/CPT2
DAG (diacylglycerol)
essential fatty acid
FABP
FAS (fatty acid synthase)
FAT/CD36
FATP
fatty acid
fatty acid synthase
FFA (free fatty acid)
glycerol

glycerol-3-phosphate acyltransferase (GPAT)
glyceroneogenesis
GPAT
HDL
HSL (hormone sensitive lipase)
ketone
LDL
linolenic acid
linoleic acid
LPL (lipoprotein lipase)
lipogenesis
lipolysis
lipoprotein
long chain fatty acid
MAG (monoacylglycerol)
malonyl CoA
MCT

Biochemistry for Sport and Exercise Metabolism, First Edition. Don MacLaren and James Morton.
© 2012 John Wiley & Sons, Ltd. Published 2012 by John Wiley & Sons, Ltd.

NEFA (non-esterified fatty acid)	stearic acid
oleic acid	steroids
omega-3 fatty acid	TAG (triacylglycerol)
omega-6 fatty acid	TCA cycle
palmitic acid	trans-fats
PDH	triglyceride
plasma membrane	unsaturated fatty acid
saturated fatty acid	VLDL

6.1 Relevance of lipids for sport and exercise

We have already seen in the previous chapter that carbohydrate is an important source of energy for high-intensity work as well as for prolonged activity. Lipids, on the other hand, cannot be used during high-intensity exercise, although they are an important source of energy in the recovery period between high-intensity bouts and, indeed, during prolonged aerobic exercise. So, lipids cannot be used anaerobically; they require aerobic processes.

Specifically, it is **fatty acids** that are the important sources of energy from lipids. There are plentiful supplies of lipids even in the leanest person, and they can be found in adipose tissue and also within intramuscular stores in the form of triglycerides or triacylglycerols. Lipids are also important in so far as they are an integral part of the plasma membrane (see Figure 6.1), and they also form the backbone of the sex hormones progesterone, oestrogen and testosterone.

Figure 6.2 demonstrates the importance of lipids as energy sources during exercise of increasing intensity. As exercise intensity increases (represented by percentage VO_{2max}), note that the contribution of lipids reaches a peak at around 60 to 65% VO_{2max} and thereafter decreases substantially – so much so that at 100% VO_{2max} there is no contribution of lipid. This reflects the fact that lipids are unable to be used as an energy source for intense bouts of activity.

On the other hand, with increasing duration of steady state exercise, lipids become more prominent in the later stages (see Figure 6.3). This is as a consequence of hormonal changes resulting in the switch from carbohydrates to lipids as a focus for energy. In particular, the hormone *insulin* acts as a regulator of fat release and, thereby, availability. When insulin is elevated (e.g. after a meal or a carbohydrate drink), there is an inhibition of fatty acid availability. However, when insulin levels in blood are low, the inhibition on fat release is removed and greater fat oxidation occurs. Endurance-trained athletes are capable of using lipids as their energy store to a greater extent than sedentary individuals or sprint-trained athletes. Indeed, they possess greater stores of intramuscular triglycerides.

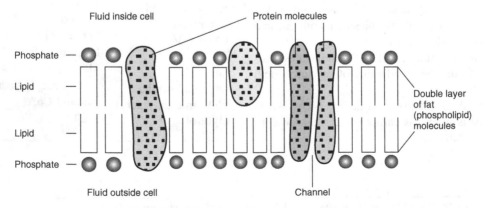

Figure 6.1 Structure of the plasma membrane

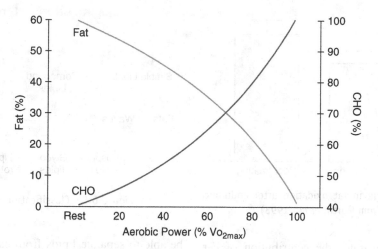

Figure 6.2 Relationship between exercise intensity and the use of carbohydrate and fat as energy sources

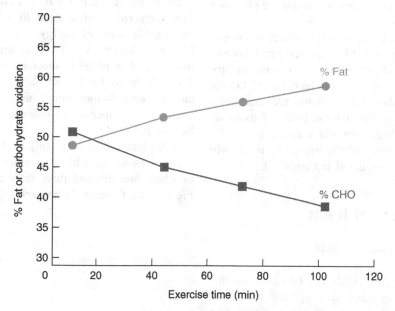

Figure 6.3 Relative contribution of carbohydrate and fat as energy source during steady state exercise lasting 100 minutes

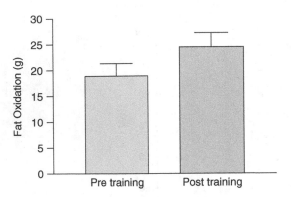

Figure 6.4 Change in fat oxidation after endurance training (adapted from Martin *et al.*, 1993)

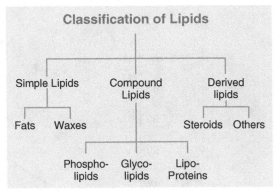

Figure 6.5 Classification of lipids

Figure 6.4 illustrates the contribution of carbohydrates and lipids during exercise before and after an endurance training programme. The use of lipids increases significantly and thereby results in lowered muscle glycogen use, i.e. muscle glycogen is spared.

Thus, far from being a useless source of energy, fats play an important role in exercise metabolism. Without fatty acids, the ability to exercise for prolonged periods of time would be difficult. On the other hand, it should be remembered that lipids cannot be used during intense bouts of exercise, where carbohydrates are likely to be used. The interaction between carbohydrates and lipids will be explored in more detail in Chapter 9.

6.2 Structure of lipids

6.2.1 Classification of lipids

So what is a lipid? Lipids can be classified into three types: simple lipids, compound lipids and derived lipids. Figure 6.5 is a schematic of their classification. From an energy perspective, and as sport scientists, we are mainly interested in the fats, although from a health perspective we are interested in lipoproteins and from a regulatory and growth perspective we are interested in the steroids. Lipids are not defined by their structure, but rather are defined by being soluble in nonpolar solvents such as ether. Therefore, we should

be able to separate lipids from carbohydrates and protein by dissolving fats in ether, wherein any carbohydrates and proteins present would fail to dissolve.

Lipids are stored in the body as **triglycerides** or **triacylglycerols** (abbreviated to TAGs), whereas the useable form of energy are the **fatty acids**. Lipids can be found as TAGs in adipose tissue, in muscle, and in blood in the form of lipoproteins. TAGs have to be broken down to fatty acids and **glycerol** before being used as an energy source. This process is known as **lipolysis** (see Section 6.3.1).

A triglyceride or triacylglycerol is in effect a glycerol molecule which provides the backbone to which are attached three fatty acyl units (see Figure 6.6). Glycerol, when released, is normally

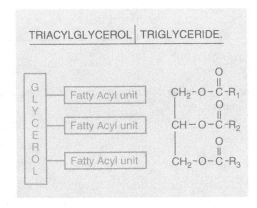

Figure 6.6 Structure of a triacylglycerol (triglyceride)

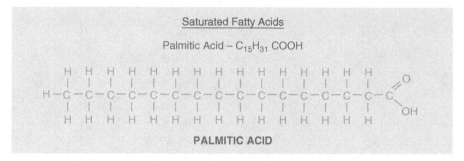

Figure 6.7   A saturated fatty acid

metabolized by the liver to produce energy, or it can be converted to glucose by gluconeogenesis, whereas fatty acids are taken up by muscle and liver, where they undergo beta-oxidation (**β-oxidation**) before entering the TCA cycle and undergoing further oxidation to carbon dioxide and water.

The fatty acids which make up triglycerides are monocarboxylic acids with a general formula is R-COOH, in which the R-group is usually an unbranched chain with an even number of carbon atoms and can be either *saturated* or *unsaturated*. If there are double bonds between the carbon atoms, then the fatty acid is unsaturated. Figure 6.7 shows the structure of *palmitic acid*, which has 15 carbons in a chain, followed by a carboxylic group that is the 16th carbon, as well as oxygen and the hydroxyl group. There are no double bonds between the 15 carbon atoms, so it is a *saturated fatty acid*.

If you now look at the structure of *oleic acid* (Figure 6.8), you will note that there is a single double bond (between the 9th and 10th carbon atoms); this makes oleic acid an *unsaturated fatty acid*. Beneath oleic acid, note that there are two further unsaturated fatty acids which have either two or three double bonds. **Linoleic acid** has two double bonds (between the 9th and 10th and between the 12th and 13th carbon atoms) whereas **linolenic acid** has three double bonds (between the 9th and 10th, between the 12th and 13th, and between the 15th and 16th).

Linolenic and linoleic acids, together with **arachidonic acid**, are known collectively as **essential fatty acids**; linolenic acid is commonly known as **omega-3 fatty acid** and linoleic acid is known as **omega-6 fatty acid**. Omega-3 fatty acids are found in fish and in some seeds (e.g. flax seed), while omega-6 fatty acids are more commonly found in meat products. Being essential fatty acids implies that these fatty acids are essential to have in the diet regularly or else a deficiency symptom arises. This is due to the body being incapable of synthesizing them (or at least making sufficient amounts for health).

Recently there has been some publicity surrounding the use of so-called '**trans-fats**' or hydrogenated fats in foods. Trans-fats have been linked to increases in coronary heart disease and some cancers, and so it is clearly not advisable to eat them if possible. So what is a trans-fat? A saturated fatty acid is a straight chain molecule, whereas an unsaturated fatty acid is usually bent. Have a look at Figures 6.7 and 6.9 to note the difference between palmitic and oleic acids. Palmitic acid, as a saturated fatty acid, is a straight chain, whereas oleic acid is bent at the double bond and this structure is the naturally occurring cis-form of oleic acid. However, oleic acid can be straightened if hydrogen is forced onto the double bonds (hydrogenation) to make it saturated. In this state, it becomes the trans-form.

If there are a number of fatty acids in the cis-form, it is difficult for them to lie next to each other structurally, but if they are in the trans-form they can lie close together. In the trans-form, they appear more like saturated fatty acids which have a high melting point. This can confer a degree of stability on the structure, and hence trans-fats are used in confectionery products as stabilizers.

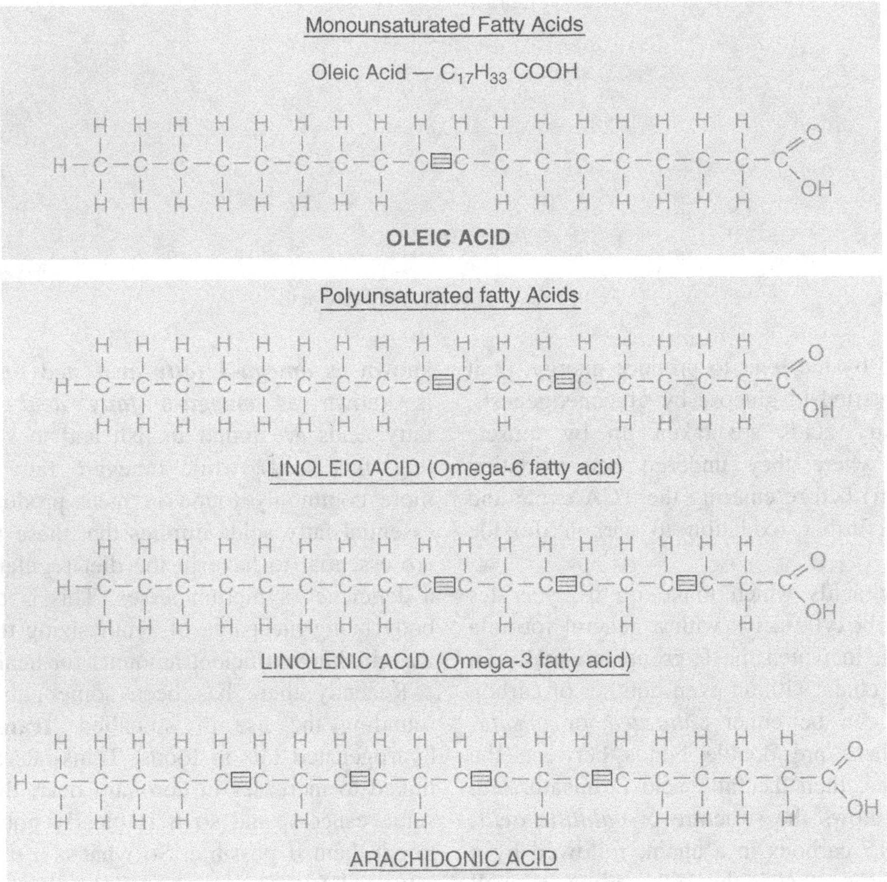

Monounsaturated Fatty Acids
Oleic Acid — $C_{17}H_{33}$ COOH
OLEIC ACID
Polyunsaturated fatty Acids
LINOLEIC ACID (Omega-6 fatty acid)
LINOLENIC ACID (Omega-3 fatty acid)
ARACHIDONIC ACID

Figure 6.8 Unsaturated fatty acids

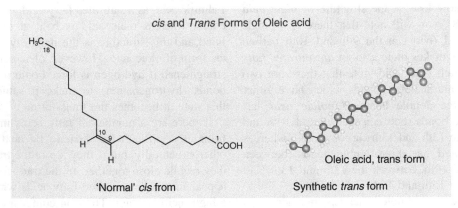

cis and *Trans* Forms of Oleic acid
H_3C
18
10
9
1
H
COOH
H
'Normal' *cis* from
Oleic acid, trans form
Synthetic *trans* form

Figure 6.9 Cis- and trans- fatty acid

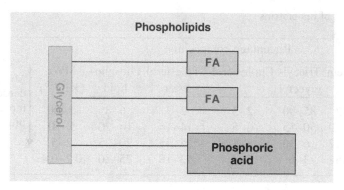

Figure 6.10   Structure of a phospholipid

6.2.2   Compound lipids

Fatty acids and glycerol thus together make up the simple lipids, in so far as they contain carbon hydrogen and oxygen only. However, if we were to incorporate a phosphate or nitrogen group to the fatty acid, we would no longer have a simple lipid – instead we would have a *compound lipid*. This can be seen in Figure 6.10 with the *phospholipids*. Phospholipids contain glycerol, fatty acids and phosphoric acid, and they form an integral part of the plasma membrane.

Other types of compound lipids include *lipoproteins*, such as *chylomicrons*, **very low density lipoprotein (VLDL)**, **low-density lipoprotein (LDL)** and **high-density lipoprotein (HDL)**. These are in effect lipids such as triglycerides and *cholesterol* surrounded by protein (see Table 6.1 and Figure 6.11). The greater the lipid content in relation to the protein content, the less dense is the lipoprotein, and so chylomicrons are the least dense and HDLs are the most dense. Furthermore in relation to their size, the less dense lipoprotein molecules (chylomicrons) are larger than the more dense lipoproteins (HDL).

Chylomicrons are formed as a result of the digestion of lipids and are produced by the intestinal cells from the absorbed fatty acids in our food before being synthesized to TAGs, which make up by far the largest constituent. Chylomicrons are then taken to the liver and to other tissues, where the triglycerides are broken down by **lipoprotein lipase** (LPL) in the blood to release the fatty acids and then transported into the cell for storage.

6.2.3   Derived lipids

The final group of lipids are the *derived lipids*, which include cholesterol and the *steroids*. From Figure 6.12, you can see that the structure of cholesterol is very similar to the steroid hormones. In fact, cholesterol is crucial for the synthesis of steroid hormones such as testosterone, progesterone, and oestrogen (the sex hormones). A diet totally lacking in cholesterol would prove problematic for sex hormone production.

6.3   Metabolism of lipids

6.3.1   Lipolysis

Lipolysis is the process whereby triglycerides are broken down to glycerol and fatty acids. This process is regulated by hormones such as insulin and the catecholamines. The process requires the activation of the enzymes adipose triglyceride lipase (ATGL), **hormone sensitive lipase (HSL)** and monoacylglycerol lipase (MGL) which, when activated, remove fatty acids from the glycerol

Table 6.1   Composition of lipoproteins

Lipoprotein	Percentage composition						More dense, more protein	More lipid
	Protein	Triacyl-glycerol	Cholesterol	Cholesterol ester	Phospho-lipid	MWt $(\times 10^{-6})$		
Chylomicrons	1–2	85–90	2–3	2–3	6–8	>400		
VLDL	8–10	50–55	6–8	14–16	16–20	5–10		
LDL	18–22	6–10	8–12	35–45	20–25	2–5		
HDL	47–52	3–6	2–4	12–18	25–30	0.2–0.4		

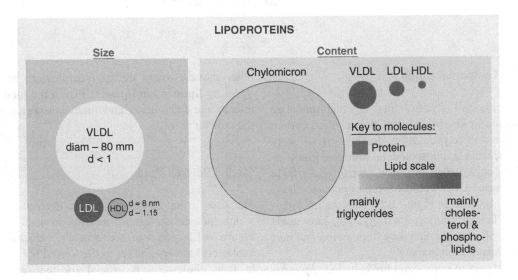

Figure 6.11   Some characteristics of lipoproteins

backbone to result in the formation of three fatty acids and a glycerol. The ATGL initiates the cleavage of the first free fatty acid whereas the HSL cleaves the second fatty acid and then the MGL completes the removal of the final fatty acid (see Figure 6.13).

The process of lipolysis takes place in adipose tissue and also in muscles, so be aware that muscle cells do contain triglycerides.

Lipoproteins, such as LDL and VLDL, also contain triglycerides which can undergo lipolysis. However, in this instance, the triglycerides are broken down by the use of a different enzyme, i.e. LPL. Lipoprotein lipase is released by the endothelial cells in the region of adipose tissue or muscle to bring about the release of fatty acids and glycerol from lipoproteins and thereby results in the uptake of fatty acids by either adipocytes (after eating) or by muscle cells (during exercise).

Lipolysis occurs during exercise and also some hours (around six hours or more) after a meal when fatty acids are needed as an energy source by various tissues. Lipolysis does not occur within a few hours (1–2 hours) after a meal; particularly if the meal is high in carbohydrates.

The fatty acids and glycerol released by adipose tissue as a result of lipolysis pass out of the adipocyte into the blood. The glycerol is soluble, whereas the fatty acids are bound to

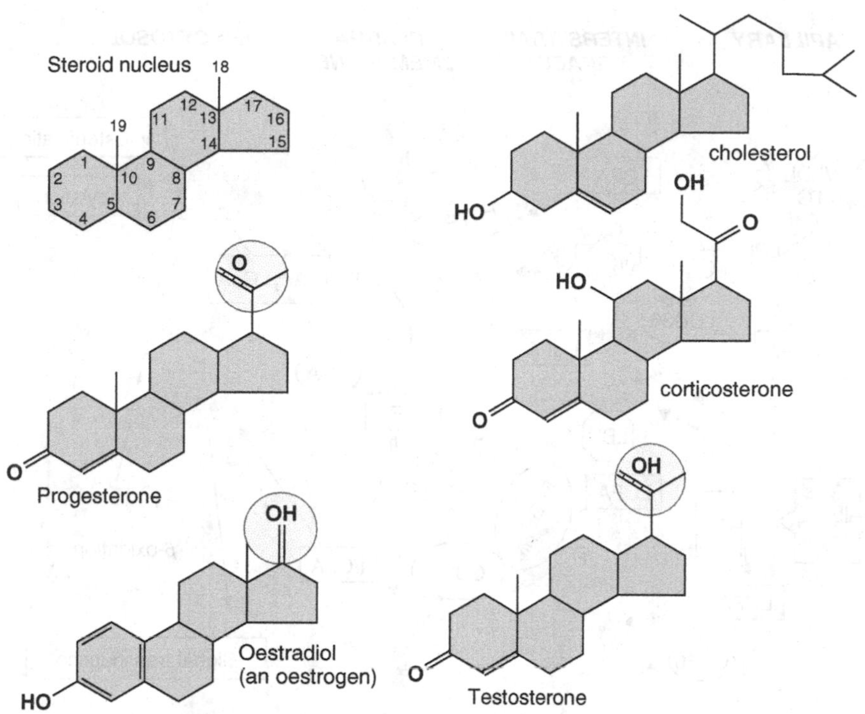

Steroid nucleus 18

cholesterol

Progesterone

corticosterone

Oestradiol
(an oestrogen)

Testosterone

Figure 6.12   Derived lipids: cholesterol and steroid hormones. Note how the steroid hormones are derivatives of cholesterol

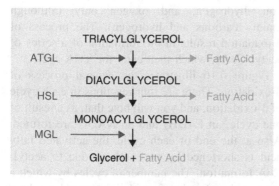

Figure 6.13   Outline of lipolysis

albumin molecules in blood. Albumin molecules are proteins and have the capacity to carry up to ten fatty acid molecules each. The amount of fatty acids delivered to muscle from adipose tissue is dependent on the blood flow through the adipose tissue and on the numbers of albumin molecules in the blood. More detail about the regulation of fat metabolism during exercise will be explored in Chapter 7.

Once the fatty acid molecules arrive at the muscle cell (carried by albumin), they are transported across the plasma membrane by various fatty acid transporters. These include *fatty acid binding protein* (**FABP**), *fatty acid transport protein* (**FATP**), and *fatty acid translocase* (**FAT** – also known as **CD36**). The greater the presence of the fatty acid transporters in the membrane, the greater the uptake of fatty acids into the cell.

As with other transporters (which are protein molecules), FABP, FATP, and FAT are inducible by exercise and diet. Endurance-trained athletes up-regulate the amount of fatty acid transporters and hence can take up and utilize greater amounts of fatty acids as an energy source. Likewise, a diet high in fat and low in carbohydrate over an extended period of time also leads to more fatty acid transporters being produced. Figure 6.14 illustrates fatty acid uptake across a muscle membrane

Once inside the cytoplasm of the muscle cell, fatty acids are bound to another fatty acid binding protein (FABP$_{cyt}$), by which they are

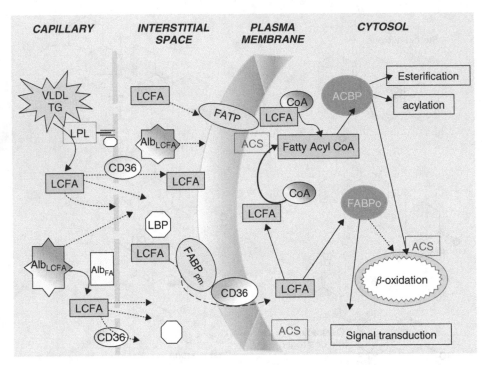

Figure 6.14   Fatty acid uptake across a muscle cell (adapted from Kiens, 2006)

transported to the mitochondria. At the outer membrane of the mitochondria, the fatty acids are activated by the enzyme ACS and CoA, and thus become 'activated' fatty acids. The activated fatty acid is attached to a **carnitine** molecule by the enzyme **carnitine palmitoyl transferase (CPT1)**. CPT-1 transports the acylcarnitine molecule across the mitochondrial membrane to the inner surface, whereby **CPT-2** removes the carnitine and leaves the activated fatty acid in the mitochondrial matrix. The carnitine is then translocated back to the outer membrane, where it can pick up another activated fatty acid. This is sometimes known as the *carnitine shuttle* (Figure 6.15) Only long chain fatty acids are transported in this manner, as medium and short chain fatty acids are capable of passing directly through the mitochondrial membrane without a transporter.

6.3.2   β-oxidation

Once in the mitochondrial matrix, the activated fatty acids then undergo β-oxidation.

Remember that the fatty acids consist of carbon, hydrogen, and oxygen only (although mainly carbons and hydrogen). The process of β-oxidation results in the formation of a series of acetyl-CoAs, which then enter the TCA cycle.

Figure 6.16 illustrates the general process of β-oxidation. There are four reactions in each cycle of β-oxidation, and you will note that, as a result of one cycle, an $FADH_2$ and an NADH are formed. Also at the end of each cycle, the activated fatty acid is shortened by two carbons due to acetyl-CoA formation. The number of cycles by which a fatty acid undertakes β-oxidation depends on how many carbon atoms are present.

A 16-carbon fatty acid would undergo seven cycles, because the last cycle results in the formation of two acetyl-CoA from a four-carbon fatty acyl-CoA. The total number of ATPs likely to result from β-oxidation of a 16-carbon fatty acid is approximately 131 (Figure 6.17). This is derived from seven NAD, which provide 21 ATPs (remember that each NAD results in three ATPs from oxidative phosphorylation) and

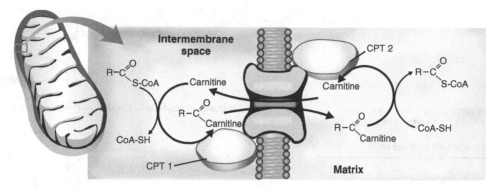

Figure 6.15 Long chain fatty acid uptake across a mitochondrial membrane

seven $FADH_2$ which provide 14 ATPs (remember that every $FADH_2$ re-oxidized from oxidative phosphorylation results in two ATPs). In addition, eight acetyl-CoA are formed, which provides 96 ATPs (remember that for every acetyl-CoA going through the TCA cycle, 12 ATPs are generated). However, we should deduct two ATPs, which are used up in the process of activating the fatty acid before it enters the mitochondria.

Two things are now apparent: first, that a great amount of energy arises from fatty acid oxidation (certainly more than from glucose); and second, that fatty acids are only used during aerobic activities since the TCA cycle and oxidative phosphorylation are involved.

6.3.3 Ketone body formation

If there is an increased availability of fatty acids to muscle and the liver as a consequence of increased lipolysis and release, the muscle can cope with this and oxidize the fatty acids. The liver, on the other hand, appears to be less capable of oxidizing the fatty acids. The liver therefore deals with the excess amounts of acetyl-CoA from β-oxidation of fatty acids by converting them to ketone bodies.

Figure 6.18 shows how the acetyl-CoA is converted to acetoacetate and that the acetoacetate can then be converted to β-hydroxybutyrate. Both acetoacetate and β-hydroxybutyrate are ketone bodies, which than pass out of the liver into the blood and can be taken up and metabolized by other tissue, such as muscle and respiratory tissue.

In order to be metabolized, the ketone bodies are reconverted to acetyl-CoA and thereafter the acetyl-CoA enters the TCA cycle for oxidation. Thus, the processes of ketone body formation from acetyl-CoA are reversible.

Increases in ketone bodies can be found as a consequence of prolonged exercise, and also as a consequence of reduced carbohydrate intake or even starvation. Ketone bodies reflect increased fat availability

6.3.4 Formation of fatty acids

Fatty acids do not only arise from digestion and absorption of lipid-containing foods, but can also be synthesized in the liver and to a lesser extent in adipose tissue from glucose. In other words, the human body has the capability of making fatty acids (and hence triglycerides) from carbohydrate, which is why too large an intake of carbohydrate in the diet leads to increases in adiposity. So, how are fatty acids synthesized?

Fatty acid synthesis occurs in the cytoplasm, unlike the oxidation of fatty acids (β-oxidation), which takes place in the mitochondria. Oxidation of fats involves the reduction of FADH and NAD, whereas synthesis of fatty acids involves the oxidation of NADH. The essential chemistry of the two processes are the reverse of one another. Both oxidation and synthesis of fatty acids involve acetyl-CoA, although the acetyl-CoA in fatty acid synthesis exists temporarily and is bound to the enzyme complex as malonyl-CoA.

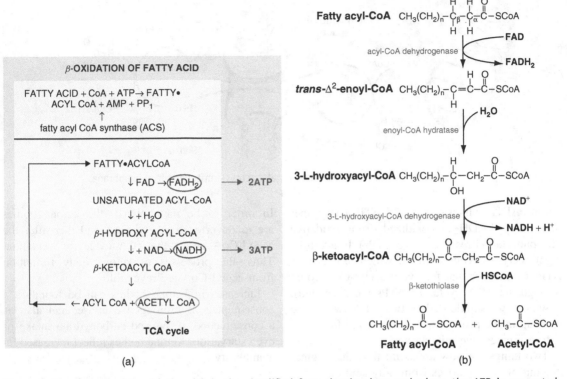

Figure 6.16 Process of β-oxidation (a) is the simplified form showing how and where the ATP is generated, whereas (b) shows the key enzymes involved in red. The enzyme β-hydroxyacyl CoA dehydrogenase (HAD) is often used as a 'marker' of β-oxidative activity.

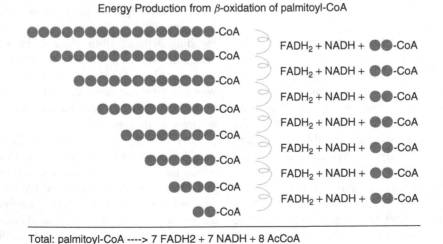

Energy Production from β-oxidation of palmitoyl-CoA

Total: palmitoyl-CoA ----> 7 FADH2 + 7 NADH + 8 AcCoA

In ATP terms: $(7 \times 2) + (7 \times 3) + (8 \times 12) = 131$

Figure 6.17 Likely energy from β-oxidation of a 16-carbon fatty acid (palmitic acid); blue circles denote carbon atoms

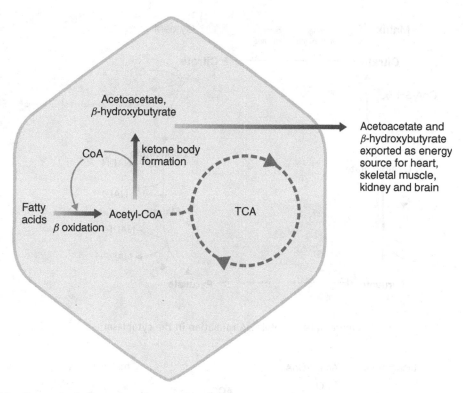

Figure 6.18 Ketone body formation. The reactions for ketone body formation take place in liver(hepatocyte) cells

The synthesis of malonyl-CoA from acetyl-CoA is the first committed step of fatty acid synthesis, and the enzyme that catalyzes this reaction, *acetyl-CoA carboxylase* (**ACC**), is the major site for the regulation of fatty acid synthesis.

The rate of fatty acid synthesis is controlled by the activation of ACC from its inactive form to its active form (this is a concept we will examine in Chapter 7). The activity of ACC is enhanced by citrate and is inhibited by long-chain fatty acids, which implies that fatty acid synthesis is reduced when there is an increase in fatty acids in the cell.

The synthesis of fatty acids from acetyl-CoA and malonyl-CoA is carried out in the cytoplasm by a large complex enzyme, *fatty acid synthase* (**FAS**). All of the reactions of fatty acid synthesis (and there are four repeating stages similar to that of β-oxidation) are carried out by the multiple enzymatic activities of FAS. In the first instance, acetyl-CoA, generated in the mitochondria from

the 'link reaction' (hence from glycolysis) and from β-oxidation of fatty acids, is required to be moved out of the mitochondria and into the cytoplasm.

The shift from fatty acid oxidation and glycolysis occurs when storage is required (as after a meal) rather than during exercise (when fatty acids are needed for energy). This results in reduced oxidation of acetyl-CoA via the TCA cycle.

Acetyl-CoA enters the cytoplasm in the form of citrate using the tricarboxylate transport system (see Figure 6.19). Once in the cytoplasm, citrate is converted to oxaloacetate and acetyl-CoA by *ATP-citrate lyase*. The resultant oxaloacetate is converted to malate, then pyruvate, which can enter the mitochondria. The acetyl-CoA formed is converted to malonyl-CoA as illustrated in Figure 6.20.

Once malonyl-CoA is formed, a repeated series of four reactions occurs on FAS to produce

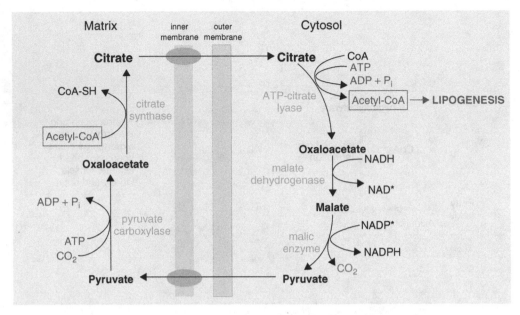

Figure 6.19   Acetyl-CoA formation in the cytoplasm

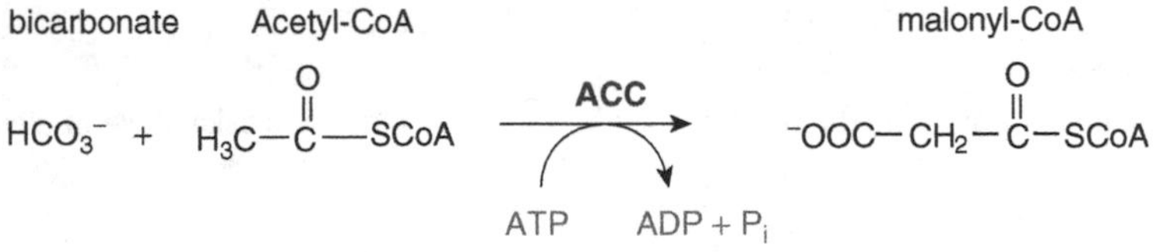

Figure 6.20   The synthesis of malonyl-CoA from acetyl-CoA

the required chain length of fatty acid. The reactions involve malonyl-CoA (formed from acetyl-CoA) reacting with another acetyl-CoA to form acetoacetyl-ACP (a four-carbon compound) and the production of carbon dioxide. A further three reactions, two of which result in NADP formation, complete the cycle with the production of butyryl-ACP (Figure 6.21). The cycle repeats itself six more times for the formation of a 16-carbon fatty acid (i.e. four butyryl-ACPs, each of which is a four-carbon compound), needed for the formation of palmitic acid (a 16-carbon fatty acid).

6.3.5 Triglyceride synthesis

Triglycerides are synthesized from glucose and fatty acids and is regulated by the hormone insulin.

Insulin promotes the uptake of glucose and fatty acids into adipose tissue. Once in the adipocyte, glucose is converted to glycerol phosphate and then to glycerol, which provides the backbone to which the fatty acids are attached. Thus, meals containing fats and carbohydrates invariably result in the formation of triglycerides in adipose tissue. Figure 6.22 illustrates this process.

The uptake of fatty acids from blood into liver, adipose tissue or skeletal muscle invariably results in the synthesis of a TAG after a meal. This is unlikely to happen during exercise, since oxidation is a more likely occurrence. The essence of TAG synthesis is the reverse of lipolysis in so far as three fatty acids need to be attached to a glycerol backbone. For this to occur, the glycerol is derived as glycerol-3 phosphate from glycolysis (hence the

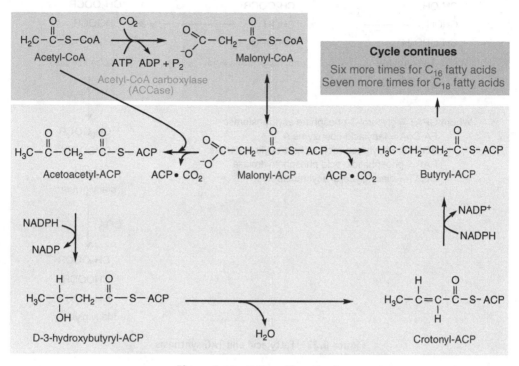

Figure 6.21 Fatty acid synthesis

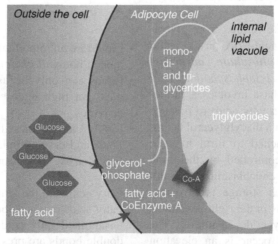

Figure 6.22 General schema for TAG synthesis. The schema highlights the use of glucose to produce the glycerol backbone of the TAG, and the fatty acids which are attached to the glycerol backbone. Both glucose and fatty acids may come from the diet or synthesized by the liver

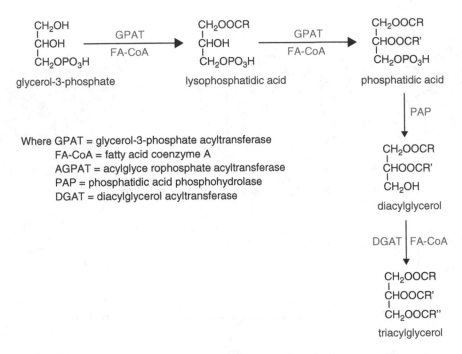

Figure 6.23   Fatty acid and TAG synthesis

link to carbohydrate metabolism), although more recently evidence has been found that *de novo* synthesis occurs through **glyceroneogenesis** (Nye *et al.*, 2008).

The glycerol-3 phosphate formed from glycolysis is esterified by fatty acid-CoA in a reaction catalysed by ***glycerol-3-phosphate acyltransferase*** (**GPAT**) to form *lysophosphatidic acid* (Figure 6.23). The next phase involves a further *esterification* (addition of a fatty acid) to produce *phosphatidic acid* and then a diacylglycerol before a third fatty acid is attached to form a TAG. All these processes are controlled by the same enzyme, i.e. GPAT, in the endoplasmic reticulum.

Any condition in which storage is favoured, such as after a meal, results in the right conditions for fatty acid and triglyceride synthesis. The key hormone for this to occur is an elevation in blood insulin concentration. Such an event typically occurs after a carbohydrate meal. Under the influence of insulin, fatty acids are taken up by adipose tissue and synthesis to TAGs occurs.

In addition, fatty acid synthesis is also stimulated, further adding to storage.

6.4 Key points

- Lipids are an important source of energy for prolonged bouts of exercise.
- Lipids can only be used during aerobic activities, not high intense or so-called 'anaerobic' activities.
- Lipids can be classified into fats, compound lipids and derived lipids.
- Fats consist of carbon, hydrogen and oxygen only.
- Fatty acids are the simplest form of lipid.
- Fatty acids can be subdivided into saturated and unsaturated fatty acids, depending on whether double bonds are present in the structure.
- Fatty acids are the useable form of lipids for energy.
- Triacylglycerols or triglycerides (TAGs) are the storage form of lipids.

- TAGs consist of a glycerol backbone and three fatty acid units.
- TAGs are found in adipose tissue, skeletal muscle and in lipoproteins.
- Compound lipids contain more than carbon, hydrogen and oxygen and often contain phosphate or nitrogen, or even carbohydrate or protein.
- Derived lipids include cholesterol and the steroid hormones.
- Lipolysis is the breakdown of a TAG to liberate three fatty acids and a glycerol, and is regulated by HSL in adipose tissue or muscle and by LPL in blood.
- Fatty acids are carried by albumin in the blood, whereas glycerol is freely soluble.
- Fatty acid transport across the plasma membrane uses three transporters, i.e. FATP, FABP, and FAT/CD36.
- Fatty acids are activated in the cytoplasm of a cell before transport across the mitochondrial membrane
- Fatty acids combine with carnitine in the presence of CPT1 before being transported across the mitochondrial membrane.
- β-oxidation of fatty acids occurs in the mitochondrial matrix, where a repeat cycle of four reactions cleaves an acetyl-CoA, so reducing the fatty acid by two carbons.
- Each cycle of β-oxidation results in the generation of five ATP and the acetyl-CoA produced then enters the TCA cycle for complete oxidation.
- Ketone bodies are produced in the liver as a consequence of elevated concentrations of acetyl-CoA due to oxidation of fatty acids.
- Fatty acid synthesis occurs in the cytoplasm from acetyl-CoA and malonyl-CoA derived in part from excess glucose availability, and under the influence of insulin and using the enzyme FAS.
- The liver is the major site for fatty acid synthesis, although adipose tissue also has the capability.
- TAG synthesis involves the 'attachment' of three fatty acids (one at a time) to a glycerol molecule. which arises from glycerol-3-phosphate from glycolysis or possibly de novo synthesis.
- The key enzyme GPAT brings about TAG synthesis and is found in the endoplasmic reticulum.

Part Three
Metabolic Regulation in Sport and Exercise

7

Principles of metabolic regulation

Learning outcomes

After studying this chapter, you should be able to:

- critically evaluate the role of hormones in regulating energy-requiring processes;
- describe how peptide hormones and neurotransmitters affect their target tissue;
- explain, specifically, how the processes of glycogenolysis, lipolysis, and glycogenesis are influenced by adrenaline and insulin;
- describe how steroid hormones affect their target tissue;
- explain the role of allosteric effectors in regulating enzyme activity;
- explain, specifically, how glycogen phosphorylase, PFK, PDH, and CPT1 are influenced by allosteric effectors;
- evaluate the role of AMPK as an 'exercise' signalling molecule.

Key words

adenylate cyclase	Akt
adipose tissue	allosteric effector
adrenaline	AMP

AMP activated protein kinase (AMPK)	lipophobic
	liver
	LPL
cortisol	MAG (mono-acylglycerol)
CPT1	
catecholamines	malonyl CoA
cyclic-AMP (cAMP)	mineralocorticoids
DAG (diacylglycerol)	muscle
dephosphorylation	myokinase
G-protein	neurotransmitter
glucagon	NO
glucocorticoids	noradrenaline
gluconeogenesis	oestrogen
GLUT4	peptide hormone
glycogen synthase	phosphorylase
glycogen synthase kinase-3 (GSK3)	phosphorylation
	PDE-3
glycogenesis	PDH
glycogenolysis	PI 3-kinase
growth hormone (GH)	PKB
	progesterone
HSL	protein degradation
insulin	protein kinase A (PKA)
insulin receptor (IRS) substrates	
	protein synthesis
IRS-1	steroid hormone
lipolysis	TAG (triacylglycerol)
lipophilic	testosterone

Biochemistry for Sport and Exercise Metabolism, First Edition. Don MacLaren and James Morton.
© 2012 John Wiley & Sons, Ltd. Published 2012 by John Wiley & Sons, Ltd.

7.1 How are catabolic and anabolic reactions controlled?

So far we have examined some key aspects of the biochemistry of macronutrients required for energy (and storage) in a sport and exercise context. Furthermore, Chapter 1 provided a taster as to how and when the energy sources are used. An important factor to realize is that enzymes are involved in all the energy-producing and energy-storing processes, and that these enzymes play an essential role in controlling how quickly the processes are turned on and off as well as how fast they actually happen.

Energy-producing processes must have the facility to be turned on (activated) rapidly, especially with regard to intense bouts activity, where an athlete moves from a sedentary or low level of activity to a sprint-type of activity. In addition, when engaged in more prolonged bouts of exercise, it is important to keep producing the appropriate amounts of ATP from aerobic sources. The question remains as to how the enzymes are activated or inactivated.

After bouts of training, the muscle needs to recover in structural terms (i.e. **protein synthesis** must be enhanced), or else muscle may continually break down. Indeed, as we shall see in the remaining three chapters, training induces enzymatic and structural changes within muscle. How is all this regulated? This chapter explores the *regulation* of enzyme activity and protein synthesis, from which you should realize the importance of both hormones and intracellular chemical compounds known as **allosteric effectors**.

7.2 Hormones

Control of the release of energy from carbohydrate and lipid stores during exercise, as well as the synthesis of glycogen and **TAGs** following meals and the resynthesis of muscle protein, are regulated in part by hormones. From the context of energy production and energy storage, we need to be aware of the role of the following hormones – **catecholamines** (**adrenaline** and noradrenaline), **insulin**, **glucagon**, **growth hormone** (**GH**), and **cortisol**. However, as muscle protein synthesis is important to maintain or increase muscle mass, this demands that an appreciation of the roles of insulin and **testosterone** is required.

Table 7.1 highlights the key processes regulated by these hormones and also their target tissue. From an energy production and storage perspective, the key tissues include **muscle**, **liver** and **adipose tissue**, while muscle remains the tissue for maintaining protein synthesis.

During exercise there is an increase in circulating catecholamines, glucagon, GH and cortisol, whereas insulin levels decrease (Figure 7.1A). As a consequence, there is an increase in **glycogenolysis** and glycolysis in muscle and liver, an increase in **lipolysis** in muscle and adipose tissue, an increase (after 20–30 minutes or more) in **gluconeogenesis** in the liver and an increase in **protein degradation** in liver and muscle. The net effect is that circulating concentrations of glucose remain fairly constant (at least for 60–90 minutes or so), whereas fatty acids, glycerol and ketones increase and amino acids increase. These are the energy sources that can be utilized by muscle.

If a carbohydrate drink, such as a sports drink, is ingested during the exercise bout, a slightly different scenario is presented (El-Sayed *et al.*, 1997). Under this circumstance, the levels of insulin increase while there are lower levels of the other hormones. The effect is reduced lipolysis, gluconeogenesis and protein degradation, whereas glycolysis is enhanced. There is thus a benefit to drink carbohydrate drinks during exercise from a protein breakdown perspective, but not from a 'fat burning' perspective.

In addition to the effects of the hormones on energy availability during exercise, it is important to appreciate that hormones also regulate the recovery process after exercise. This includes not only resynthesis of muscle glycogen stores ready for the next training session, but also promotion of protein synthesis in muscle – so muscle structure can recover. Additionally, when meals are consumed after training, the products of digestion and absorption have to be incorporated into body

Table 7.1   Hormones, the major tissue secreted from, their target tissue, and their effect on various biochemical processes

Hormone	Target tissue	Processes influenced
Insulin (β-cells of pancreas)	Muscle	↑glycogenesis; ↓ lipolysis; ↑ protein synthesis
	Adipose tissue	↑lipogenesis; ↓ lipolysis
	Liver	↑glycogenesis
Glucagon (α-cells of pancreas)	Muscle	↑glycogenolysis; ↑ protein degradation
	Adipose tissue	
	Liver	↑glycogenolysis; ↑ gluconeogenesis; ↑ protein degradation
Adrenaline (adrenal medulla)	Muscle	↑glycogenolysis; ↑ lipolysis
	Adipose tissue	↑lipolysis
	Liver	↑glycogenolysis
Noradrenaline (adrenal medulla)	Muscle	↑glycogenolysis; ↑ lipolysis
	Adipose tissue	↑lipolysis
	Liver	↑glycogenolysis
Growth Hormone (hypothalamus)	Muscle	↑protein synthesis; ↑ lipolysis
	Adipose tissue	↑lipolysis
	Liver	↑gluconeogenesis
Cortisol (adrenal cortex)	Muscle	↑protein degradation
	Adipose tissue	↑lipolysis
	Liver	↑gluconeogenesis
Testosterone (testes)	Muscle	↑protein synthesis
	Adipose tissue	↑lipolysis
	Liver	
Oestrogen (ovaries)	Muscle	
	Adipose tissue	↑lipolysis
	Liver	
Progesterone (ovaries)	Muscle	↑glycogenesis
	Adipose tissue	↑lipolysis
	Liver	↑gluconeogenesis

tissue, such as the storage of carbohydrate and lipids, and of course protein in muscle. Once again, hormones help to regulate these post-prandial (after a meal) events.

What we now need to explore is how the hormones affect their target tissue in order to mobilize energy substrates as illustrated in Figure 7.1A, aid recovery and promote storage.

The hormonal regulation of cells invariably concerns either the activation of inactive enzymes (as produced by peptide hormones and catecholamines) or the formation of new enzymes

(*de novo* synthesis) from protein synthesis (as for **steroid hormones**). Most of the enzymes involved in the energy-producing and energy-storage processes exist in two forms, i.e. an active form and an inactive form. The active form is required to 'drive' the process.

For example, glycogen **phosphorylase** needs to be in its active form to promote breakdown of glycogen during exercise, and so would PFK for glycolysis or ATGL and **HSL** for lipolysis. During rest periods, these enzymes would be present in the cells in their inactive form.

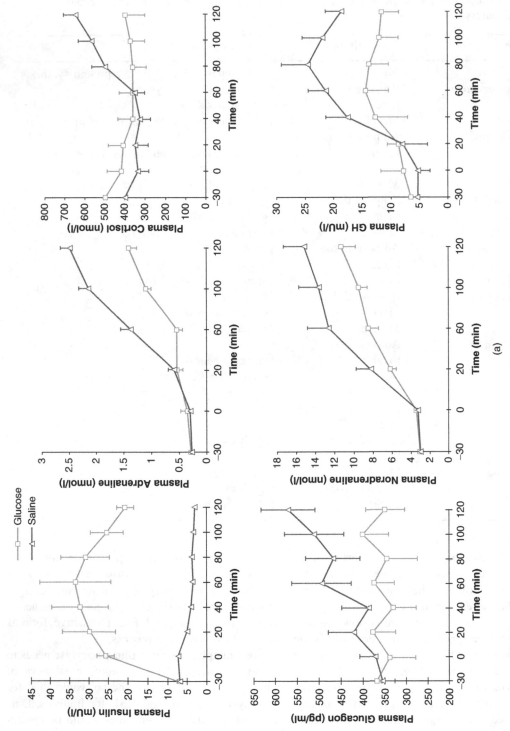

Figure 7.1 Changes in circulating concentrations of hormones (a) and metabolites (b) during cycling exercise at 70% VO$_{2max}$ for two hours with and without glucose infusion (adapted from MacLaren et al., 1999)

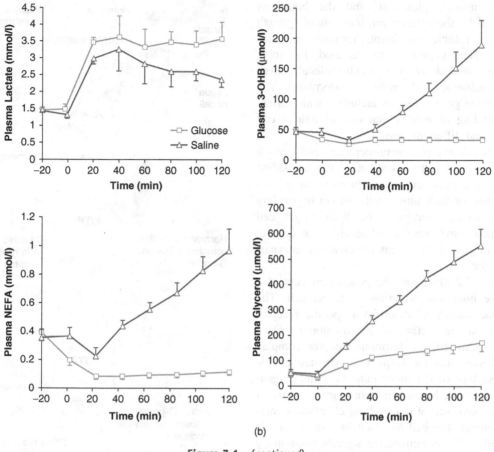

(b)

Figure 7.1 (*continued*)

Hormones have the capacity to affect the activity of these enzymes, and so can 'turn on' a cell. From a hormone action perspective, there are two ways by which hormones influence their target cells:

- *Peptide hormones* (in effect polypeptides) and the catecholamines are **lipophobic** and so are unable to pass through the plasma membrane due to the internal domain of the membrane consisting of fatty acid chains. Consequently, they affect their target cells by attaching to receptors on the surface of the cell membrane and thereby influencing the cell. Peptide hormones include insulin, glucagon, and growth hormone (GH).

- *Steroid hormones* are **lipophilic** and are thereby capable of passing through the target cell

membrane and attaching to a receptor molecule in the cytoplasm, from which protein synthesis is stimulated. Examples include cortisol, testosterone, oestrogen, and progesterone.

7.3 Peptide hormones, neurotransmitters and regulation

The widest variety of signalling molecules in animals are peptides, ranging in size from only a few to more than a hundred amino acids. This group of signalling molecules includes peptide hormones, *neuropeptides* and an array of polypeptide growth factors. Peptide hormones include insulin, glucagon, and the hormones produced by the anterior *pituitary gland* (growth hormone, follicle-stimulating hormone and pro-lactin). Neuropeptides are secreted by some neurons instead of the small-molecule **neu-rotransmitters**, and include endorphins. The polypeptide growth factors include a wide variety of signalling molecules that control animal cell growth and differentiation.

Peptide hormones, neuropeptides and growth factors, as well as the neurotransmitters adrenaline and noradrenaline, are unable to cross the plasma membrane of their target cells, so act by binding to the surface receptors on their target cell membrane, and thereby influencing the activity of the target cell by means of activating enzymes within the cell.

Figure 7.2 illustrates the general concept of a **peptide hormone** affecting its target cell. The hormone must first attach to a specific receptor protein on the surface of the membrane. Once that is achieved, the hormone-receptor complex activates an inactive **G-protein**, situated on the inner surface of the membrane. G-proteins (gua-nine nucleotide-binding proteins) are a family of proteins involved in transmitting chemical signals from outside the cell to result in changes inside the cell. They communicate signals from many hormones, neurotransmitters, and other signaling factors. Signal molecules bind to a domain located outside the cell. An intracellular domain activates a G-protein. The G-protein activates a cascade of further compounds, and finally causes a change downstream in the cell.

G-proteins function as molecular switches. When they bind guanosine triphosphate (GTP), they are 'on', and when they bind guanosine diphosphate (GDP), they are 'off'. G-proteins regulate metabolic enzymes, ion channels, trans-porters, and other parts of the cell machinery, controlling transcription, motility, contractility, and secretion. Once activated, the G-protein activates an inactive **adenylate cyclase**, which then converts ATP to **cyclic-AMP** (**cAMP**). Cyclic-AMP is a signalling molecule capable of activating a range of inactive enzymes, one example being *protein kinase A* (**PKA**).

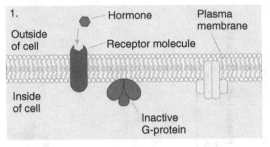

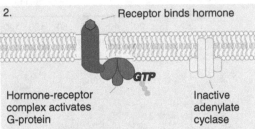

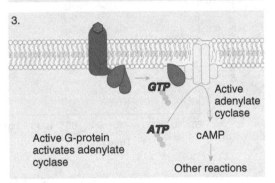

Figure 7.2 General schema showing stages of cAMP formation from a hormone

We shall examine three key examples as to how production of cAMP via activation of the G-protein and adenylate cyclase in the follow-ing sections. These include the activation of glycogenolysis through activation of phosphory-lase, of lipolysis through the activation of HSL, and of, glycogen synthesis via the activation of glycogen synthase.

7.3.1   Adrenaline activation of glycogenolysis

Adrenaline, a hormone secreted from the adrenal medulla during exercise, as well as being a neu-rotransmitter secreted by neurons, attaches to its receptor on a muscle cell membrane, from where

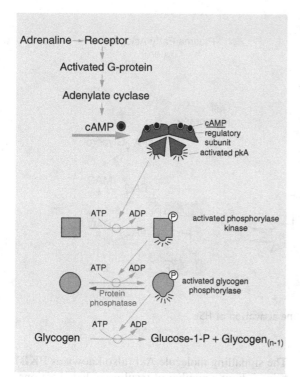

Figure 7.3   Activation of glycogen phosphorylase as in a muscle cell or in a liver cell

it activates a G-protein, which then activates adenylate cyclase, which converts ATP to cAMP in the cytoplasm of the cell. Hence, a molecule on the outside influences processes inside the cell without actual entering the cell (typical of peptide hormone action). Figure 7.3 illustrates this process.

The cAMP then activates an inactive PKA and the active PKA then activates phosphorylase kinase. which in turn activates glycogen phosphorylase, the enzyme responsible for cleaving a glucose molecule from glycogen. Note that the active phosphorylase kinase and the active glycogen phosphorylase are phosphorylated, i.e. they contain a phosphate group from an ATP. It is also worth noting that the active glycogen phosphorylase is inactivated (by **dephosphorylation**) by the enzyme protein phosphatase.

Regulation of the activities of phosphorylase kinase and protein phosphatase thereby promotes or diminishes the formation of active glycogen phosphorylase. Adrenaline, through its effect on

increasing cAMP, enhances glycogen breakdown, while insulin, through its effect on protein phosphatase, has an antagonistic effect.

7.3.2   Adrenaline activation of lipolysis

During exercise, an increase in circulating adrenaline also targets skeletal muscle cells and adipocytes, resulting in the breakdown of TAGs to release fatty acids and glycerol, both of which can be oxidized in muscle and liver. Figure 7.4 illustrates how this process of lipolysis occurs. Adrenaline attaches to its receptor on the membrane, activating a G-protein, which activates adenylate cyclase, which converts ATP to cAMP, which then activates PKA. The PKA then activates HSL.

The activated HSL is the phosphorylated form, which cleaves a fatty acid from the DAG to form a free fatty acid and a **monoacylglycerol** (**MAG**). You should be aware that the DAG has arisen due to the activation of ATGL. This is not shown in Figure 7.4 since the regulation of ATGL has not yet been clearly established, and we wished to focus on activation of HSL. The final stage of breakdown to release the third fatty acid and the glycerol involves a monoacylglycerol lipase (MGL). It is also worth noting that insulin is a potent anti-lipolytic hormone, which inhibits HSL activation by stimulating the activity of phosphodiesterase (Figure 7.7). Phosphodiesterase converts cAMP to the inactive form, AMP, resulting in lack of PKA and activated HSL.

So far we have seen how hormones such as adrenaline and insulin affect a muscle or a fat cell by activating or inactivating key enzymes (in these instances through **phosphorylation** and **dephosphorylation**). We shall now explore the effect of a hormone, insulin, on glycogen synthesis, and note that the key enzyme in this case is activated by becoming dephosphorylated.

7.3.3   Insulin activation of glycogen synthase

During recovery from exercise, and after consuming a meal containing carbohydrate, insulin

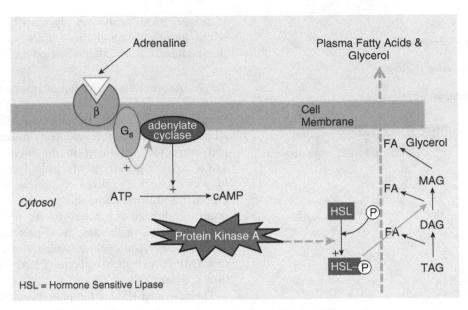

Figure 7.4   Adrenaline activation of HSL

concentrations become elevated in response to an increase in blood glucose levels. As with adrenaline, insulin attaches to a specific receptor on its target cells and thereby modifies activities within the cell. However, the situation is different to what we have seen for adrenaline. The membrane-bound receptor for insulin is a protein consisting of four subunits. Two subunits protrude out from surface of the cell and bind insulin, and two subunits span the membrane and protrude into the cytoplasm (Figure 7.5). These receptors range from fewer than 100 in most cells in our body to more than 1,00,000 in some liver cells.

The binding of insulin to the outer subunits of the receptor causes a conformational change in the membrane-spanning subunit, which is also an enzyme (a tyrosine kinase). The activated subunits add phosphate groups to the cytoplasmic domain of the receptor, as well as a variety of **insulin receptor substrates (IRS)**. The activated IR then phosphorylates **IRS-1** and other substrates. IRS-1 then serves as a docking protein for *PI 3-kinase*, which is activated by this interaction. The cascade initiated by PI 3-kinase involves activation of PI 3-K-dependent kinases (PDK) and then **Akt**.

The signalling molecule Akt (also known as **PKB**) brings about a number of insulin-mediated actions, i.e. activation of **glycogen synthase**, translocation of **GLUT4** from vesicles to the membrane for glucose transport, and stimulation of protein synthesis (Figure 7.5).

Once insulin has attached to its receptor and brought about an increase in Akt within the cell, there is an increase in the activity of the enzyme glycogen synthase. This is achieved by dephosphorylation of the enzyme, which is in contrast to the phosphorylation exhibited by phosphorylase (Figure 7.6). The enzyme *glycogen synthase kinase-3* (**GSK3**) regulates glycogen synthase activity by phosphorylating it and so causing inactivation, and in turn is regulated by Akt i.e. Akt inactivates GSK3 and hence the inhibition of glycogen synthase is removed, so enabling it to increase glycogen storage. In addition, Akt stimulates translocation of the glucose transporter, GLUT4, to move from vesicles within the cytoplasm to the membrane and hence promote glucose uptake into the cell. Consequently, the increase in glucose and the activation of glycogen synthase leads to greater glycogen synthesis.

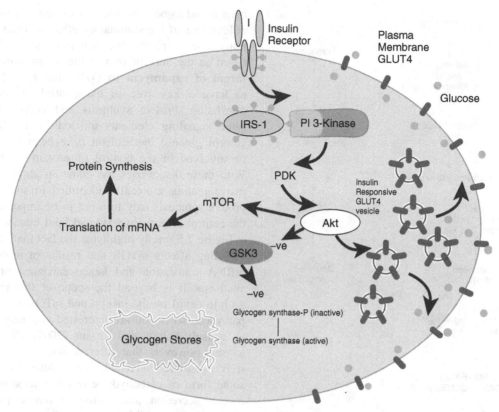

Figure 7.5   Insulin action showing activation of glycogenesis. Note how insulin activates Akt, which in turn inactivates GSK3 (an inhibitory enzyme for activation of glycogen synthase). In other words, glycogen synthase becomes activated

7.3.4   Insulin inhibition of lipolysis

Insulin is an anabolic hormone, i.e. it promotes synthesis rather than degradation. To this end, insulin is potently anti-lipolytic and favours storage of lipids rather than breakdown. It achieves this through activation of Akt, which then activates phosphodiesterase (**PDE-3**), an enzyme which converts cAMP to **AMP** (Figure 7.7). If cAMP levels are reduced in adipose tissue, the consequences are that HSL is not activated and hence lipolysis does not take place. This is just what insulin does. So, if an athlete wishes to 'fat burn', they should attempt to keep insulin concentrations low, or else they may be wasting their time! This means not ingesting carbohydrates before or during an exercise session.

7.3.5   Insulin stimulation of protein synthesis

The stimulation of protein synthesis is a classic, though maybe to some surprising, action of insulin. Remember that insulin is an anabolic hormone, and so it should not be a surprise that insulin, as well as promoting fat storage (lipogenesis) and carbohydrate storage (**glycogenesis**), should also promote protein storage (protein synthesis). Loss of the stimulatory effect of insulin on protein synthesis contributes to the cessation of growth and to weight loss.

The effect of insulin on protein metabolism is complex and involves changes in both synthesis and degradation. In some cell types an increase in rate of protein synthesis may be detected within minutes of insulin treatment. This response to

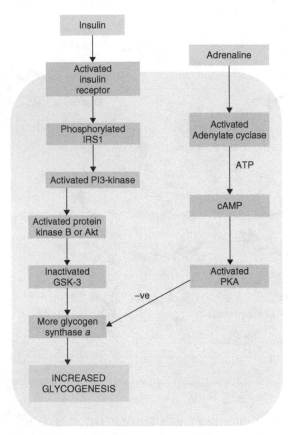

Figure 7.6 Effect of insulin (and adrenaline) on glycogen synthase

insulin occurs within a timeframe comparable to that of other acute actions of the hormone, such as the activation of glucose transport and glycogen synthase activation. The rapid effects of insulin on protein synthesis involve increases in mRNA translation, the process through which the genetic code transcribed in the mRNA template is translated into protein. Translation takes place on ribosomes in a complex series of reactions that can be segregated into three phases – initiation, elongation and termination (review section 4.5.5). Although the effects of insulin on mRNA translation have received less attention than those on carbohydrate and lipid metabolism, recent studies have increased our understanding of the mechanisms involved in the control of protein synthesis. The activities of several translation factors have

been found to be controlled by insulin, explaining at least in part the stimulatory effect of insulin on translation. A newly discovered signaling system based on the Ser/Thr protein kinase, **mammalian target of rapamycin (mTOR)**, has been found to have a key role in the control of mRNA translation. Protein synthesis and many of the same signaling elements utilized by insulin to control glucose metabolism have been found to be involved in the control of protein synthesis. With these discoveries has come an appreciation that signaling molecules identified in studies of protein synthesis may turn out to be important in the control of carbohydrate and lipid metabolism.

Figure 7.5 briefly highlights the fact that insulin signaling affects mTOR and results in increased mRNA translation and hence enhanced protein synthesis. It is beyond the scope of this text to go into detail on the insulin and mTOR signaling pathways, so if you are interested you may wish to consult Saltiel and Pessin (2007). Needless to say however, that after a bout of exercise it is considered advisable for athletes to ingest some form of carbohydrate in order to stimulate insulin secretion and thereby promote protein synthesis. The addition of some form of protein too is necessary in order to provide the amino acids required for building up protein. Indeed, there is a case for the addition of branched chain amino acids (in particular leucine) to stimulate the recovery process.

7.4 Steroid hormones and regulation

We have seen that peptide hormones act by attaching to a specific receptor on the cell membrane. Steroid hormones, on the other hand, are hydrophobic molecules capable of passing through the cell membrane and thereby attaching to their specific receptor in the cytoplasm. The steroids include the sex hormones (**testosterone, oestrogen, and progesterone**), **glucocorticoids and mineralocorticoids,** and they are all synthesized from cholesterol (see Chapter 6). Testosterone, oestrogen, and progesterone are the

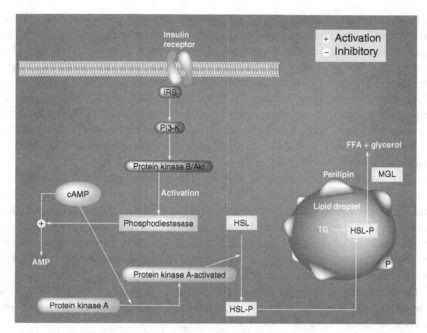

Figure 7.7   Insulin inhibition of lipolysis – major effect is on removal of cAMP to AMP and so lack of PKA

sex steroids and are produced by the gonads. The corticosteroids (e.g. cortisol) are produced by the adrenal cortex and include the glucocorticoids, which act on a variety of cells to stimulate production of glucose, and the mineralocorticoids, which act on the kidney to regulate salt and water balance.

Although thyroid hormone, vitamin D3 and retinoic acid are structurally and functionally distinct from the steroids, they share a common mechanism of action in their target cells. Thyroid hormone plays important roles in development and regulation of metabolism, while vitamin D3 regulates Ca^{2+} metabolism and bone growth, and retinoic acid (synthesized from vitamin A) is important for development.

Because of their lipophilic character, the steroid hormones, thyroid hormone, vitamin D3 and retinoic acid are able to enter cells by diffusing across the plasma membrane (Figure 7.8). Once inside the cell, they bind to intracellular receptors that are expressed by the hormonally responsive target cells. These receptors, which are members of a family of proteins known as the steroid receptor superfamily, are transcription factors that

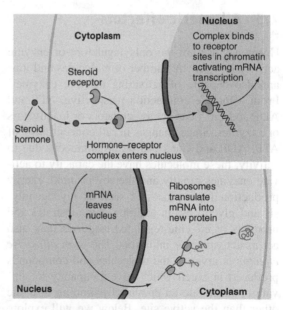

Figure 7.8   Steroid hormone action

contain related domains for DNA binding and for transcriptional activation. The steroid hormones and related molecules directly thus regulate gene expression.

Since this process involves transcription and then translation before a new protein is produced, it takes longer for new enzymes (or maybe structural proteins) to be available for energy production or storage, in contrast to the peptide hormones, which have an immediate impact.

Some members of the steroid receptor superfamily, such as the oestrogen and glucocorticoid receptors, are unable to bind to DNA in the absence of hormones. The binding of a hormone induces a conformational change in the receptor, allowing it to bind to regulatory DNA sequences and activate transcription of target genes. In other cases, the receptor binds DNA in either the presence or absence of hormone, but hormone binding alters the activity of the receptor as a transcriptional regulatory molecule. For example, thyroid hormone receptor acts as a repressor in the absence of hormone, but hormone binding converts it to an activator that stimulates transcription of thyroid hormone-inducible genes.

7.5 Allosteric effectors

Hormones are not the only regulators of enzyme activity in a cell. A number of molecules and ions are also capable of activating inactive enzymes. From a muscle contraction perspective, ATP and ADP and Ca^{2+} can act as activators or inactivators of enzymes. Since changes in cell concentration of ATP, ADP and Ca^{2+} can be instantaneous due to activity, these molecules have the capacity to activate enzymes rapidly and thereby promote energy production from processes such as glycogenolysis and glycolysis. In addition, the substrates and products of enzyme-regulated reactions may also act as activators or inhibitors. The term *allosteric effector* is given to the molecules and compounds produced in a cell which have a capacity to activate or inactivate an enzyme by binding to a site other than the active site. Below we will explore some key examples of allosteric regulation.

7.5.1 Regulation of glycogen phosphorylase

As we have already seen, glycogen phosphorylase is activated via the cAMP cascade from

hormones such as adrenaline. However, during intense 'sprint' bouts of exercise when the energy required in a muscle (from glycogenolysis) goes from rest to explosive bouts within a matter of seconds, the cAMP cascade mediated by adrenaline is too slow, and the available evidence (Chapter 8) highlights that glycogenolysis is activated within 1 second. So how does glycogen phosphorylase become activated so rapidly?

The answer lies in the presence of Ca^{2+} in the cytoplasm due to release from the *sarcoplasmic reticulum* during muscle contraction. A slight increase in Ca^{2+} directly activates phosphorylase kinase, which in turn activates phosphorylase and hence bypasses the cAMP cascade. Of course, the latter will help regulation as the exercise duration increases. Figure 7.9 illustrates the allosteric regulation of glycogen phosphorylase by Ca^{2+}.

7.5.2 Regulation of PFK

The key regulatory enzyme for glycolysis is PFK. When going from a rest or starting position as in a 60 or 100 metre sprint, where the level of glycolysis is low, to the actual sprint, where glycolytic activity is maximal, necessitates allosteric regulation in order to rapidly activate PFK. Figure 7.10 highlights that PFK activity is promoted by increased cellular levels of AMP and P_i, as would be expected at the start of a bout of exercise. Furthermore, PFK is inactivated when levels of ATP are high (as is expected at rest or low levels of exercise), and also when citrate concentrations are high. Citrate moves out from the mitochondria when the TCA cycle is working rapidly, probably due to greater fat oxidation, leading to increases in acetyl-CoA formation and hence rapid throughput into the TCA cycle.

7.5.3 Regulation of PDH

PDH plays a pivotal role in the formation of acetyl-CoA from pyruvate. Since acetyl-CoA is

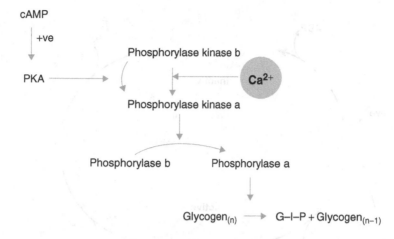

Figure 7.9 Allosteric regulation of phosphorylase by Ca^{2+}

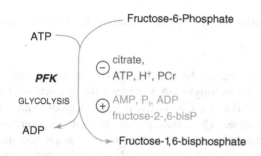

Figure 7.10 Allosteric regulation of PFK

formed from pyruvate via glycolysis and as the end result of β-oxidation of fatty acids, PDH is recognized to be important in the regulation of carbohydrate and lipid oxidation. Inactivation of PDH would reduce carbohydrate oxidation, since the pyruvate from glycolysis could not be converted to acetyl-CoA and result in glycolysis itself being inhibited. Figure 7.11 illustrates the allosteric effectors which activate and inhibit PDH.

It is clear that in order for PDH to be activated it is necessary that PDH kinase becomes inactivated. This happens when mitochondrial levels of pyruvate, NAD^+, CoASH, ADP, and Ca^{2+} are elevated. On the other hand, PDH kinase becomes activated (and hence inactivates

PDH) when ATP, NADH, and acetyl-CoA are increased. If you think about what happens during exercise, you will appreciate that pyruvate levels become elevated in the mitochondria due to enhanced glycolysis and so cause activation of PDH. Likewise, ADP concentrations become elevated during exercise as ATP hydrolysis occurs and hence another factor in promoting activation of PDH. You should also note that on the right hand side of Figure 7.11 the enzyme PDH phosphatase, when active, promotes activation of PDH. Allosteric effectors which cause activation of PDH phosphatase are Mg^{2+} and Ca^{2+}, both of which are made available during muscle contraction. Furthermore, an important inhibitor of PDH activity is the product of the reaction i.e. acetyl-CoA. It is quite common to observe what is termed **'product inhibition'** of an enzyme i.e. the product formed from an enzyme-regulated reaction, if not removed, will inhibit the enzyme. So any build-up of acetyl-CoA causes product inhibition of PDH. The latter may occur if both glycolysis and beta-oxidation occur rapidly and thereby result in significant build up of acetyl-CoA. The regulation of PDH has become an area of significant amounts of research over the years because it appears to be at the crossroads for both carbohydrate and lipid metabolism.

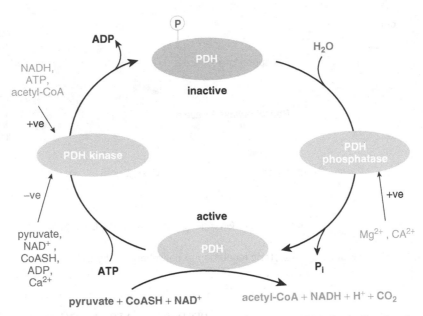

Figure 7.11 Allosteric regulation of PDH. Note that the active form of PDH is dephosphorylated whereas the inactive form is phosphorylated

7.5.4   Regulation of CPT1

In order for long chain fatty acids to enter the mitochondria and undergo β-oxidation, they have to pass across the inner mitochondrial membrane via a transporter (see Chapter 5). The enzyme **CPT1** plays a pivotal role in this transport process, so any factor that diminishes or enhances the activity of CPT1 is likely to diminish or increase the uptake of long chain fatty acids into the mitochondrial matrix.

It has been shown that *malonyl-CoA* is an inhibitor of CPT1 activity, i.e. increased cytoplasmic levels of malonyl-CoA inhibit CPT1, while reduced levels remove the inhibition. Figure 7.12 illustrates the role of malonyl-CoA and shows that increased malonyl-CoA occurs when concentrations of acetyl-CoA in the cytoplasm are elevated. This happens when there is an increase in carbohydrate availability in the cell such as glycogen loading or enhanced carbohydrate oxidation and may be maintained when more fatty acids are oxidized. Note that the stimulus of exercise elevates cytoplasmic **AMPK**, which in turn inhibits the enzyme ACC, thereby resulting in less malonyl-CoA and hence the removal of the inhibition on CPT1. Clearly this happens during exercise. The consequence is that as exercise duration progresses and more fatty acids become liberated and available, the exercise-stimulated increase in AMPK promotes activation of CPT1 and thereby enables greater uptake (and oxidation) of the fatty acids.

7.5.5   AMPK as a metabolic regulator

In addition to the hormonal regulation and allosteric regulators discussed thus far, AMP is a particularly important metabolite which can modulate cellular responses. It is well known that AMP is produced during muscle contraction, particularly in intense bouts of exercise (through the **myokinase** reaction in the intermembrane space – see below).

$$ADP + ADP \rightarrow ATP + AMP$$

An increase in cytoplasmic AMP results in activation of both glycogen phosphorylase and

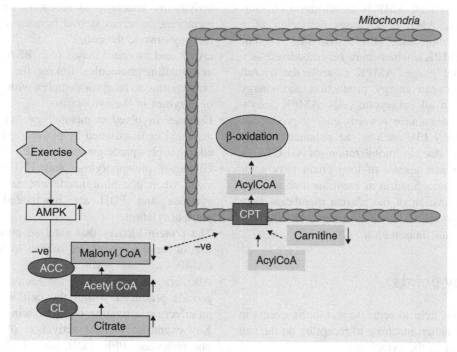

Figure 7.12   Regulation of CPT1 (adapted from Kiens, 2006)

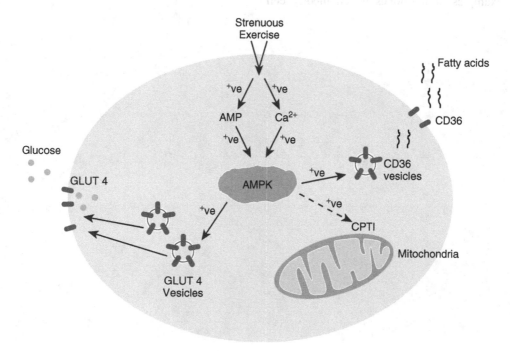

Figure 7.13   AMPK activation and consequences

PFK so, in effect, AMP is an allosteric effector. In addition, AMP also causes activation of a signalling molecule, ***AMP activated protein kinase*** (**AMPK**), which may be considered as a cellular fuel gauge. AMPK controls the overall balance between energy production and energy utilization in all eukaryotic cells. AMPK activation tilts the balance towards energy production (see Figure 7.13), such as an enhanced uptake of glucose due to mobilization of GLUT4 or may be greater uptake of long chain fatty acids across the mitochondria as mentioned above, and even mobilization of the plasma membrane fatty acid transporter, CD36. For in depth reading you should consult Jensen *et al.*, (2009).

7.6   Key points

- Hormones help to regulate metabolic events in cells by either attaching to receptors on the cell surface or in the cytoplasm.
- Peptide hormones, as well as catecholamines, are examples of hormones which modify cell activity by attaching to receptors on the cell membrane, whereas steroid hormones attach to receptors inside the cell.
- cAMP and protein kinases (e.g. PKA, Akt) act as signalling molecules, linking the cell membrane hormone-receptor complex with activation of enzymes in the cytoplasm.
- Enzymes involved in metabolism can be either activated or inactivated by phosphorylation, i.e. adding a phosphate group via ATP.
- Glycogen phosphorylase and HSL are activated when phosphorylated, whereas glycogen synthase and PDH are inactivated through phosphorylation.
- The protein kinases that catalyse phosphorylation of these enzymes are subject to control by cAMP, Ca^{2+} and AMP.
- Allosteric effectors are molecules or compounds produced within the cell which have an effect on activating or inactivating enzymes. Key examples include activation of glycogen phosphorylase, PFK, PDH, and CPT1.

8

High-intensity exercise

Learning outcomes

After studying this chapter, you should be able to:

- outline the main sites of control which potentially underpin the regulation of metabolism during high-intensity exercise;
- critically evaluate the effects of exercise duration on metabolic regulation of substrate utilization during high-intensity exercise;
- critically evaluate the effects of CHO feeding on HIE;
- outline the potential nutritional ergogenic aids that have a positive impact on HIE performance;
- critically evaluate the effects of training on substrates and enzyme activity relating to HIE;
- critically discuss potential metabolic causes of fatigue associated with HIE.

Key words

acidosis	allosteric regulation
adenylate kinase	AMP
ADP	ATP
β-alanine	caffeine
alkalinizer	cAMP
alkalosis	carnosine

creatine	metabolic alkalosis
CS	MCT
extracellular K^+	muscle biopsy
glycogen	myokinase
glycogen	Na^+/K^+ pump
phosphorylase	oxygen deficit
H^+	PCr
HAD	PFK
lactate	pH
LDH	sarcolemma
Magnetic Resonance	sarcolemmal
Spectroscopy	depolarization
(MRS)	sarcoplasmic
maximal accumulated	reticulum
oxygen deficit	sodium bicarbonate
(MAOD)	sodium citrate
metabolic acidosis	supra-maximal

8.1 Overview of energy production and metabolic regulation in high-intensity exercise

8.1.1 Definition of high-intensity exercise

High-intensity exercise (HIE) can be defined as a maximal bout of activity which lasts for less than a second (as in a kick, jump, punch, or

Biochemistry for Sport and Exercise Metabolism, First Edition. Don MacLaren and James Morton.
© 2012 John Wiley & Sons, Ltd. Published 2012 by John Wiley & Sons, Ltd.

throw) or as long as 1–2 minutes, and in which the major sources of energy are derived from anaerobic processes. This could encompass events such as sprint track cycling, maximal running of distances between 60–200 metres, swimming 50–100 metres, most field events in athletics, sprint ice-skating and so on.

Maximal efforts demand not just the use of anaerobic energy sources but also that all muscle fibre types are recruited – in particular, the type IIx or FG fibres. The consequence is the generation of large amounts of **ATP** at a very rapid rate. Indeed, the rate at which ATP is generated determines how much force or velocity can be produced and for how long.

The energy continuum observed in Chapter 1 provides an idea of the likely sources of energy during HIE. Once significant amounts of energy are derived from aerobic energy sources, then we move into the domain of prolonged exercise (see Chapter 9). This can be illustrated by the example of a well-trained cyclist who achieves a VO_{2max} at a power output of 400 W and is able to produce a peak power output (PPO) of 1200 W in a 10 second maximal test (Calbet *et al.*, 2003). In this instance, VO_{2max} is obtained at $\approx$33% of PPO. The remaining $\approx$67% represents an exercise intensity above the maximal aerobic power and thereby can be termed **supra-maximal** exercise. For the purposes of this chapter, HIE is equivalent to supra-maximal exercise, and where the predominant energy supply is derived from anaerobic processes.

Cycling, running and the use of maximal voluntary contractions (MVC) are the predominant modes of exercise employed in research studies, mainly due to the comparative ease of accessing major muscle groups for biopsy samples and for blood sampling. The more recent developments in **Magnetic Resonance Spectroscopy (MRS)** have enabled 'real time' measures of phosphorus-containing metabolites (**ATP, ADP, AMP**, and P_i) as well as changes in **pH** within the active muscle, albeit using isometric contractions in the main.

Since most forms of HIE are dynamic rather than static, the value of findings from MRS or from biopsies following MVC should be treated with a degree of caution. Having said that, valuable changes in metabolites have been elucidated by Hultman and colleagues using MVC and biopsy data (Hultman *et al.*, 1981).

8.1.2   Energy production during high-intensity exercise

Since HIE demands a 100-fold increase in the rate of ATP use as compared with rest, it is important to consider the fact that the rate of ATP required is very high. Indeed, the rate of ATP production necessary is so high that it is unlikely (at least in the early stages) for the oxygen supply to the muscle to match the energy required (i.e. ATP demand). If the actual oxygen uptake is plotted against time from rest to a steady state bout of exercise (Figure 8.1), there is a time lag before steady state is reached. The difference between the amount of oxygen required for the exercise bout and the actual oxygen consumed is known as the *oxygen deficit* (O_2 deficit). During this lag phase, the energy for muscle contraction comes from anaerobic sources, compensating for the inability of the cardiovascular system to provide sufficient oxygen immediately to the muscle as well as for the activation of the PDH complex. Once steady state is reached, the oxygen uptake is then equivalent to the oxygen demand.

But what if the exercise bout is an intense bout of HIE in which steady state is unlikely to be achieved because during HIE the major energy sources are supra-maximal (i.e. above 100% VO_{2max})? In this situation, the O_2 deficit is

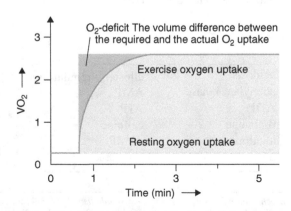

Figure 8.1   Oxygen deficit during steady state exercise

much greater and cannot be paid back during the exercise bout because the cardiovascular system is incapable of delivering enough oxygen to the muscle as well as the ability of the muscle to fully utilize the oxygen. The consequence is an inability to fully sustain the energy required.

Figure 8.2 highlights the O_2 deficit during an HIE bout, and from which you will note that steady state cannot be reached. Calculations of the energy demand can be made based on the actual O_2 consumed and the required O_2 for the level of HIE. This is known as the **maximal *accumulated oxygen deficit*** (**MAOD**). For further information on MAOD, see Winter & MacLaren (2009).

It would be useful now for you to recap how energy is derived during a bout of HIE (you should re-examine Chapter 1 if you wish at this point). Examination of Figure 8.3 provides an overview of the energy sources likely to be employed, i.e. **ATP**, **PCr**, anaerobic glycogenolysis and glycolysis. All of these reactions take place in the cytoplasm, since the oxygen-requiring processes of aerobic metabolism are unlikely to produce energy in these events. This is not merely because of a lack of oxygen getting into muscle but also because allosteric effectors will have activated a number of key reactions, such as glycogenolysis, glycolysis

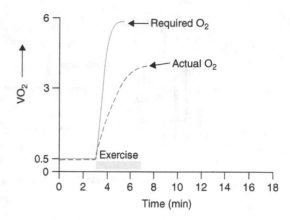

Figure 8.2 Oxygen deficit during HIE

and PCr degradation, and so will have 'started the ball rolling' in energy production terms.

One noteworthy reaction which has, to date, not been described in this text is that of the ***myokinase*** or ***adenylate kinase*** reaction. During HIE, sufficient levels of ADP in the cytoplasm trigger the activation of the enzyme myokinase (also known as adenylate kinase). The enzyme converts two molecules of ADP to an ATP and an AMP:

$$ADP + ADP \rightarrow ATP + AMP$$
$$myokinase$$

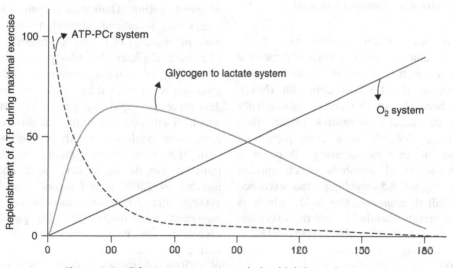

Figure 8.3 Primary energy sources during high intensity exercise

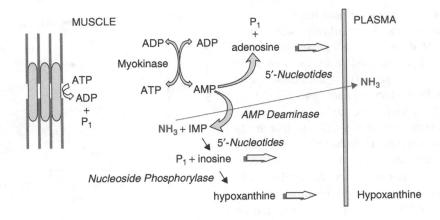

Figure 8.4 Purine nucleotide cycle

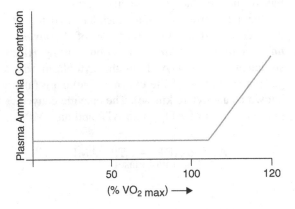

Figure 8.5 Ammonia threshold

The ATP is used for muscle contraction, while the AMP is removed via the Purine-Nucleotide Cycle (PNC) which is shown in Figure 8.4. One end product of the PNC is ammonia (NH_3), which has been shown to increase substantially in plasma at exercise intensities greater than 100% VO_{2max}. Indeed, as a consequence of an increase in exercise intensity, there is a greater production of ammonia which appears in plasma. Figure 8.5 highlights the existence of the so-called *ammonia threshold*, which is akin to the **lactate** threshold with the exception that it occurs at intensities above 100% VO_{2max}. For further reading you should consult Robergs *et al.* (2004).

8.1.3 Evidence of energy sources used in HIE

An early study using electrical stimulation and **muscle biopsy** over a period of 1.68 to 5 seconds highlighted the fact that PCr is rapidly decreased and that lactic acid is produced within 1.68 seconds (Figure 8.6). It should, however, be mentioned that this study had the muscle blood supply occluded in order to have an enclosed system, so is not typical of normal exercise events which are dynamic and with an intact blood flow.

Cheetham *et al* (1986) investigated the changes in muscle metabolites during 6 and 30 seconds of sprint cycling. Their data (Figure 8.7) demonstrates the significant depletion (and therefore use) of muscle PCr and **glycogen**. Levels of PCr were depleted by nearly two thirds after 30 seconds of intense exercise, while muscle glycogen was depleted by nearly one third. These data represent rapid changes in key metabolites which, if allowed to continue at this rate, would ensure total depletion in a short time frame.

In the same investigation, the concentrations of muscle lactic acid were observed to increase by 250% after 6 seconds and by nearly 1000% after 30 seconds, thereby reflecting the important contribution of glycogenolysis and glycolysis for energy provision. It is worth noting that ATP stores are reduced to a level of ≈50% of resting values. This is possibly

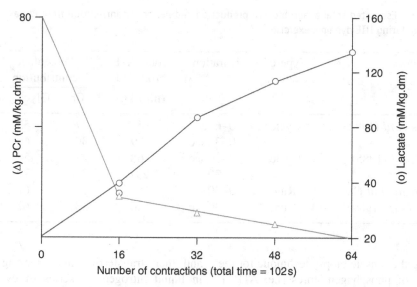

Figure 8.6   Muscle PCr depletion and lactate increase during electrical stimulation (adapted from Hultman *et al.*, 1990)

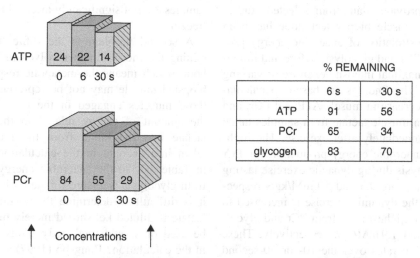

% REMAINING		
	6 s	30 s
ATP	91	56
PCr	65	34
glycogen	83	70

Figure 8.7   Changes in muscle phosphagens and glycogen after maximal exercise lasting 6 and 30 seconds (adapted from Cheetham *et al.*, 1986)

an inbuilt safety margin to ensure that muscle is never completely devoid of ATP (only found in rigor mortis!).

Bogdanis *et al.* (1996) examined the metabolic response when repeating two 30-second maximal cycling bouts separated by 4 minutes of rest. Examination of the data after the initial 30-second bout revealed that muscle pH decreased from 7.05

to 6.69, muscle lactate concentration increased from 5 to 108 mmol.kg dry weight^{-1}, muscle PCr decreased from 84 to 40 mmol.kg dry weight^{-1}, muscle glycogen decreased from 327 to 228 mmol.kg dry weight^{-1}, and that PCr, glycolysis and aerobic metabolism accounted for 21, 50 and 29%, respectively, of the total energy production.

Table 8.1   Estimated total anaerobic ATP production and per cent contribution from PCr and glycolysis during HIE dynamic exercise

Reference	Type of exercise	Duration	Total ATP produced (mM/kg)	PCr	Glycolysis
Boobis *et al* (1983)	Cycle	0–6 sec	63	47	53
		0–30 sec	189	30	64
Jones *et al* (1985)	Cycle	0–10 sec	168	42	58
		0–30 sec	291	21	79
Cheetham *et al* (1986)	Run	0–30 sec	183	38	62
Nevill *et al* (1989)	Run	0–30 sec	186	33	67

When using the muscle biopsy technique for the determination of phosphagen stores (i.e. ATP + PCr) following high-intensity exercise, speed of sampling and freezing the muscle tissue is necessary since some resynthesis is possible.

Table 8.1 provides data from selected studies in which the muscle biopsy technique has been used for the estimation of anaerobic energy production from PCr and glycolysis before and immediately after maximal intensity exercise of varying time periods. The findings are based on calculations of the decrease in muscle ATP and PCr, and the increase in muscle lactate from samples taken at rest and immediately after exercise. The highest rates of anaerobic energy production for PCr and for glycolysis during dynamic exercise lasting up to 10 seconds are 9.3 and 5.1 mM/kg/s respectively. When the dynamic exercise is increased to 30 seconds, the highest rates from PCr and glycolysis are 5.9 and 1.9 mM/kg/s respectively. These values are mean rates over the 10- or 30-second bouts, and the actual peak rates would be expected to occur within the first second or so. Indeed, the change in power output during the 30-second Wingate test reflects the maximal rates of ATP being used within the muscle from these anaerobic sources as well as any aerobic contribution.

There are problems with the estimations calculated from the biopsy data. First, there is the time delay in getting the muscle sample frozen following exercise. This procedure involves stopping the exercise, immobilizing the limb, taking the biopsy and then transferring and freezing the sample in liquid nitrogen – a series of events that can take between 10 and 20 seconds. Nevertheless, Soderlund & Hultman (1986) have shown that ATP and PCr concentrations from muscle biopsy samples are not significantly affected by a delay in freezing.

A second problem is the difficulty in determining the muscle mass involved in the exercise bout, which means the metabolic response of the biopsied muscle may not be representative of all those muscles engaged in the exercise. Finally, the amount of energy related to the release of lactate into the blood from the muscle is not taken into account in the calculations presented in Table 8.1, so the anaerobic energy production from glycolysis is underestimated. This is because it is difficult to determine the volume in which lactate is diluted i.e. should merely blood volume be used or should total body fluids be involved in the calculation? Bangsbo (1997) suggested that the likely underestimation for a 75 kg individual is between 5.2 and 25.6% for maximal exercise of 30 seconds. The lower value is based on a dilution volume of 6 litres (i.e. blood volume), whereas the higher discrepancy is based on a dilution volume of 30 litres (i.e. total body fluids). Having said that, even these calculations do not take account of the lactate metabolized by inactive or other nearby type I fibres muscles. You should remember that lactate produced in a working muscle can be oxidized by other nearby muscle fibres without getting into the blood (especially nearby type I fibres).

In spite of these limitations, there is a consistency in the data on the rates of anaerobic ATP production during maximal-intensity exercise from the various studies. Indeed, the data from a study employing 20 electrically evoked maximal isometric actions of the anterior tibialis muscle using both MRS and muscle biopsy demonstrated that there was little difference in the muscle concentrations of PCr, although differences were observed in the estimates of ATP and changes in lactate (Constantin-Teodosiu *et al.*, 1997). The significantly higher muscle lactate concentrations estimated using MRS accounted for ≈30% greater estimation of ATP turnover.

All the studies reported above have documented the metabolic response of mixed muscle to maximal intensity exercise without recourse to possible variations in fibre type responses. Conclusions from investigations using single fibres which have measured ATP, PCr and glycogen of one fibre type

at rest, during muscle action and in recovery have demonstrated greater rates of PCr degradation and glycolysis in type IIx compared with type I fibres (Soderlund *et al.*, 1992; Greenhaff *et al.*, 1994; Casey *et al.*, 1996).

Does aerobic energy production play any part in high intensity exercise? Indirect estimates of the anaerobic and aerobic contribution to intense isolated knee extension exercise of 30 seconds are 80% and 20% respectively (Bangsbo *et al.*, 1990). These values change to 45:55% and 30:70% anaerobic:aerobic as the exercise duration increases from 60 to 90 sec and 120 to 180 sec. During the first 10 seconds of a 30-second Wingate test, the estimated contribution from aerobic metabolism is 3% (Serresse *et al.*, 1988), whereas the mean values of the aerobic contribution for the 30 s Wingate test have been reported as being between 16% and 28% (Serresse *et al.*, 1988; Smith & Hill, 1991). Even if the participant does not breathe, myoglobin and haemoglobin stores can provide oxygen for aerobic energy.

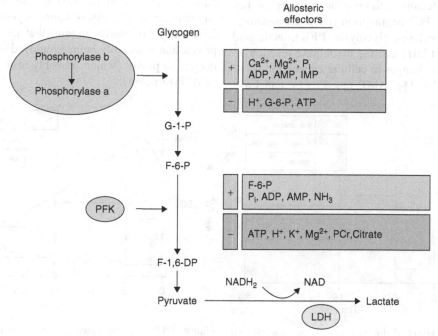

Figure 8.8   Allosteric effectors and enzyme activation during HIE. Note the green blocks contain +ve effectors whereas the red blocks contain the −**ve** or inhibitory allosteric effectors (adapted from Bangsbo, 1996)

8.1.4 Metabolic regulation during high-intensity exercise

Since generation of energy for HIE is required immediately and quickly, the intervention of hormones to trigger activation of key regulatory enzymes is unlikely. You have to remember that hormones have to be secreted into blood, then transmitted to the muscle, then have to attach to a receptor molecule, then activate signalling molecules before appropriate enzymes are activated. Such a series of events would be comparatively slow when the evidence suggested above is that the production of energy (even via the formation of lactic acid from anaerobic glycolysis) is observed within one second. Therefore, we can rule out hormonal regulation of regulatory enzyme activity during HIE. So what *does* regulate enzyme activation?

The answer surely must be **allosteric regulation**. In this regard, changes in intracellular concentrations of **ATP**, **ADP**, **AMP**, and **Ca^{2+}**, which happen in an instant, are more likely controlling agents. Figure 8.8 summarizes how allosteric effectors influence the activity of key enzymes for PCr degradation (CK), glycogenolysis (phosphorylase), glycolysis (**PFK**), lactic acid production (**LDH**) and the myokinase reaction.

Immediate changes in cellular concentrations of ATP ($\downarrow$), ADP ($\uparrow$), AMP ($\uparrow$), P$_i$ ($\uparrow$), and Ca^{2+} ($\uparrow$) are likely as soon as muscles are engaged in contraction and, as we have seen previously, these are all allosteric effectors. Therefore, there is no need for hormonal control at the onset of HIE.

8.2 Effects of exercise duration

Parolin *et al.* (1999) measured energy sources during HIE of 6, 15 and 30 seconds' duration and calculated the ATP turnover rate as well as the contribution from hydrolysis of PCr, from glycolysis and from aerobic oxidation (Figure 8.9). Note that as the exercise duration increases, the contribution of energy from PCr and glycogenolysis declines but oxidative processes increase. The resultant effect is that there is an observed decrease in the rate of ATP turnover.

Examination of the power profile for a Wingate test shows a peak being achieved within the first few seconds (normally the first 5 seconds), which is followed by a steady decline in power over the subsequent 30 seconds (Figure 8.10). This profile may be explained by the switch from predominant use of PCr in the first 0–5 seconds before an increase in glycolysis happens over the next 25 seconds, but bearing in mind that aerobic energy production is steadily being employed – hence the decline in power (which probably mirrors the rate of ATP turnover).

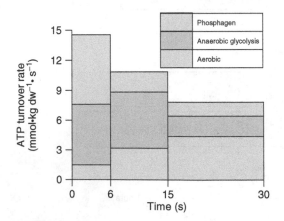

Figure 8.9 Effect of duration of maximal exercise on substrate use and rate of ATP turnover (adapted from Parolin *et al.*, 1999)

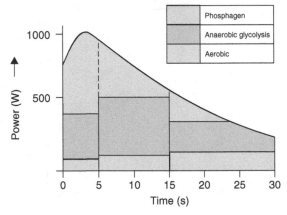

Figure 8.10 Typical power profile from a 30-second Wingate test and the likely contribution from PCr, glycolysis, and aerobic processes

Table 8.2 Effects of carbohydrate status on HIE performance

| Endurance time (min) | | | | | |
Normal	Low-CHO	High-CHO	n	PE	Reference
4.87 ± 1.07	3.32 ± 0.93	6.65 ± 1.39	6	Yes	Maughan & Poole (1981)
5.13 ± 2.00	3.68 ± 0.97	5.75 ± 3.12	11	Yes	Greenhaff et al. (1987a)
3.95 ± 0.48	3.33 ± 0.38	3.80 ± 0.27	7	No	Greenhaff et al. (1987b)
3.50 ± 1.08	2.98 ± 1.05	3.65 ± 1.15	6	No	Greenhaff et al. (1988a)

8.3 Effects of nutritional status

The nutritional status of participants plays a significant role in the ability to perform prolonged exercise as a result of affecting metabolic factors (see Chapters 9 and 10). A high-intensity exercise bout uses carbohydrate at a very high rate, but the total use is limited due to the brief duration of exercise. Reduction of muscle glycogen during a single 30-second sprint is likely to be in the range of 25–35% of the total glycogen store in the active muscles.

Muscle glycogen is depleted more rapidly from type IIx than from type I fibres during high-intensity exercise. Thus, even when glycogen depletion in mixed muscle fibres is modest, extensive glycogen use by type IIx fibres may precipitate fatigue. Performance of a single sprint or of repeated sprints is usually superior after a high-carbohydrate compared to a low-carbohydrate diet, whereas the benefit of a high-carbohydrate vs. moderate-carbohydrate diet for performance of HIE has not been clearly demonstrated.

Maughan & Poole (1981) observed that participants who consumed a high carbohydrate diet had a greater time to fatigue at 100% VO_{2max} compared to a normal and a low carbohydrate diet (High CHO: 6.65 min; low CHO: 3.32 min; normal CHO: 4.87 min). This significant finding was later supported by Greenhaff et al. (1987a) although, in two subsequent studies, Greenhaff et al. (1987b; 1988) found that, although a high CHO diet provided the longer times to fatigue, the results were not statistically significant.

Table 8.2 highlights the findings from these studies. What is of interest is that whereas a high CHO status may not necessarily provide an advantage for HIE, in all likelihood a low CHO status may prove detrimental to performance. The benefit of consuming a moderate-CHO diet versus that of a low-CHO diet several days before high-intensity sprint exercise was supported by Langfort et al. (1997), in which three days of carbohydrate intake (50%; approximately 4.5 g/kg body mass per day) compared with a low CHO intake (5%; less than 1 g/kg body mass per day) resulted in an 8% higher peak power in a 30-second Wingate test. One has to say, however, that it is unlikely that any person would wish to take a carbohydrate intake as low as 5% of total daily energy consumed.

Most studies do not observe a benefit of a high CHO versus a moderate-CHO diet on high-intensity sprint performance. For example, Vandenberghe et al. (1995) found no difference in cycling time to exhaustion at 125% VO_{2max} between participants on a 50% CHO diet and a 70% CHO diet. Likewise, Hargreaves et al. (1997) found no difference in mean or peak power for cyclists exercising supra-maximally for 75 seconds after a high CHO (80% CHO) versus a low CHO (25% CHO) diet. For further studies you may wish to read a review by Maughan et al. (1997).

In some of the studies reported above, the authors focused on the fact that a high CHO diet engendered a more alkaline status in the blood (i.e. *metabolic alkalosis*) and that a low CHO (high fat/protein) diet resulted in a more acid status in the blood (i.e. *metabolic acidosis*). Examination of research by Maughan et al. (1997) confirms this likelihood. Since HIE results in elevated lactic acid concentrations, it may be of some concern to start HIE in an acidotic condition. Hence, reasonable amounts of carbohydrate in a diet not only ensure adequate levels of muscle glycogen for HIE performance but also produces a more alkaline environment, which is useful when significant amounts of lactic acid are likely to be produced.

Although the evidence appears promising, Ball *et al.* (1996) found that correction of the acidotic condition does not normalize performance. In that study, consumption of **sodium bicarbonate** (0.3 g/kg body weight) by subjects who had consumed a low carbohydrate diet normalized blood acidosis but failed to improve performance of a cycle sprint at 100% VO_{2max}.

In summary, most, but not all, studies reported a superior performance of a single, high-intensity exercise bout lasting 30 s to 5 min in subjects consuming a high-carbohydrate diet versus a low-carbohydrate diet. However few athletes actually consume a 'low-carbohydrate' diet. There is little evidence for the value of increasing dietary carbohydrate to higher than moderate ($\approx$50% of energy which equates to approximately 6 g/kg BM/day) levels.

8.3.1   Can nutritional ergogenic aids help HIE?

Although it is beyond the scope of this text to provide detail about nutritional ergogenic aids, it may be useful to gain further understanding about energy provision and fatigue (see Section 8.5) by noting what ergogenic aids may be helpful for HIE and how they may work. Examination of the literature highlights that the following ergogenic aids, on balance of evidence, have a positive effect: **creatine**, **alkalinizers** (**sodium bicarbonate** and **sodium citrate**), **caffeine**, and **β-alanine**. Further details about their efficacy can be seen by reading MacLaren (2011) and Chester (2011).

Creatine

As we have already seen, PCr is an important energy source for very intense bouts of exercise and that stores maybe be depleted rapidly. Creatine ingestion (5–20 g/day for 1–5 days respectively) has been shown to boost total creatine concentrations in skeletal muscle and thereby enhance HIE performance – notably repeated bouts rather than single bouts (MacLaren, 2011).

Alkalinizers

Sodium bicarbonate and sodium citrate are alkalinizers, which have been observed to result in metabolic alkalosis, i.e. an increase in HCO_3 levels from 24 mM to 29 mM and thereby an increase in blood pH from 7.4 to 7.8. Since lactic acid production during HIE is inevitable and may be a fatiguing factor, ingestion of 3–5 g/kg body mass 2–3 hours before HIE has resulted in improved capacity and performance, so long as the duration of the exercise is greater than 30 seconds (Castell *et al.*, 2010; MacLaren, 2011) – in other words, during exercise which significantly stresses anaerobic glycolysis.

Caffeine

The release of Ca^{2+} is necessary for intense bouts of activity, and indeed is essential for muscle contraction. One of the purported effects of caffeine ingestion (3–5 mg/kg body mass 30–60 minutes before exercise) is to enhance Ca^{2+} availability for strong muscle contraction. However, it has been suggested that in order to achieve an enhanced Ca^{2+} within muscle would require caffeine to be present in supra-physiological doses. Evidence for the beneficial effects of caffeine on HIE are now substantial (Chester, 2011; Stear *et al.*, 2010). Caffeine also stimulates the CNS and enhances brain activity.

β-alanine

Skeletal muscle has intracellular buffers which attempt to buffer the acidity caused by decreases in pH resulting from lactic acid and other acids during HIE. One such (major) buffer is **carnosine**. Recent evidence has shown that ingesting 4 g/day of **β-alanine** over a period of four weeks or more increases the muscle carnosine content. In some instances it leads to an improvement in HIE performance (Castell *et al.*, 2010; MacLaren, 2011).

8.4 Effects of training

Sprint training normally results in an increase in the ability to perform maximal intensity exercise. Figure 8.11 highlights changes observed in a 30-second Wingate test before and after an 8-week sprint training programme. Both peak and mean power are significantly improved.

Are these performance changes reflected in an enhanced capacity for generation of energy from anaerobic processes? Boobis *et al* (1983) trained subjects for eight weeks by means of sprinting on a cycle ergometer and analyzed muscle samples at rest before and after the training. Power output was increased by 8%, and the change was mirrored by an increase in anaerobic energy production from glycolysis, although energy produced from the phosphagens was not significantly affected. Similar results were obtained in a study in which recreational athletes were sprint trained for eight weeks; a 6% increase in mean power was observed as well as a 20% increase in anaerobic energy production from glycolysis, but not from phosphagens (Nevill *et al*, 1989).

An important factor in examining data from studies on the effects of HIE training concerns

whether trained or untrained participants are employed. A recent, excellent review by Iaia & Bangsbo (2011) provides some comprehensive findings from a plethora of investigations in this field, and it is worth reading.

Although HIE training results in an enhanced performance, the exact regulatory mechanisms are controversial. Indeed, HIE training enhances the capacity for glycolysis but not for PCr hydrolysis (at least in relatively trained participants). But a question remains as to what extent can muscle fibres be changed – i.e. can type I (slow twitch) fibres be converted to type IIx (fast twitch) fibres in humans? Although the data are equivocal, the proportion of type I fibres has been shown to decrease and the relative number of type IIx has been demonstrated to increase or remain unaltered with high intensity training. For example, a recent study observed a significant increase in FT_x fibres when high-intensity training was accompanied by a severe reduction in training volume (Iaia *et al.*, 2009).

There are equivocal findings in relation to resting levels of ATP following HIE-trained subjects. The difference may be related to the type of HIE training protocol used (i.e. relatively long or short sprint bouts) as well as the length of the recovery period (Iaia & Bangsbo, 2011). On the other hand, sprint training of untrained participants has been shown to decrease the resting levels of skeletal muscle ATP, notably if the training is frequent and very intense. The apparent reduction in resting ATP levels does not appear to have a major negative impact on work capacity, as all training studies have shown increases in exercise performance. The muscle concentration of PCr does not appear to be affected by HIE training.

Whether HIE training increases muscle glycogen concentration is equivocal. It appears that untrained individuals, in general, increase resting muscle glycogen, whereas this may not be the case for more trained individuals. It is not easy to examine the effects of training on muscle glycogen in athletes, as the control level may be influenced by the frequent training sessions. Nevertheless, it is doubtful whether a change in muscle glycogen plays a role in the improvement

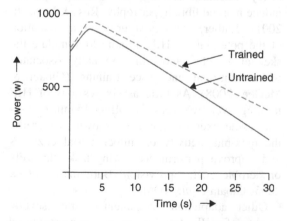

Figure 8.11 Changes in the power profile of a 30-second Wingate test after eight weeks of sprint training (adapted from Nevill *et al.*, 1989)

in performance during a single HIE bout, as muscle glycogen does not appear to be a limiting factor in short-term intense exercise (Bangsbo *et al.*, 1992).

The effect of HIE training on the activity of enzymes related to the anaerobic metabolism of trained individuals is not clear. Roberts *et al.* (1982) found that the maximal activity of glycolytic enzymes and CK was increased by high intensity training. However, the participants in this study were regularly active but not well trained, and studies employing trained subjects have not shown changes (Iaia *et al.*, 2008; Bangsbo *et al.*, 2009).

It is traditionally believed that in order to enhance the activity of metabolic enzymes, it is fundamental to use an exercise mode that produces high flux through the relevant pathways in the contracting muscles. The CK activity was reported to be higher when a group of untrained subjects performed a sprint-training program consisting of 6-second maximal runs separated by 1 minute of recovery, whereas it remained unchanged for another group performing 30-second runs at a speed eliciting $\approx 130\%$ VO_2 max. This suggests that a high rate of PCr breakdown is an important stimulus for CK adaptation (Mohr *et al.*, 2007).

In agreement, a number of studies on untrained people have shown improvements in anaerobic enzymes activity after periods of training including very short maximal or near maximal exercise bouts (5–30 seconds) interspersed with relatively long resting periods (Parra *et al.*, 2000; Rodas *et al.*, 2000).

On the other hand, studies using training protocols of 30 seconds sprints with 3–4 minutes of rest found the activity of CK and PFK remained unaltered in trained participants (Iaia *et al.*, 2008; Bangsbo *et al.*, 2009). Thus, the higher fitness level, together with longer exercise periods (i.e. 30 seconds), may explain why no changes were seen. Nevertheless, pronounced changes in performance were observed, despite unaltered levels of enzymes related to anaerobic energy production, suggesting that the changes in the activity of these enzymes are not crucial for work capacity

improvements during exercise lasting 30 seconds to 2 minutes.

The activity of oxidative enzymes in trained subjects does not appear to be elevated with HIE training, which is in contrast to a number of studies of untrained subjects (Burgomaster *et al.*, 2005; 2008; Gibala *et al.*, 2006; Parra *et al.*, 2000; Rodas *et al.*, 2000). This difference may be related to the lower level of enzyme activity in untrained, as compared with already trained, individuals, and to the fact that untrained subjects respond to almost all types of training stimuli by increasing a large number of muscle proteins.

It is interesting to note, however, that in a study with a 65% reduction in training volume, the levels of citrate synthase (**CS**) and 3-hydroxyacyl-CoA dehydrogenase (**HAD**) were maintained with regular HIE training, indicating that this type of training in trained humans stimulates the mitochondrial oxidative proteins (Iaia *et al.*, 2009). Shepley *et al.* (1992), investigating highly trained runners during a week of reduced training combined with speed endurance training, found an 18% increase in the CS level in association with improved performance. Thus, it appears that HIE training is a powerful stimulus to induce mitochondrial protein synthesis. Whether it leads to net synthesis depends on the training status as well as on the frequency and amount of training.

Although sometimes equated with strength or heavy resistance training, HIE training does not induce marked fibre hypertrophy (Ross & Leveritt, 2001). Rather, there is a growing appreciation of the potential for HIE training to stimulate the skeletal muscle remodelling normally associated with traditional endurance training (Gibala & McGee, 2008). As little as six sessions of HIE training over two weeks, totalling 15 min of 'all-out' cycle exercise, has been shown to increase the maximal activity of mitochondrial enzymes and improve performance during tasks that rely on aerobic energy provision (Burgomaster *et al.* 2005; Gibala *et al.* 2006).

Other adaptations documented after several weeks of HIE training include an increased muscle content of proteins associated with the transport and oxidation of glucose and fatty acids and reduced non-oxidative energy provision during matched-work exercise (Burgomaster *et al.* 2008). For a more comprehensive review of the molecular adaptations to HIE training, you should consult Gibala (2009).

Among the wide range of potential candidates involved in the fatigue processes, **sarcolemmal depolarization** due to **extracellular K^+** accumulation has been suggested to be of primary importance for development of fatigue during HIE (Sejersted & Sjogaard, 2000). This hypothesis is based on observations that during dynamic exercise the contracting muscles lose K^+, which progressively accumulates in the extracellular space, leading to a depolarization of the membrane potential. A lower membrane potential has been shown to cause reduced membrane excitability and tetanic force (Sejersted & Sjogaard, 2000).

The evidence of K^+ being of importance for fatigue development in humans is related to the findings that muscle interstitial K^+ during intense exercise is elevated to levels from $4\,mM$ to $10\,mM$ (Nielsen *et al.*, 2004), and that training leads to reduced interstitial K^+ accumulation (Nielsen *et al.*, 2004) in association with improved exercise performance and a change in the amount of Na^+/K^+ **pumps** (Clausen, 2003). HIE training of trained subjects elevates the expression of the Na^+/K^+ pump subunits (Iaia & Bangsbo, 2011). The changes reported in the subunits were 29% and 68%.

These adaptations occurred despite the fact that the trained subjects may already have had an elevated protein content before the training, as endurance training has been demonstrated to increase the Na^+/K^+ pump subunits. The augmented Na^+/K^+ pump subunits may result in a high number of functional pumps and play an important role for the increases in work capacity during HIE performance. Indeed, a higher Na^+/K^+ pump maximum activity reduces the net loss of K^+ from the contracting muscles, preserving the cell excitability and force production (Sejersted & Sjogaard, 2000).

In trained people, isoforms of the muscle monocarboxylate transporters (**MCT**) have been shown to be unchanged with HIE training (Iaia

et al., 2008), whereas data from untrained subjects demonstrates an increase of MCT1 (Mohr *et al.*, 2007). Apparently, improved short-term performance can occur without changes in MCT and buffering capacity (Iaia & Bangsbo, 2011). Messonnier *et al.* (2007) observed that trained participants, with elevated levels of HIE performance compared with untrained individuals, were less dependent on the muscle content of proteins involved in buffering, as well as for lactate/H^+ transport. As such, it appears reasonable to assume that for trained individuals, mechanisms other than changes of pH regulatory systems may predominate in delaying fatigue and enhancing work capacity during HIE.

8.5   Mechanisms of fatigue

Muscle fatigue may be defined as an exercise-induced reduction in the ability of muscle to produce force or power, whether or not the task can be sustained (Bigland-Ritchie & Woods, 1984). This may be demonstrated by examining the power output profile of an individual undergoing a 30-second Wingate test. The profile shows a peak in the first few seconds, followed by a steady decline over the subsequent 25 seconds or so. Why is the muscle unable to support energy production at a sufficient rate to maintain a continuous peak power? Indeed, why can an individual not sprint supra-maximally for two minutes or longer? There are a number of reasons for this, and although this section will briefly describe some of the factors, for a more detailed exploration of muscle fatigue you should read Allen *et al.* (2008) or Enoka & Duchateau (2008).

Examination of Figure 8.12 shows various sites which may contribute to fatigue in skeletal muscle. These include the action potential along the sarcolemma and the T-tubule, the release of Ca^{2+} and the re-uptake of Ca^{2+} from the endoplasmic reticulum, contractile events at the crossbridge and enzyme activation. This section will not explore changes associated with muscle glycogen or hydration, but will briefly report on factors such as reduced levels of ATP and PCr,

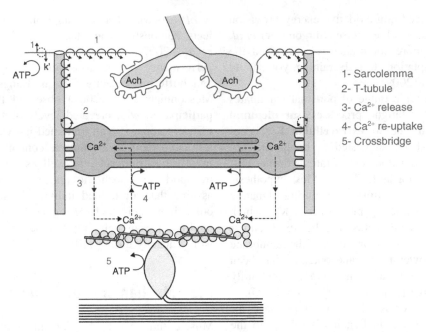

Figure 8.12   Possible sites of fatigue during HIE (adapted from Green, 1990)

increased cellular concentrations of P_i and ADP, reduced pH and changes in K^+ and Na^+.

8.5.1   Reduced ATP

Many studies have reported that cytoplasmic ATP concentration does not drop below $\approx$60% of the resting level during either electrical stimulation or dynamic exercise during HIE at the point of fatigue. ATP may decline from 24 to 12 mM, while ADP may increase from 10 to 200 μM, yet maximum force production in skinned fibres is not reduced unless the concentration of ATP is $\approx$20 μM (lower than normally found in intake fibres), and the rate of relaxation is reduced 2.5-fold when lowered to 0.5 mM. This is not due to an effect on the contractile apparatus, but instead is due to reduced Ca^{2+} uptake by the SR. ATP also has a regulatory action on the pump at the SR such that if ATP decreases from 5 to 0.25 mM, the Ca^{2+} affinity of the pump is reduced $\approx$10-fold.

Having said that, it is possible that there may be ATP reduction in certain localized areas of

a muscle. One possible site of localized ATP depletion is the space between the T-tubule and the SR. ATP consumption in this region is substantial, due to the presence of calcium pumps on the SR terminal cisternae just outside the junction and Na^+/K^+ pumps and other ATPases in the T-system membrane. Approximately 50% of all Na^+/K^+ pumps are in the T system.

Glycolytic enzymes associated with this so-called triad junction support localized synthesis of ATP. The glycolytic enzymes are well placed to utilize glucose entering the fibre via the T system, as well as the glucose-6-phosphate from adjacent glycogen stores. Na^+/K^+ pumps in muscle fibres preferentially use ATP derived from glycolysis. In view of the high density of ATP-consuming and -generating processes in the vicinity of the triad junction, as well as the comparatively small percentage of the cell volume it encompasses, ATP in the triad junction quite likely differs considerably from that in the cytoplasm as a whole. This could therefore allow the triad region to play a major role in sensing and responding to changes in cellular energy status, particularly

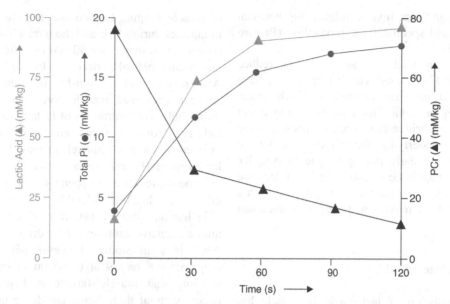

Figure 8.13 Depletion of muscle PCr and increases in lactate and P_i during intense exercise (adapted from Hultman *et al.*, 1990)

given that the triad junction is the key transduction zone regulating Ca^{2+} release and contraction.

Therefore, in HIE, the triad junction may play a key role by sensing depletion of cellular ATP levels and respond by reducing Ca^{2+} release. This will decrease the rate of ATP use by reducing both crossbridge cycling and SR Ca^{2+} uptake, the two main sources of ATP hydrolysis. The cost of this is a reduction in power output, or muscle fatigue, but the benefit is that it ultimately prevents complete exhaustion of all cellular ATP and consequent rigor development and cellular damage.

8.5.2 Reduced PCr

We have already noted that PCr levels decrease significantly in response to HIE. Indeed, muscle PCr concentrations have been reported to decrease from 80 to 15 mM in a single strenuous bout of HIE. Figure 8.13 shows changes in PCr due to a series of maximal muscle contractions over a period of 102 seconds, and it reflects almost total depletion (Hultman *et al.*, 1990).

However, other evidence is available that has observed a dissociation between the rate of

recovery of PCr and the force-generating capacity of the muscle (McCartney *et al.*, 1986). In other words, PCr recovery is faster than the recovery of muscle force. Furthermore, as ATP levels can remain high at the point of fatigue, it does not appear that PCr limits performance by limiting ATP resynthesis.

8.5.3 Increased P_i

The exchange of phosphate between ATP and PCr is catalysed by CK. During periods of high energy demand, the ATP concentration initially remains almost constant, while PCr breaks down to Cr and P_i. While Cr has little effect on contractile function, P_i may cause a decrease of myofibrillar force production and Ca^{2+} sensitivity, as well as SR Ca^{2+} release (Allen *et al.*, 2008). Accordingly, increased P_i is considered to be a major cause of fatigue.

A causative role of increased P_i has also been implied in other situations with impaired muscle function. For instance, in a study where participants were followed during rehabilitation after immobilization in a cast, there was an observed significant inverse relationship between resting P_i and specific force production (Pathare *et al.*, 2005).

A fatigue-induced increase in P_i can reduce myofibrillar Ca^{2+} sensitivity, which may a have large impact on force production. Furthermore, increased P_i can inhibit force production by direct action on crossbridge function, and this is a likely mechanism underlying the decrease in tetanic force occurring early during fatigue in type IIx fibres. The magnitude of this P_i-induced decrease in crossbridge force production is probably rather small ($\approx$10% of maximum force) in mammalian muscle.

8.5.4 Lactate and H^+

The accumulation of lactic acid in muscle has historically been suggested to be the major cause of muscle fatigue. Lactate and H^+ are produced in muscles during HIE and the intracellular lactate concentration may reach 30 mM or more while the intracellular pH (pH_i) decreases by $\approx$0.5 pH units. A close temporal relationship is often observed between decreased muscle force and increased intracellular concentrations of lactate, and particularly H^+. However, such correlations break down in many cases, and although increased intracellular levels of H^+ may reduce muscle performance to some degree, it now appears that its deleterious effects have been considerably overestimated.

In humans, muscle pH_i at rest is $\approx$7.05, and after exhaustive exercise it may drop to as low as $\approx$6.5. In some studies, however, pH_i decreases only to $\approx$6.8 or 6.9 at the point of exhaustion, showing that muscle fatigue in humans often occurs without there being any large increase in concentration of $H^+{}_i$. Importantly, in cases where

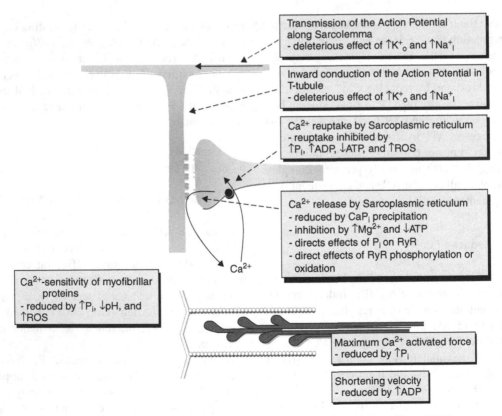

Figure 8.14   Possible fatigue sites and likely causes (adapted from Allen, 2008)

pH_i does drop to low levels in a fatigued muscle, then upon ceasing the exercise or stimulation, force typically recovers much faster than pH_i (Allen *et al.*, 2008).

Another way in which low pH previously was thought to reduce force responses was by inhibiting Ca^{2+} release from the SR. Low pH does reduce direct activation of the Ca^{2+} release channel to stimulation by Ca^{2+} and caffeine. However, activation of Ca^{2+} release, the normal physiological mechanism, is not noticeably inhibited even at pH 6.2. Therefore, when pH_i is lowered in intact fibres, maximum tetanic force is reduced by no more than the amount expected.

In summary, under physiological circumstances, low pH has a far less inhibitory effect on the activation of the contractile apparatus and Ca^{2+} release than previously assumed, and its effects on the SR Ca^{2+} pump actually favour force development. Therefore, raised H^+_i is not *per se* the main cause of muscle fatigue, with its direct effects on force production being quite small.

Having said that, could a reduction in pH_i cause decreased activation of key enzymes associated with energy production, i.e. phosphorylase, PFK, CK and even ATPases? This premise is based on the fact that all enzymes have an optimum pH for maximum activity, and invariably in cells this optimum pH is ≈ 7.0. Since skeletal muscle pH can decrease to values as low as 6.4, there is some suggestion that this lowering of pH by ≈ 0.5 units is sufficient to inhibit the above key enzymes and thereby reduce ATP production (MacLaren *et al.*, 1989). Although this is an interesting point, the findings are not conclusive and so, although this remains a consideration, muscle fatigue during HIE could be (in part) due to enzyme activity affected by pH.

In conclusion, in intense exercise, the triad junction may play a key role by sensing depletion of cellular ATP levels and respond by reducing Ca^{2+} release. This will decrease the rate of ATP usage by reducing both crossbridge cycling and SR Ca^{2+} uptake, the two main sources of ATP hydrolysis. The cost of this is a reduction in power output, or in other words muscle fatigue, but the benefit is that it ultimately prevents complete exhaustion of all cellular ATP and consequent rigor development and cellular damage. Figure 8.14 summarizes these points.

8.6 Key points

- High intensity exercise typically refers to non-steady state exercise performed for durations between >1 second to 1–4 minutes.
- O_2 deficit and MAOD result from an imbalance between O_2 delivery and O_2 requirement. In the case of MAOD, the O_2 delivery is never able to compensate for the amount needed. Anaerobic energy provision occurs during these phases.
- Phosphagens (ATP and PCr), as well as anaerobic glycolysis and the myokinase reaction, provide the energy for HIE.
- Evidence is available from studies on electrical stimulation, isometric and dynamic exercise (normally using biopsy samples pre- and post-event) to highlight the levels of depletion of ATP, PCr and glycogen, as well as the increase in lactic acid.
- The relative contribution of anaerobic and aerobic processes during HIE is available and, in general, the contribution of the latter increases with duration of HIE.
- Dietary intervention in relation to ingesting high amounts of CHO do not result in improved HIE performance when compared with an adequate intake, although a really low intake of CHO over a number of days may lead to impaired performance.
- Ingesting a diet high in CHO increases the likelihood of ensuring an alkalotic environment in the body, whereas a high fat/protein diet is more likely to promote an acidotic scenario.
- Nutritional ergogenic aids such as creatine, caffeine, alkalinizers and β-alanine are, if used correctly, likely to enhance HIE performance.
- HIE training improves HIE performance.
- HIE training of untrained individuals is likely to result in increased levels of resting muscle glycogen, no change in phosphagens, and increased levels of phosphorylase, PFK, LDH,

and CK, whereas there are less likely/marked changes when using trained individuals.

- Maybe surprisingly, HIE results in enhanced levels of aerobic enzymes such as CS and HAD. This may not be found for trained participants.

- HIE training of trained subjects elevates the expression of the Na^+/K^+ pump subunits, which results in a high number of functional pumps and plays an important role for the increases in work capacity during HIE performance.

- Fatigue during HIE could be due to accumulation of extracellular K^+, localized ATP depletion, reduced Ca^{2+} release and uptake from and into the SR and acidity-induced inactivation of key enzymes.

9

Endurance exercise

Learning outcomes

After studying this chapter, you should be able to:

- outline the main sites of control which potentially underpin the regulation of metabolism during endurance exercise;
- critically evaluate the effects of exercise intensity on metabolic regulation of substrate utilization during endurance exercise;
- critically evaluate the effects of exercise duration on metabolic regulation of substrate utilization during endurance exercise;
- critically evaluate the effects of muscle glycogen availability on metabolic regulation of substrate utilization during endurance exercise;
- critically evaluate the effects of fat loading on metabolic regulation of substrate utilization during endurance exercise;
- critically evaluate the effects of pre-exercise CHO feeding on metabolic regulation of substrate utilization during endurance exercise;
- critically evaluate the effects of acutely elevating pre-exercise plasma FFA availability on metabolic regulation of substrate utilization during endurance exercise;
- critically evaluate the effects of training status on metabolic regulation of substrate utilization during endurance exercise;

- critically discuss potential metabolic causes of fatigue during endurance exercise.

Key words

acetyl-CoA carboxylase	fat adaptation
adipose tissue	GLUT4
adipose triglyceride lipase (ATGL)	glycogen
ADP	glycogen phosphorylase
alanine	H$^+$
allosteric regulation	heparin
AMP	high glycemic
BCKAD	HSL
BCKAD kinase	IMP
Ca^{2+}	indirect calorimetry
carnitine	insulin
cAMP	intramuscular triglyceride (IMTG)
caffeine	
catecholamines	knee extensor
covalent modification	lactate
citrate	lactate threshold
CPTI	liver
cycling	low glycemic
deamination	liver glycogenolysis
FAT/CD36	malonyl-CoA
FABPpm	mitochondria
FATP	

Biochemistry for Sport and Exercise Metabolism, First Edition. Don MacLaren and James Morton.
© 2012 John Wiley & Sons, Ltd. Published 2012 by John Wiley & Sons, Ltd.

muscle biopsy	PDH kinase
muscle glycogen	PDH phosphatase
Na^+/K^+ ATPase	phosphodiesterase
pump	PFK
oleate	plasma FFA
octanoate	plasma glucose
running	protein kinase A
P_i	stable isotope tracers
palmitate	steady state
PDH	transamination

9.1 Overview of energy production and metabolic regulation in endurance exercise

9.1.1 Definition and models of endurance exercise

By definition, endurance exercise can typically be defined as prolonged steady-state exercise performed for durations between four minutes and four hours (Whyte, 2006). This could therefore encompass middle distance events (e.g. track cycling, rowing, and swimming) through to marathon running and extended stages of road cycling such as those of the Tour de France (exercise of durations beyond four hours, such as 'Ironman triathlons' are classified as *ultra-endurance*). While there are undoubtedly pacing strategies which athletes utilize in these events, the exercise intensity is usually considered as *steady state* (i.e. constant intensity), as the athlete aims to exercise at the highest power output for as long as they can.

The most common modes of endurance exercise and the most frequently studied within the literature are *cycling* and *running*. Cycling appears to be the predominant mode of exercise utilized in research studies, probably due to the methodological control which it offers the experimenter. For example, the vastus lateralis is heavily recruited during cycling and, as such, this muscle offers an appropriate sampling site to study local adaptations to exercise. This is in contrast to running, where muscles of the lower limb such as the gastrocne-

mius and soleus are more active compared with the vastus lateralis (Morton *et al.*, 2009). Furthermore:

- the exercise intensity during cycling can be easily controlled and energy expenditure (i.e. work done) can be readily quantified by using an ergometer to measure the power output of the subject when pedalling;
- because the subject's arms are in a relatively fixed position (as opposed to running), venous blood samples can be easily obtained during exercise, therefore allowing detailed studies of substrate kinetics to occur *during* exercise;
- many investigators have utilized knee extensor models to study metabolic regulation, which is advantageous as it minimizes the effects of hormonal responses and blood flow limitations, and essentially isolates the metabolic responses to contraction *per se*.

Students of exercise biochemistry should appreciate, however, that the absolute active muscle mass recruited and, indeed, the energy cost, hormonal and metabolic responses to exercise, are different between these exercise modes (Arkinstall *et al.*, 2001). It is therefore important to keep these considerations in mind when interpreting the data from the research studies that are discussed in this chapter.

9.1.2 Energy production in endurance exercise

At this stage of your study of exercise metabolism, you should now fully appreciate that the majority of ATP production during exercise is fuelled by metabolism (and in the case of endurance exercise, the *oxidative* metabolism) of carbohydrates and lipids. Both fuel sources can be provided from extra-muscular sources such as **plasma FFAs** (derived from **adipose tissue lipolysis**) or **plasma glucose** (provided from **liver glycogen** or glucose originating from the gastrointestinal tract). Alternatively, substrates can be provided from intra-muscular sources such as **muscle glycogen** or **intra-muscular triglyceride**

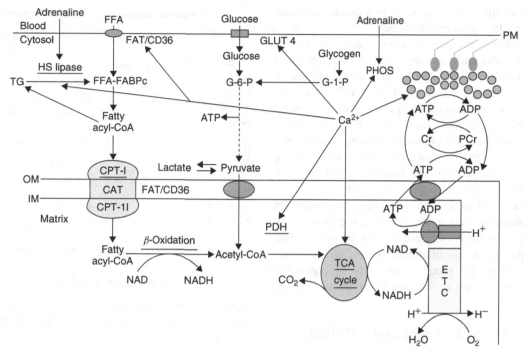

Figure 9.1 Schematic overview of energy producing pathways in skeletal muscle related to CHO and lipid metabolism. PM denotes plasma membrane, OM denotes outer mitochondrial membrane and IM denotes inner mitochondrial membrane (adapted from Spriet, 2007)

(IMTG). A schematic overview of the main sources and pathways involved in the metabolism of CHO and lipids is shown in Figure 9.1.

Protein (i.e. amino acids) can also contribute a small proportion of ATP production during exercise (usually around 5% of ATP production), and the regulation of amino acid metabolism during endurance exercise is discussed separately later in this chapter.

9.1.3 Overview of metabolic regulation in endurance exercise

Examination of Figure 1.1 suggests there are a number of potential sites of control which can regulate the interaction of CHO and lipid metabolism during endurance exercise. These include availability of intra-muscular and extra-muscular substrate (controlled by diet and the action of key hormones such as the **catecholamines** and

insulin), the abundance of transport proteins involved in transporting substrates across both the plasma and mitochondrial membranes and, of course, the activity of the key regulatory enzymes involved in the metabolic pathways.

As discussed in previous chapters, the activity of enzymes can be modified acutely through **covalent modification** (i.e. phosphorylation and dephosphorylation) and/or **allosteric regulation** via important signalling molecules that are produced in the muscle as a result of contraction (e.g. **ADP, AMP, IMP, P_i, Ca^{2+}, H^+**, etc.). Enzyme activity could also be modified through substrate activation or product inhibition, such that increasing the substrate concentration increases catalysis, whereas increased product concentration may inhibit the reaction. Finally, enzyme activity can be regulated in the long term through increasing the muscle cell's content of the actual enzyme protein (i.e.

more of the enzyme is actually present), as would occur with endurance training.

Clearly, our muscle cells possess a highly coordinated and regulatory network of signalling and feedback pathways which function to ensure ATP demand is matched by ATP synthesis. From a physiological perspective, important overriding factors such as *exercise intensity, duration, nutritional status, training status*, etc. can all regulate substrate utilization during exercise, largely through influencing the potential regulatory control points discussed above. This chapter will outline the metabolic regulation of substrate utilization during endurance exercise by discussing each of these factors in turn, where we pay particular attention to what are *currently* considered the predominant sites of regulation that are relevant to the specific situation.

9.2   Effects of exercise intensity

Classical studies, using a range of methodology such as ***indirect calorimetry, stable isotope tracers*** and ***muscle biopsies***, have quantified the varying contribution of CHO and lipids to ATP production across a range of sub-maximal exercise intensities (Romijn *et al.*, 1993; Van Loon *et al.*, 2001). Data from one of these studies is shown in Figure 9.2, where it can be clearly seen that as exercise intensity (and therefore energy expenditure) increases, the contribution of CHO metabolism to ATP production increases while the contribution of lipid sources to ATP production decreases.

Typically, as exercise intensity progress from moderate (i.e. 65% VO_{2max}) to high-intensity (85% VO_{2max}), muscle glycogenolysis and glucose uptake increases, such that CHO metabolism predominates. In contrast, there appears to be reduction in whole body lipid oxidation due to a reduction in both plasma FFA and **intramuscular triglyceride** oxidation. Maximal rates of lipid oxidation are considered to occur around 65% VO_{2max}, though this is dependent on a number of other factors such as training status, gender and diet (Achten & Jeukendrup, 2004). In what follows, we discuss the regulatory mechanisms

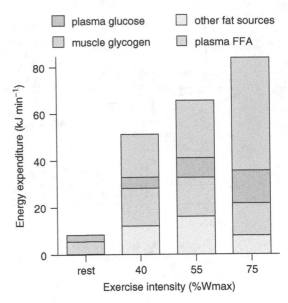

Figure 9.2 Effects of exercise intensity on substrate utilization during exercise (adapted from Van Loon *et al.*, 2001)

underpinning the up-regulation of CHO and down-regulation of lipid oxidation as exercise intensity increases.

9.2.1   CHO metabolism

Muscle glycogenolysis

The breakdown of muscle glycogen to glucose 1-phosphate is under the control of **glycogen phosphorylase**, and this reaction requires both glycogen and P_i as substrates. Phosphorylase, in turn, exists as a more active *a* form (which is under the control of phosphorylation by phosphorylase kinase) and also as a more inactive *b* form (which exists in a dephosphorylated form due to the action of the protein phosphatase 1). Given that phosphorylase can be transformed via covalent modification (i.e. phosphorylation by phosphorylase kinase), it would be reasonable to expect that greater phosphorylase transformation from *b* to *a* may be one mechanism to explain increased glycogenolysis evident with increasing exercise intensity. This would also be logical given that sarcoplasmic Ca^{2+} levels would be

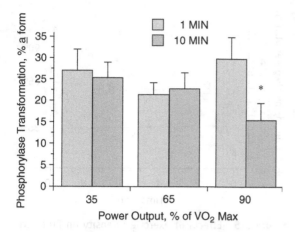

Figure 9.3 Effects of exercise intensity on phosphorylase transformation, expressed as percentage of the enzyme in the a-form (adapted from Howlett *et al.*, 1998)

increased with high-intensity exercise (given the need for more rapid crossbridge cycling), and that Ca^{2+} is a potent positive allosteric regulator of phosphorylase kinase through binding to the calmodulin subunit.

However, the percentage of phosphorylase in the more active *a* form does not appear to be increased with exercise intensity and, in fact, is decreased after only ten minutes of high intensity exercise (see Figure 9.3), which may be related to the reduced pH associated with intense exercise (Howlett *et al.*, 1998). Whereas this mechanism of transformation (mediated by Ca^{2+} signalling) may be in operation within seconds of the onset of contraction (Parolin *et al.*, 1999), it appears that *post-transformational* mechanisms are in operation during more prolonged periods of high-intensity exercise, given that glycogenolysis still occurs despite reduced transformation. In this regard, vital signals related to the energy status of the cell play a more prominent role.

In keeping with this line of thinking, we should remember that as we progress from moderate to high-intensity exercise, the rate of ATP hydrolysis increases so much so that there is greater accumulation of ADP, AMP and P_i (see Figure 9.4). In this way, the increased accumulation of P_i as a result of increased ATP hydrolysis can

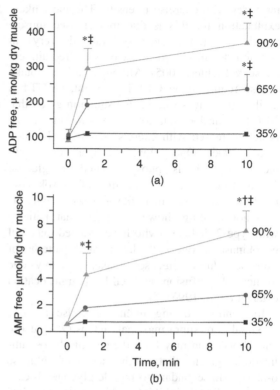

Figure 9.4 Effects of exercise intensity on muscle free AMP and ADP concentration (adapted from Howlett *et al.*, 1998)

increase glycogenolysis as it provides increased substrate required for the reaction. Furthermore, greater accumulations of free ADP and AMP can also subsequently fine-tune the activity of phosphorylase *a* through allosteric regulation (Howlett *et al.*, 1998). Finally, although it is well documented that phosphorylase is under the hormonal control of adrenaline, infusion of adrenaline to levels beyond that of endogenous production during high-intensity exercise does not augment glycogenolysis (Chesley *et al.*, 1995), probably due to already sufficient activation of phosphorylase through the local mechanisms discussed above.

Plasma glucose utilization, muscle glucose uptake and glycolysis

In addition to muscle glycogen, the contribution of plasma glucose to ATP production also increases with exercise intensity. The most likely explanation for this is due to increased muscle blood flow (and hence substrate delivery) in addition to increased muscle fibre recruitment (Rose & Richter, 2005). Although glucose uptake is also regulated by **GLUT4** content, GLUT4 is unlikely to play a role in this situation given that GLUT4 translocation to the plasma membrane is not increased with exercise intensity (Kraniou *et al.*, 2006). Once glucose is transported into the cytosol, it is phosphorylated to glucose 6-phosphate under the control of hexokinase. Evidence suggests that hexokinase activity is also not limiting, however, given that patients with type 2 diabetes (who have reduced maximal hexokinase activity) display normal patterns of exercise-induced glucose uptake, probably due to normal perfusion and GLUT4 translocation (Martin *et al.*, 1995).

In contrast, during intense exercise at near maximal or supra-maximal intensity, glucose phosphorylation may limit the rate of glucose utilization, given that high rates of glucose 6-phosphate secondary to muscle glycogen breakdown can directly inhibit hexokinase activity (Katz *et al.*, 1986). Once glucose enters the glycolytic pathway, the rate limiting enzyme to glycolysis is considered to be **PFK**. PFK is allosterically activated by ADP, AMP and P_i, and this mechanism is likely to explain high rates of glycolysis during intense exercise, even in the face of metabolic acidosis, when PFK could be inhibited.

Carbohydrate oxidation

Glucose 6-phosphate (which has originated either from glycogenolysis or phosphorylation of glucose) is eventually converted to pyruvate through the reactions of glycolysis. Before pyruvate can be oxidized, it must be converted to acetyl-CoA, a reaction which is under the regulation of **PDH**. PDH is, in turn, inactivated through phosphorylation by **PDH kinase** and activated through dephosphorylation by **PDH phosphatase**.

Unlike glycogen phosphorylase, PDH transformation to its more active form is actually increased with exercise intensity (Howlett *et al.*, 1998) and appears to be an accurate reflection of CHO flux

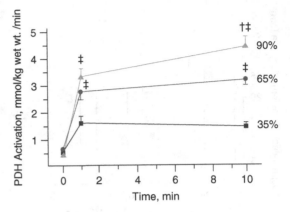

Figure 9.5 Effects of exercise intensity on PDH activation (adapted from Howlett *et al.*, 1998)

into the mitochondria and, hence, CHO oxidation (see Figure 9.5). This increased PDH activation is mediated by an increase in substrate (i.e. pyruvate) as a result of increased glycolytic flux, and also by increased Ca^{2+}, which allosterically activates PDH phosphatase, which in turn dephosphorylates (i.e. activates) PDH. Increased pyruvate and ADP also inactivate PDH kinase, thus rendering PDH less susceptible to phosphorylation (i.e. deactivation). Collectively, as a result of this shift in balance towards activation of PDH phosphatase and deactivation of PDH kinase, PDH transformation is increased with exercise intensity and CHO oxidation is concomitantly increased as well.

9.2.2 Lipid metabolism

It is well documented that the contribution of lipid sources to ATP production is inversely related to exercise intensity and that it declines beyond intensities greater than 65% VO_{2max}. There are a number of potential mechanisms underpinning this intensity-induced shift from lipid to CHO oxidation, and we will now discuss the potential sites involved in regulating these processes.

Adipose tissue lipolysis and FFA availability/delivery

The first stage of failure in lipid oxidation rates with increased exercise intensity is often cited as a reduction in adipose tissue lipolysis. However, there is strong evidence to suggest that it is not a failure in lipolysis *per se*, which is the limitation, but rather an inability to deliver FFA to the exercising muscles primarily as a result of inadequate adipose tissue blood flow.

Indeed, Romijn *et al.* (1993) assessed plasma FFA (remember, FFA is non-soluble and requires albumin for transport) and glycerol (which is water soluble) during exercise at 25, 65 and 85% VO_{2max} (see Figure 9.6). These authors observed that plasma FFA declined during exercise at 85% VO_{2max}, although these data should be not be interpreted as a reduction in lipolysis, given that plasma glycerol increased during exercise.

The use of plasma glycerol per se as an indicator of lipolysis is, of course, not without limitations, as glycerol may also be taken up by other tissues, namely the liver. Nevertheless, stable isotope methodology demonstrated that the *rate of appearance* of glycerol (considered an accurate indication of the rate of lipolysis) was not reduced at 85% VO_{2max}, compared to 65% VO_{2max}. It was therefore suggested that the reduced plasma FFA availability was not to due to reduced lipolysis, but rather a reduction in adipose tissue blood flow (given that more blood is now being directed to the active muscles) and, as such, there was less albumin available to transport FFA. In such cases, FFA may become re-esterified within the adipocyte due to this inadequate perfusion (Frayn, 2010).

Evidence supporting this theory of blood flow limitation is also provided in the recovery period after exercise, where it can be seen that as soon as exercise terminates (and blood flow is thus available for adipose tissue again), plasma FFA suddenly increases, whereas plasma glycerol (and, indeed, rate of appearance) actually declines, therefore indicating reduced lipolysis post-exercise (see Figure 9.6).

In a subsequent study, Romijn *et al.* (1995) tested the hypothesis that reduced plasma FFA availability is limiting to lipid oxidation rates during high-intensity exercise by intravenous infusion of lipid and **heparin** during exercise at 85% VO_{2max}. In this way, plasma FFA was artificially maintained above $1 \, mmol.L^{-1}$, which

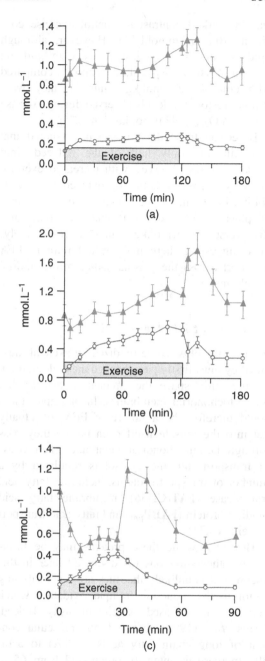

Figure 9.6 Plasma glycerol (red symbols) and FFA (green symbols) during and in recovery from exercise at (a) 25, (b) 65 and (c) 85% VO_{2max} (adapted from Romijn *et al.*, 1993)

was in marked contrast to control exercise conditions $(0.2–0.3\,\text{mmol.L}^{-1})$. However, although lipid oxidation rates were increased with lipid and heparin infusion $(34\,\mu\text{mol.kg}^{-1}.\,\text{min}^{-1})$ compared with control $(26\,\mu\text{mol.kg}^{-1}.\,\text{min}^{-1})$, they were still not restored to levels observed during exercise at 65% $\text{VO}_{2\text{max}}$ $(43\,\mu\text{mol.kg}^{-1}.\,\text{min}^{-1})$.

Based on these data, it can be assumed that approximately only half of the reduced lipid oxidation rates observed with increased exercise intensity can be explained by reduced FFA availability. Furthermore, the actual rate of appearance of plasma FFA exceeded lipid oxidation rates (61 versus $34\,\mu\text{mol.kg}^{-1}.\,\text{min}^{-1}$, respectively) thus suggesting there may be a failure in FFA transport across the plasma and/or mitochondrial membranes.

FFA transport into the cytosol

In order for FFAs to be oxidized by skeletal muscle, they must firstly pass through the endothelium, the interstitial space, the sarcolemma and, finally, the mitochondrial membranes. In principle, there could therefore be a failure of FFA to actually get into the muscle itself even before they pass through the mitochondrial membrane. The process of transport into the cytosol is regulated by a number of transport proteins, including fatty acid translocase (**FAT/CD36**), membrane fatty acid binding protein (**FABP$_{pm}$**) and fatty acid transport protein (**FATP**).

However, while these proteins may be limiting in other situations (as discussed later in this chapter), it is unlikely that they are a contributing factor to the reduction in lipid oxidation which occurs with increased exercise intensity. Indeed, Kiens *et al.* (1999) observed intra-muscular content of long chain fatty acids (LCFA) to actually increase as intensity progressed from 65 to 90% $\text{VO}_{2\text{max}}$, despite reductions in lipid oxidation rates. Such data therefore point to a failure of the mitochondria to increase lipid utilization, either through a failure in transport across mitochondrial membranes and/or metabolic oxidation.

FFA transport across mitochondrial membranes

In recapping what we discussed in Chapter 6, you should remember that, once in the cytosol, fatty acids combine with CoA to form fatty acyl-CoA through the action of acyl-CoA synthase. The *activated* fatty acid can now pass through the outer mitochondrial membrane by combining with **carnitine** to form acylcarnitine in a reaction catalysed by **CPTI**. Acylcarnitine is, in turn, transported through the inner mitochondrial membrane via the acylcarnitine/carnitine translocase system. Once on the matrix side, the fatty acyl group is transferred back to CoA, thus reforming fatty acyl-CoA in a reaction catalysed by CPTII. In this way, the free carnitine that has been cleaved from acylcarnitine can be transported back to the outer mitochondrial membrane to participate in the initial reaction involving CPTI.

Of the various components in this transport shuttle system, CPTI activity is thought to be rate limiting. It is important to note that only LCFAs (i.e. those with carbon chain lengths of 12 to18) are transported using this mechanism, whereas the medium and short chain fatty acids can freely diffuse into the mitochondrial matrix.

To test the hypothesis that FFA transport across mitochondrial membranes is limiting during high-intensity exercise, Sidossis *et al.* (1997) conducted a study using isotope methodology during which **oleate** (a LCFA) and **octanoate** (an MCFA which does not require facilitated transport) were infused during exercise at both 40 and 80% $\text{VO}_{2\text{max}}$. Lipid and heparin were also infused during high-intensity exercise, in order to offset the reduction in plasma FFA that occurs at these intensities and therefore to ensure that plasma FFA was similar between trials. Interestingly, the percentage of oleate uptake that was oxidized during exercise was significantly decreased during exercise at 80% $\text{VO}_{2\text{max}}$, compared with 40% $\text{VO}_{2\text{max}}$, whereas octanoate oxidation did not change with exercise intensity (see Figure 9.7). These data therefore suggest that an inhibition of LCFA entry into the mitochondria

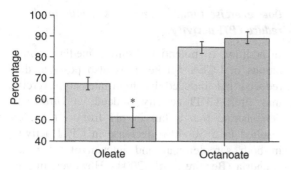

Figure 9.7 Percentage of oleate and octanoate tracer uptake oxidized during exercise at 40 (blue bars) and 80% VO_{2max} (pink bars) (adapted from Sidossis *et al.*, 1997)

is a contributing factor to the reduction in lipid oxidation rates with high-intensity exercise.

Does malonyl-CoA regulate LCFA uptake?

The mechanisms underpinning the reduction in LCFA entry to the mitochondria likely involve CPTI activity. In this regard, early attention focused on **malonyl-CoA**, which is a potent inhibitor of CPTI under resting conditions and light exercise. Indeed, under these conditions, muscle malonyl-CoA decreases, thus relieving the inhibition on CPTI and permitting LCFA mitochondrial uptake. In contrast, if malonyl-CoA inhibits LCFA uptake during high-intensity exercise, then muscle malonyl-CoA content should progressively increase with increments in exercise intensity.

Malonyl-CoA is formed from acetyl-CoA in a reaction catalysed by *acetyl-CoA carboxylase* (ACC). Given that acetyl-CoA would be increased with high-intensity exercise (due to increased glycolytic flux), it is reasonable to suggest that an increased formation of malonyl-CoA may coordinate the down-regulation of lipid and the up-regulation of CHO metabolism. However, evidence supporting this mechanism during high-intensity exercise is limited. ACC is under control through allosteric activation by **citrate** and is also deactivated through phosphorylation through 5' AMP activated protein kinase (AMPK). AMPK

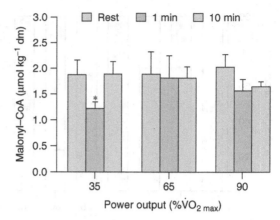

Figure 9.8 Skeletal muscle malonyl-CoA content at varying exercise intensities (adapted from Odland *et al.*, 1998a)

activity is greater with high-intensity exercise compared with moderate intensity exercise, and thus ACC activity is lower, favouring decreased malonyl-CoA production. Accordingly, muscle malonyl-CoA remains unchanged during exercise at 90% VO_{2max}, compared with 65 VO_{2max} (see Figure 9.8).

Does free carnitine availability regulate LCFA uptake?

Carnitine is required as a substrate for CPTI and is therefore required for the transport of an activated LCFA across the inner mitochondrial membrane. If acetyl-CoA formation from the oxidation of pyruvate exceeds the rate of utilization by the Krebs cycle, PDH activity could be reduced due to product inhibition. As a result, exercise intensity would be reduced and performance impaired. In such situations, carnitine can also act as a buffer for excess acetyl-CoA production by combining with acetyl-CoA to form acetylcarnitine through the action of carnitine acetyl transferase (CAT). In this way, PDH activity and Krebs cycle flux can continue, thereby allowing exercise to continue at high-intensity.

However, the down side of this is that the use of carnitine in this way reduces the amount of free carnitine available to act as a substrate for CPTI,

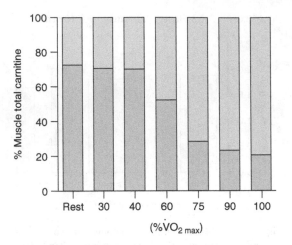

Figure 9.9 The percentage of carnitine present in free (pink bars) form or as acetylcarnitine (blue bars) in relation to exercise intensity (adapted from Stephens *et al.*, 2007)

and hence its activity is reduced. Indeed, the amount of free carnitine is reduced and acetylcarnitine is increased in accordance with increases in exercise intensity (see Figure 9.9). Furthermore, there is a strong positive and negative correlation with acetyl carnitine concentration and RER and fat oxidation rate, respectively, as shown in Figure 9.10. Based on these data, a proposed model for carnitine mediated regulation of lipid oxidation is outlined in Figure 9.11.

Does exercise-induced decreases in muscle pH reduce CPTI activity?

In addition to potential carnitine mediated limitations in LCFA uptake, it is also possible that reduced pH induced by high-intensity exercise may limit CPTI activity. Indeed, *in vitro* data demonstrate that a fall in pH from 7.1 to 6.8 resulted in a 30–40% decrease in CPTI activity in both sarcolemmal and inter-myofibril mitochondria (Bezaire *et al.*, 2004). However, further studies to test this hypothesis in exercising human skeletal muscle are warranted.

9.3 Effects of exercise duration

In contrast to exercise intensity, prolonged steady state exercise lasting several hours is characterized by a shift towards increased lipid oxidation and reduced carbohydrate oxidation rates (see Figure 9.12). This shift in oxidation rates is accompanied by an increased contribution of plasma FFA towards energy expenditure and a decreased reliance on both muscle glycogen and IMTGs (see Figure 9.13).

Studies examining the regulatory mechanisms underpinning this shift in substrate utilization have suggested that a reduction in muscle glycogen availability (due to progressive glycogen

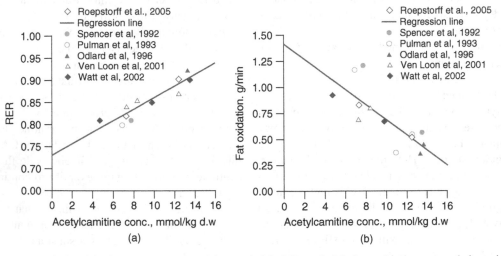

Figure 9.10 Relationship between acetylcarnitine and (a) RER and (b) fat oxidation rates (adapted from Kiens, 2006)

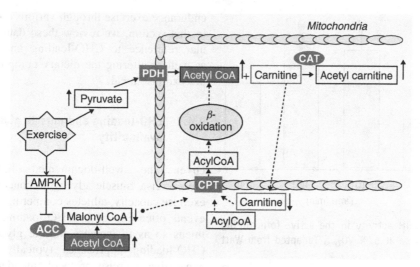

Figure 9.11   Schematic illustration of the potential regulation of lipid oxidation in conditions where glycolytic flux is elevated such as increasing exercise intensity, CAT denotes carnitine acetyltransferase (adapted from Kiens, 2006)

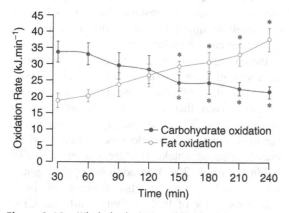

Figure 9.12   Whole body CHO and lipid oxidation rates during prolonged exercise at 57% VO_{2max} (adapted from Watt *et al.*, 2002)

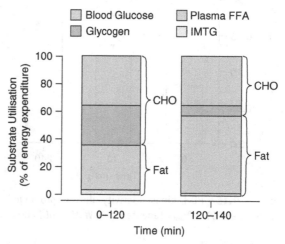

Figure 9.13   Relative contribution of muscle and blood-borne substrates to energy production during prolonged exercise at 57% VO_{2max} (adapted from Watt *et al.*, 2002)

depletion), and hence a reduced glycolytic flux, down-regulate PDH activity, thereby leading to reduced CHO oxidation. In addition, progressive increases in plasma FFA availability (due to continual lipolysis in adipose tissue) stimulate lipid oxidation. The down-regulation of PDH activity as exercise duration progresses (see Figure 9.14) may be due to reduced pyruvate flux, therefore reducing substrate production required for the PDH reaction. In addition, more recent

data demonstrate an up-regulation of PDH kinase activity during exercise, which would therefore directly inhibit PDH activity (see Figure 9.15).

Taken together, these data are consistent with the many observations that increasing or decreasing substrate availability is one of the most potent regulators of fuel utilization patterns

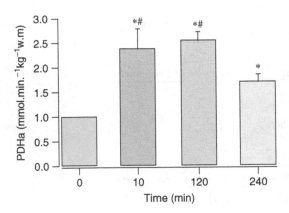

Figure 9.14 PDH activity in the active form during prolonged exercise at 57% VO_{2max} (adapted from Watt *et al.*, 2002)

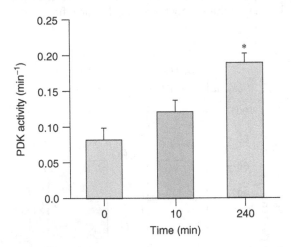

Figure 9.15 PDH kinase activity during prolonged exercise at 55% VO_{2max} (adapted from Watt *et al.*, 2004)

during exercise, and this concept is discussed in the next section.

9.4 Effects of nutritional status

Modifying substrate availability through dietary manipulation (such as loading regimens, pre-exercise meals or providing enhanced substrate availability during exercise) has consistently been shown to alter metabolic regulation during endurance exercise through various control points. In this section, we review these data with particular reference to CHO-loading and fat-loading, as well as altering the dietary composition of the pre-exercise meal.

9.4.1 CHO-loading and muscle glycogen availability

Given the well-documented link between pre-exercise muscle glycogen concentration and exercise capacity, athletes competing in endurance events often engage in CHO-loading dietary regimens so as to increase muscle glycogen stores. CHO-loading approaches typically involve an exhaustive exercise protocol intended to deplete glycogen stores, followed by a high-carbohydrate diet in order to induce high glycogen resynthesis rates which have been augmented by the prior exercise. In addition to CHO-loading, athletes are also advised to consume daily diets high in carbohydrate intake to ensure that high training intensities can be maintained.

Increasing muscle glycogen concentration enhances glycogenolysis during exercise (Hargreaves *et al.*, 1995) by enhancing phosphorylase activity, given that glycogen is a substrate for phosphorylase. The enhanced glycogenolysis with elevated glycogen stores does not appear to affect muscle glucose uptake (Hargreaves *et al.*, 1995; Arkinstall *et al.*, 2004). In addition to glycogenolysis, muscle glycogen also appears to be a potent regulator of PDH activity (and thus CHO oxidation) during exercise. Indeed, commencing exercise with reduced muscle glycogen attenuates the exercise-induced increase in PDH activity and vice versa (Kiilerich *et al.*, 2010), probably due to reduced glycolytic flux as well as increased resting content of PDK4 (the kinase responsible for deactivating PDH) when glycogen concentration is low. PDH regulation appears particularly sensitive to nutritional status even at rest. In fact, just three days of a low CHO (but increased fat diet) up-regulates PDH kinase activity and down-regulates PDH activity (Peters *et al.*, 1998).

Although we documented the effects of exercise intensity on substrate utilization in section 9.1,

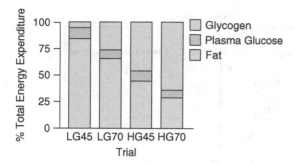

Figure 9.16 Relative contribution of glycogen, glucose and fat oxidation to 60 minutes of exercise undertaken at 45 or 70 with low (LG) or high pre-exercise glycogen (HG) concentrations (adapted from Arkinstall *et al.*, 2004)

it appears that muscle glycogen availability can influence fuel metabolism over and above that of exercise intensity. Indeed, Arkinstall *et al.* (2004) observed that glycogen utilization was enhanced during exercise at 45% VO$_{2max}$ that was commenced with high glycogen (591 mmol.kg dw^{-1}), as opposed to exercise at 70% VO$_{2max}$ commenced with low glycogen concentration (223 mmol/kg dw), despite the higher intensity. In contrast to glycogen utilization and CHO oxidation rates, lipid oxidation was highest when exercise was commenced with reduced glycogen stores (see Figure 9.16).

The shift towards fat oxidation when pre-exercise muscle glycogen is low is likely mediated by a number of contributing factors. First, reduced glycogen availability is associated with increased plasma FFA availability as well as adrenaline concentrations, thus favouring conditions for augmented lipid oxidation and lipolysis, respectively, compared with conditions of high glycogen concentration (Arkinstall *et al.*, 2004). However, when a pre-exercise meal is ingested and glucose infused during glycogen-depleted exercise, such that minimal differences exist between plasma FFA and adrenaline, lipid oxidation is still augmented (Roepstorff *et al.*, 2005).

In such circumstances, available evidence points to regulation within the muscle cell itself and, more specifically, a carnitine mediated increase in lipid oxidation. Indeed, these researchers

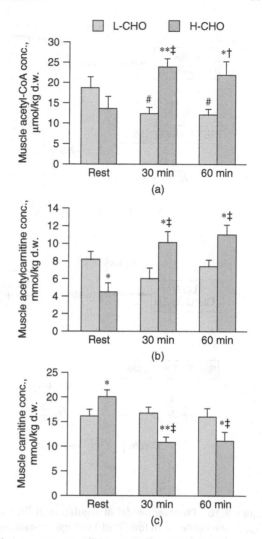

Figure 9.17 Muscle acetyl-CoA, acetylcarnitine and carnitine concentration during 60 minutes of exercise at 65% VO$_{2max}$ commenced with low (LCHO) or high pre-exercise glycogen (HCHO) concentrations (adapted from Roepstorff *et al.*, 2005)

observed lower PDH activity, acetyl-CoA and acetylcarnitine content and increased free carnitine concentrations during exercise when glycogen-depleted, compared with glycogen-loaded, conditions (see Figure 9.17). Interestingly, ACC phosphorylation increased and malonyl-CoA decreased similarly in both conditions, despite higher AMPK activity when glycogen was reduced. Such data provide further evidence that

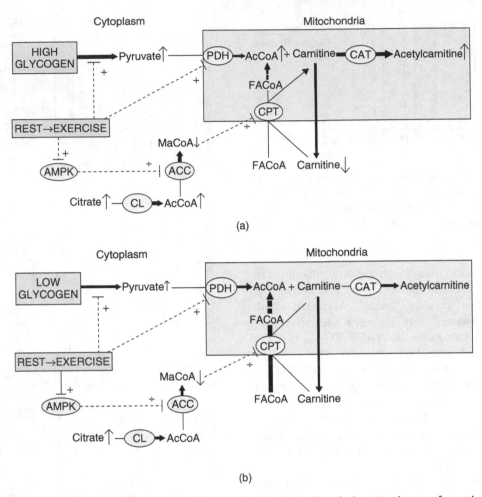

Figure 9.18 Proposed model of regulation of lipid and CHO metabolism during 60 minutes of exercise at 65% VO_{2max} commenced with low (LCHO) or high pre-exercise glycogen (HCHO) concentrations, CL denotes citrate lysase (adapted from Roepstorff *et al.*, 2005)

malonyl-CoA is not involved in regulating lipid metabolism during exercise but they provide further support (similar to the discussion on exercise intensity) for a critical role of carnitine. A proposed model for metabolic regulation under these circumstances is shown in Figure 9.18.

9.4.2 Fat-loading strategies

Given that it is well documented that performance in prolonged endurance events is limited by endogenous carbohydrate stores, many exercise scientists have become interested in strategies which could increase FFA availability and lipid oxidation, thereby sparing glycogen utilization. One such strategy is *fat adaptation*, a nutritional approach in which athletes consume a high-fat (and low-CHO) diet for a period of up to two weeks, during which they perform their normal intensity and volume of training, followed by 1–3 days of a high-CHO diet and a taper in training volume (Yeo *et al.*, 2011).

Research examining fat adaptation typically involves repeated measures crossover designs

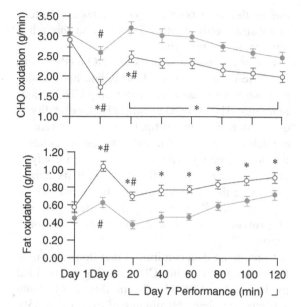

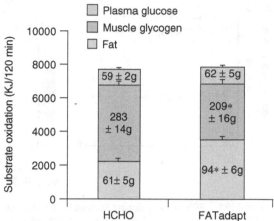

Figure 9.20 Estimated contribution of plasma glucose, muscle glycogen and fat oxidation to energy expenditure during 120 min at 70% VO_{2max} performed after 5 days of fat adaptation followed by 1 day of CHO restoration (adapted from Burke *et al.*, 2000)

Figure 9.19 CHO and lipid oxidation during fat adaptation protocol on day 1 (20 min at 70% VO_{2max}), day 6 (20 min at 70% VO_{2max}) and day 7 (120 min at 70% VO_{2max}) performed after 1 day of CHO restoration. Red line denotes Fat-Adapt, green line denotes High CHO (adapted from Burke *et al.*, 2000)

in which subjects either perform the fat-adapt protocol or consume a daily diet that is high in carbohydrate. Data from one such study is shown in Figure 9.19, where it is evident that five days of fat adaptation increases lipid oxidation and reduces CHO oxidation during exercise undertaken on both day 6 and 7, despite CHO restoration on day 6 (Burke *et al.*, 2000). While the restoration of muscle glycogen is of obvious benefit, it is remarkable that lipid oxidation is still enhanced under these conditions, considering the impact of muscle glycogen on substrate utilization as outlined in the previous sections. The increased reliance on lipid oxidation induced a sparing of muscle glycogen utilization but did not affect plasma glucose utilization (see Figure 9.20).

The mechanisms underpinning this shift in substrate utilization with fat adaptation are likely to be due to a combination of control points. For example, Burke *et al.* (2000) observed that exercise at 70% VO_{2max} is associated with

greater increases in plasma glycerol and FFA (thus suggesting increased rates of whole body lipolysis), though they were unable to identify the potential sources of fat.

More recent data suggest that fat adaptation increases intra-muscular triglyceride content (Yeo *et al.*, 2008) as well as resting muscle **HSL** activity (Stellingwerff *et al.*, 2006). Such data suggest that fat adaptation through chronic increases in plasma FFA availability (due to consumption of high fat diets) increases the muscle's capacity to synthesize triglycerides, as well as the capacity to metabolize them. In addition, it has also been hypothesized that fat adaptation may alter the capacity to transport FFAs and glucose, though further work is needed to test this theory, specifically in relation to the *sub-cellular* location of FAT/CD36, $FABP_{pm}$ and GLUT4, both at rest and during exercise (Yeo *et al.*, 2011).

In terms of reducing CHO oxidation rates, available data suggest PDH as a major control point. Indeed, fat adaptation reduces PDH activity at rest, as well as during, both sub-maximal and supra-maximal exercise (see Figure 9.21). This attenuation of PDH activity could, of course, be problematical for those events where periods of high intensity exercise (requiring high CHO

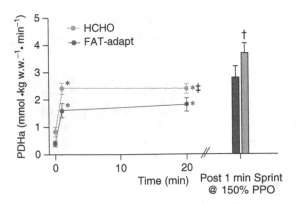

Figure 9.21   PDH activity during 20 minutes of exercise at 70% VO_{2max} and 1 minute sprint at 150% of peak power output (PPO) performed after 5 days of fat adaptation followed by 1 day of CHO restoration (adapted from Stellingwerff *et al.*, 2006)

oxidation rates) are needed, such as 'sprint finishes', etc. Reduced accumulation of free ADP and AMP during near maximal or supra-maximal exercise could also explain reduced rates of glycogenolysis, given the role of these intermediates in regulating phosphorylase activity (Stellingwerff *et al.*, 2006).

Although the effects of fat adaptation on substrate oxidation are well documented, further research is needed to elucidate the precise control points that coordinate shifts in substrate utilization. Interested readers are directed to a recent review by Yeo *et al.* (2011) for further discussion on metabolic regulation with this dietary approach to endurance exercise.

9.4.3   Pre-exercise and during-exercise CHO ingestion

When compared with exercise after overnight fasting, ingestion of carbohydrate-rich meals within the hours before exercise (as well as carbohydrate ingestion during exercise) has been shown to enhance endurance performance (Wright *et al.*, 1991). Consequently, it is common practice for athletes to adopt such dietary approaches to competition. However, it is now well documented that pre- and during-exercise CHO ingestion is

one of the most potent ways to alter the pattern of substrate utilization during exercise through a number of control points.

One of the main responses to CHO feeding is to attenuate plasma FFA availability and lipid oxidation, while simultaneously increasing CHO oxidation rates. The reduced plasma FFA availability is due to an attenuation of lipolysis which, in turn, is regulated by increased circulating insulin concentrations caused by CHO feeding. The anti-lipolytic effect of insulin is mediated through its ability to activate the enzyme **phosphodiesterase**, which degrades **cAMP** and thereby attenuates activation of **protein kinase A** and, eventually, hormone-sensitive lipase.

Convincing data confirming that lipolysis limits fat oxidation following CHO feeding is provided by Horowitz *et al.* (1997). In this study, male subjects completed 60 minutes of exercise at 45% VO_{2max} in fasted conditions or one hour after consuming 0.8 g/kg of glucose (to induce a high insulin response), 0.8 g/kg fructose (to induce a low insulin response) or an additional glucose trial during which intralipid and heparin were infused so as to maintain plasma FFA availability in the face of high insulin (see Figure 9.22). In accordance with the insulin response, lipolysis (as indicated by rate of appearance of glycerol) was reduced with CHO feeding and plasma FFA availability was reduced in these conditions (see Figure 9.23). In addition, rates of lipolysis exceeded lipid oxidation rates during fasted exercise whereas, in the CHO conditions, rates of lipolysis appeared to equal lipid oxidation rates, thus implying that lipolysis limits fat oxidation (see Figure 9.24).

However, when intralipid and heparin was infused during an additional glucose trial, lipid oxidation rates were enhanced by 30% ($4.0\,\mu mol.kg^{-1}.min^{-1}$) compared with the glucose-only trial ($3.1\,\mu mol.kg^{-1}.min^{-1}$), but they were still not restored to levels occurring during fasted exercise ($6.1\,\mu mol.kg^{-1}.min^{-1}$). Taken together, while these data suggest that only small elevations in insulin can attenuate lipolysis (i.e. $10-30\,\mu U/ml$), they also demonstrate a limitation within the muscle cell itself

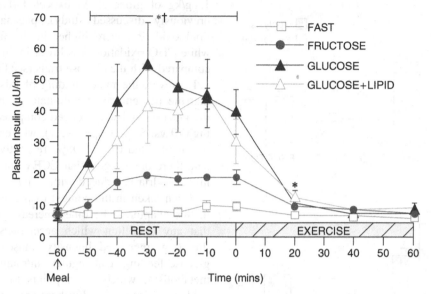

Figure 9.22   Plasma insulin concentration after feeding and during exercise (adapted from Horowitz *et al.*, 1997)

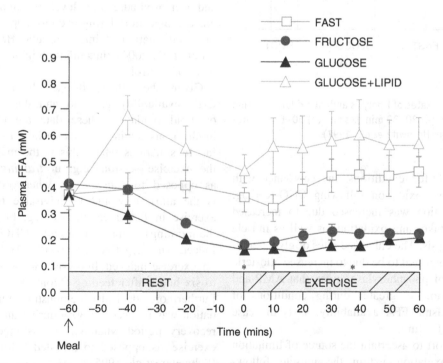

Figure 9.23   Plasma FFA concentration after feeding and during exercise (adapted from Horowitz *et al.*, 1997)

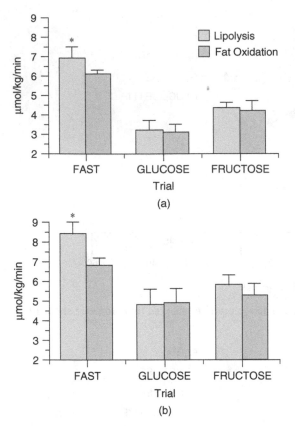

Figure 9.24 Rates of lipolysis and fat oxidation during exercise from (a) 20–30 minutes and (b) 50–60 minutes (adapted from Horowitz *et al.*, 1997)

during CHO-fed conditions. In accordance with reduced lipid oxidation following CHO-feeding, CHO oxidation was increased due to increased glucose uptake (and oxidation) as well as muscle glycogenolysis. The enhanced rates of glycogenolysis was suggested to be due to increased allosteric activation of phosphorylase, given that AMP and P_i production is greater during conditions of reduced plasma FFA availability, as is the case with CHO feeding.

In an effort to ascertain the source of limitation to lipid oxidation within the muscle following CHO feeding, Coyle *et al.* (1997) infused **octanoate** (an MCFA) or **palmitate** (an LCFA) during 40 min of exercise at 50% VO_{2max} after an overnight fast or 60 minutes after ingesting

1.4 g/kg of glucose. As expected (based on the previously discussed study), plasma FFA and lipid oxidation were higher in the fasted trials, while CHO oxidation was lower in this condition, compared with the glucose trials (see Figure 9.25).

However, the major finding of this study was that the percentage of palmitate oxidized during the glucose trial was reduced compared with fasting (70 vs. 86%, respectively), whereas octanoate was unaffected (99 vs. 98%, respectively). These data therefore suggest that LCFA uptake into the mitochondria is reduced with CHO feeding.

When taken in the context of previous sections in this chapter, it becomes increasingly apparent that any condition which accelerates glycolytic flux (e.g. increased intensity, muscle glycogen, glucose feeding) can regulate intramuscular lipid metabolism, which again points to a carnitine-mediated limitation. Furthermore, more recent data has demonstrated that the increased insulin and decreased adrenaline levels which accompany glucose ingestion during exercise appear to result in an attenuation of intra-muscular HSL activity (Watt *et al.*, 2004), thus highlighting an additional point of control.

Given the effects of acutely manipulating CHO availability prior to and during exercise on lipid oxidation, these data are of obvious implications for individuals wishing to lose body fat. In situations where this is the main goal of the exercise session (e.g. in *training* sessions, as opposed to *competition*, where performance is the aim), it would be advisable to perform exercise in fasted conditions (e.g. first thing in the morning) or many hours after CHO ingestion. Indeed, the negative effects of CHO ingestion on exercise-induced lipolysis can persist for up to six hours after feeding (Montain *et al.*, 1991). Furthermore, data also demonstrate that fat oxidation was reduced by 30% during an eight-hour recovery period when CHO was ingested after exercise, as opposed to ingested before exercise (Schneiter *et al.*, 1995).

Over the last few years, many researchers have also observed that training in conditions of reduced endogenous and exogenous carbohydrate availability enhances oxidative

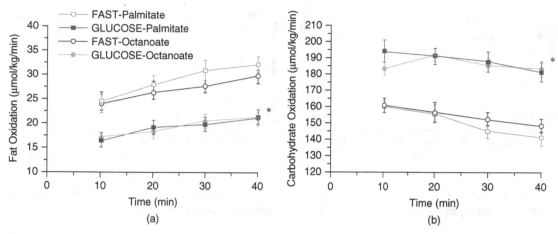

Figure 9.25   Rates of fat and CHO oxidation during exercise in fasted and glucose trials (adapted from Coyle *et al.*, 1997)

adaptations of skeletal muscle and augments the training response. Such data are particularly interesting as they appear to challenge traditional sports nutrition guidelines advising that athletes should consume carbohydrate before, during and after daily training sessions. Interested readers are directed to recent reviews summarizing these exciting new findings (Hawley & Burke, 2010).

Given that insulin is a potent inhibitor of lipolysis, one nutritional strategy to minimize this suppression is to consume *low glycemic carbohydrate* (LGI)-based foods in the hours prior to exercise, as opposed to those that are *high glycemic* (HGI). LGI foods do not produce as big an insulin response, so, as a result, plasma FFA availability and glycerol are higher during exercise undertaken in the hours after LGI meals, as opposed to HGI meals (see Figure 9.26). Consequently, lipid oxidation during exercise is higher with LGI CHO ingestion, compared with HGI ingestion, and muscle glycogen utilization is reduced (Wee *et al.*, 2005).

For this reason, athletes are typically advised to consume LGI foods as the pre-competition meal (such feeding strategies are also associated with better maintenance of plasma glucose levels during exercise), although it should be noted that effects of GI on substrate utilization during exercise appear to be minimal when large

amounts of CHO are ingested during exercise, as is typically the case in prolonged endurance events (Burke *et al.*, 1998). Where athletes are concerned with maximizing body fat loss (such as those in weight-making sports), it is advised that LGI carbohydrates should form the majority of the CHO input to the daily diet (Morton *et al.*, 2010).

9.4.4   Pre-exercise FFA availability

Research examining the effects of acutely elevating plasma FFA levels in the hours before exercise has typically used infusion of intralipid and heparin. Such approaches have proved to be advantageous, as they have clearly demonstrated that availability of lipid can alter substrate utilization, during both moderate and intense exercise. Indeed, Dyck *et al.* (1996) observed muscle glycogen utilization to be reduced by approximately 50% during 15 minutes of exercise at 85% of VO_{2max}.

The activation of PDH and transformation of phosphorylase to its more active *a* form was unaffected by lipid infusion, thus suggesting that the reduction in glycogenolysis was due to post-transformational regulation involving allosteric modulators and substrate provision. In this regard, exercise with intra-lipid infusion was associated with smaller increases in AMP, ADP

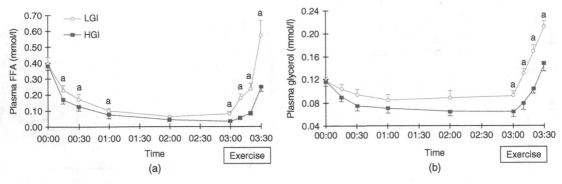

Figure 9.26   Plasma FFA and glycerol during the three-hour postprandial period after consuming a LGI or HGI breakfast and during 30 minutes of exercise at 70% VO$_{2max}$ (adapted from Wee *et al.*, 2005)

and P$_i$, which was suggested to have resulted in reduced phosphorylase *a* activity.

More recent data also demonstrated that glycogen utilization is spared (to a lower extent) even during moderate intensity exercise when undertaken with intralipid and heparin infusion (Odland *et al.*, 1998b, 2000). In the first of these studies, Odland *et al.* (1998b) observed reduced flux through phosphorylase and PFK, which was suggested to be caused by increased cytoplasmic citrate (which inhibits PFK) and reduced free AMP, ADP and P$_i$ accumulation (see Figures 9.27 and 9.28). In addition, PDH activity was also reduced during exercise (see Figure 9.29), which was suggested to be due to reduced pyruvate accumulation during the intralipid trial. Although these authors also observed reduced PDH activity in their follow-up study (Odland *et al.*, 2000), the precise mechanisms underpinning this reduction in the face of increased plasma FFA availability are not currently well understood (Spriet and Watt, 2003).

While these studies have unequivocally shown that increased lipid availability can modulate substrate utilization (probably by influencing key enzymes involved in CHO metabolism such as phosphorylase, PFK and PDH), the approach of artificially elevating plasma FFA levels is not practical in the athletic setting. Consequently, researchers have also focused on nutritional strategies such as high fat meals or ergogenic aids (e.g. **caffeine**) to acutely increase plasma FFA availability. In relation to the latter, caffeine is proposed to exert its influence by increasing

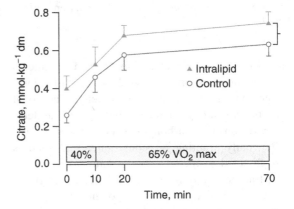

Figure 9.27   Muscle citrate content at rest and during 70 minutes of exercise at 40 and 65% VO$_{2max}$ with intralipid infusion or control (adapted from Odland *et al.*, 1998b)

adrenaline concentrations, as well as antagonizing adenosine receptors in the adipocyte. However, whether or not caffeine enhances lipid oxidation during exercise remains a contentious issue, and interested readers are directed to relevant reviews in the area (Graham *et al.*, 2008).

Regarding pre-exercise high-fat meals, there is some evidence that this feeding strategy can alter substrate utilization, albeit not as pronounced as the fat-loading strategy discussed earlier. Indeed, data from our group demonstrated that a high-fat meal administered four hours prior to 90 minutes of exercise at 70% VO$_{2max}$ only increased lipid oxidation during the initial

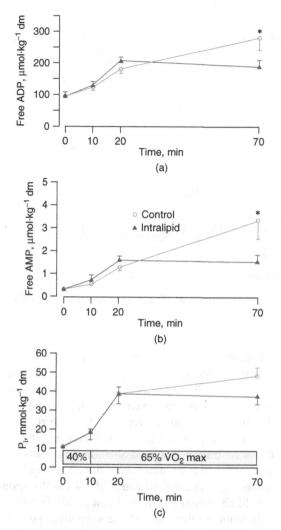

Figure 9.28 Muscle free ADP, AMP and P$_i$ content at rest and during 70 minutes of exercise at 40 and 65% VO$_{2max}$ with intralipid infusion or control (adapted from Odland *et al.*, 1998b)

15 minutes of exercise (Whitley *et al.*, 1998). Furthermore, exercise performance (a 10 km time trial undertaken after the 90 minutes of steady state exercise) was not increased by the high-fat meal, compared with an isoenergetic high-CHO meal. Athletes should also be aware of adopting high fat pre-exercise meals owing to the problems associated with digestion following consumption of meals that largely consist of long-chain triglycerides (Horowitz & Klein, 2000).

9.5 Effects of training status

Endurance training results in a number of profound physiological and metabolic adaptations which function to reduce the degree of perturbations to homeostasis for a given exercise intensity and, ultimately, delay the onset of fatigue. Adaptations to endurance training are most recognized functionally by an increase in maximal oxygen uptake, as well as a rightward shift in the **lactate threshold**.

From a metabolic perspective, the most prominent adaptation is an increase in the size and number of mitochondria (i.e. mitochondrial biogenesis), which essentially permits a closer matching between ATP requirements and production via *oxidative metabolism*. The adaptive response of muscle mitochondria is also accompanied by increases in capillary density and substrate transport proteins and increased activity of the enzymes involved in the main metabolic pathways. In addition, endurance training increases the capacity for skeletal muscle to store glycogen and triglycerides, thereby increasing substrate availability.

In relation to substrate utilization during exercise following endurance training, the most notable response is a reduction in CHO utilization with a concomitant increase in lipid oxidation (Henriksson *et al.*, 1977). In this section, we thus review the potential mechanisms underpinning this alteration in fuel utilization patterns.

9.5.1 CHO metabolism

For a given exercise intensity, glycogen utilization is reduced with exercise training (LeBlanc *et al.*, 2004), as shown in Figure 9.30. In accordance with earlier observations (Chesley *et al.*, 1996), these authors also observed that the reduced glycogenolysis observed after training was not due to any change in transformation but to allosteric mechanisms. Indeed, exercise in the trained state was associated with reduced content of ADP, AMP and P$_i$, thereby providing a mechanism leading to reduced phosphorylase activity.

The above authors also observed reduced pyruvate and lactate production during exercise

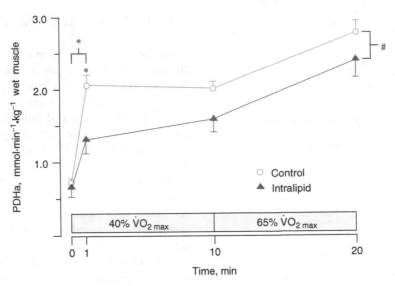

Figure 9.29   Muscle PDH activity at rest and during 10 minutes of exercise at 40 and 65% VO2max with intralipid infusion or control (adapted from Odland *et al.*, 1998b)

undertaken in the trained state (see Figure 9.31), as well as reduced PDH activity (see Figure 9.32). As a result of the reduced CHO flux, it is therefore likely that the attenuated pyruvate production (in addition to reduced ADP accumulation) may have attenuated PDH activity.

In addition to training-induced reductions in muscle glycogenolysis, several investigators have observed that training reduces exercise-induced *liver glycogenolysis*, as demonstrated by the rate of appearance of glucose in the circulation (see Figure 9.33). There is some evidence (although this is not consistent within the literature) that endurance training also reduces gluconeogenesis, which may be due to reduced release of **lactate** and **alanine** (gluconeogenic precursors) from skeletal muscle following training (Coggan *et al.*, 1995). In accordance with reduced rates of glucose production, muscle glucose uptake is reduced when exercise is undertaken at the same absolute workload following a period of endurance training (Bergman *et al.*, 1999).

Despite the fact that training increases total muscle GLUT4, the reduction in exercise-induced muscle glucose uptake is most likely caused by a reduced *translocation* of GLUT4 to the

sarcolemma following training, thereby reducing the capacity to transport glucose (Richter *et al.*, 1998). This particular study utilized a knee extensor training and exercise model, where only one limb was trained, yet both limbs performed the exercise protocol before and after training. In this way, training-induced alterations in hormonal and cardiovascular status were minimized and the reduced glucose uptake and GLUT4 translocation was likely mediated by local contractile factors.

In summarizing the link between liver glucose production and muscle glucose uptake, it is generally accepted that training-induced changes in hormone concentrations such as adrenaline, insulin and glucagon are unable to explain all of the effects (Phillips *et al.*, 1996). Rather, it is possible that the actual rate of muscle glucose uptake acts as a feedback signal to regulate glucose output from the liver (Phillips *et al.*, 1996).

9.5.2   Lipid metabolism

While it has been consistently demonstrated that endurance training results in a shift from CHO to lipid oxidation for a given absolute exercise

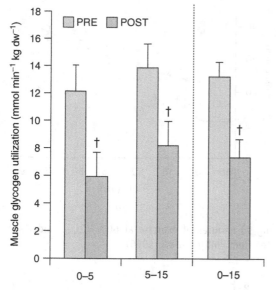

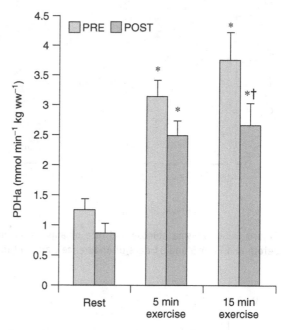

Figure 9.30 Muscle glycogen utilization during 15 minutes of exercise at 80% VO_{2max} undertaken before and after seven weeks of endurance training (adapted from LeBlanc *et al.*, 2004)

Figure 9.32 PDH activity at rest and during 15 minutes of exercise at 80% VO_{2max} undertaken before and after seven weeks of endurance training (adapted from LeBlanc *et al.*, 2004)

intensity, the precise source and mechanisms underpinning increased lipid oxidation rates is not precisely understood. In theory, this shift in substrate utilization could result from increased rates of adipose tissue lipolysis and increased FFA

delivery to muscle, increased transport of fatty acids across the sarcolemma and also increased transport of LCFA across the mitochondria. In addition, increased activity of the key enzymes

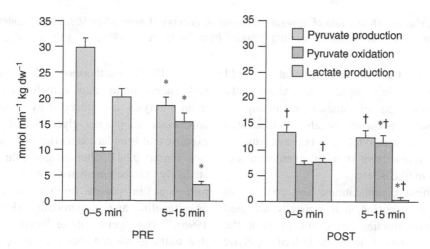

Figure 9.31 Comparison of the fate of pyruvate produced during 15 minutes of exercise at 80% VO_{2max} undertaken before (pre) and after (post) seven weeks of endurance training (adapted from LeBlanc *et al.*, 2004)

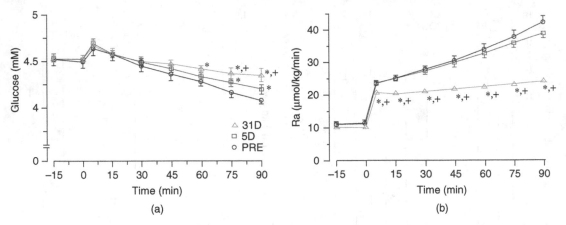

Figure 9.33 Plasma glucose and rate of appearance during 90 minutes of exercise at 60% VO_{2max} undertaken before and after 5 and 31 days of endurance training (adapted from Phillips *et al.*, 1996)

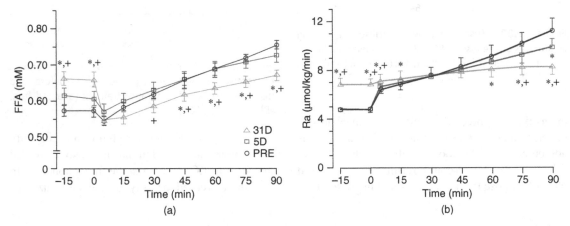

Figure 9.34 Plasma FFA and rate of appearance during 90 minutes of exercise at 60% VO_{2max} undertaken before and after 5 and 31 days of endurance training (adapted from Phillips *et al.*, 1996)

involved in the TCA cycle and β-oxidation would increase the muscle's capacity to oxidize fatty acids. Interpretation of studies attempting to address these hypotheses is also complicated by variations in methodologies between studies, e.g. duration/intensity of training, exercise mode, biochemical methods, etc.

Despite these complications, and contrary to what might be expected, it is generally accepted that endurance training does not increase the rate of adipose tissue lipolysis. Indeed, lipolytic rates are similar in trained and untrained subjects exercising at the same absolute intensity (Klein *et al.*, 1994). Furthermore, data suggests that endurance training may actually reduce adipose tissue lipolysis, as evidenced by reduced rates of appearance of plasma glycerol and FFA during exercise that is undertaken after short-term training (see Figure 9.34). The reduced rate of lipolysis is likely to be mediated by training-induced reductions in potent lipolytic hormones such as adrenaline and noradrenaline (Phillips *et al.*, 1996). Taken together, these data therefore suggest that training-induced increases in lipid oxidation is due to increased utilization of non-plasma derived lipid sources, most likely IMTGs.

Although training does not increase adipose tissue lipolysis, there is some evidence (at least from knee extensor training and exercise models) that exercise-induced muscle FFA uptake is increased following training (Turcotte *et al.*, 1992; Kiens *et al.*, 1993), despite similar FFA delivery in both trained and untrained muscle (see Figure 9.35). Such data suggest that there is a saturation to muscle FFA uptake, given that FFA uptake appeared to plateau during prolonged exercise in the untrained leg. In this regard, it has been shown that endurance training increases FABPpm and FAT/CD36 protein content, which collectively could be the mechanism underpinning increased muscle FFA uptake in trained muscle (Kiens *et al.*, 1997; 2004; Tunstall *et al.*, 2002). While an increase in protein mediated transport of FFA across the sarcolemma may be occurring following training in an isolated knee extensor model, it is difficult to ascertain if this occurs with whole body exercise, given the differences in hormonal and blood flow responses between exercise modes.

Although controversial, there is some evidence that the main underlying contributing factor to training-induced up-regulation of lipid oxidation is an increased reliance upon IMTG oxidation and, to a lesser extent, plasma triglyceride metabolism (Hurley *et al.*, 1986; Martin *et al.*, 1993; Phillips *et al.*, 1996). Cross-sectional studies have also demonstrated increased IMTG utilization when comparing trained and untrained humans (Klein *et al.*, 1994; Coggan *et al.*, 2000). Interpretation of data in this area is complicated, however, by variations in the analytical methods used to quantify lipid oxidation (for review, see van Loon, 2004).

Given that adrenaline can regulate IMTG lipolysis (similar to that in adipose tissue), it is somewhat surprising that IMTG utilization is increased with training, given that training attenuates adrenaline release. Furthermore, the hydrolysis of IMTG is also controlled by the muscle-specific isoform of hormone-sensitive lipase, yet trained muscle does not appear to express higher levels of this enzyme (Helge *et al.*, 2006) However, more recent data has characterized an additional lipase that can also

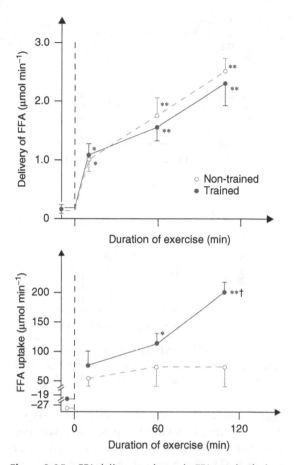

Figure 9.35 FFA delivery and muscle FFA uptake during prolonged knee extensor exercise in an untrained and trained leg (adapted from Kiens *et al.*, 1993)

increase IMTG lipolysis in skeletal muscle, known as *adipose triglyceride lipase* (**ATGL**) (Watt & Spriet, 2010), which is in fact increased by endurance training (see Figure 9.36). These authors therefore speculated that the training-induced increase in this protein may mediate, in part, the increased IMTG oxidation that is evident in the trained state (Alsted *et al.*, 2009).

In addition to increased lipolysis of IMTG triglycerides, trained subjects also appear to exhibit an increased capacity to transport LCFAs into the mitochondria. Indeed, Sidossis *et al.* (1998) observed that the percentage of oleate taken up and oxidized was higher in trained subjects, compared with untrained subjects,

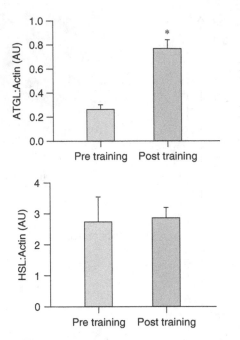

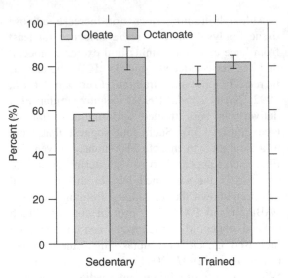

Figure 9.37 Percentage of oleate and octanoate tracer taken up and oxidized during cycling at an oxygen cost of 2 L.min^{-1} in sedentary and trained subjects (adapted from Sidossis *et al.*, 1998)

Figure 9.36 ATGL and HSL protein content in the vastus lateralis muscle before and after eight weeks of endurance training. (adapted from Alsted *et al.*, 2009)

during exercise at the same absolute oxygen cost. In contrast, octanoate uptake and oxidation was not different between training status (see Figure 9.37). The apparent increase in fatty acid uptake and oxidation into the mitochondria is likely to be due to the fact that endurance training increases CPT1 activity (Jong-Yeon *et al.*, 2002) (given that this enzyme is rate limiting for LCFA uptake), as well as increased activity of enzymes involved in the oxidation of fatty acids, such as β-hydroxyl-CoA-dehydrogenase and citrate synthase (Burgomaster *et al.*, 2008).

Finally, it should also be noted that many studies have demonstrated that training enhances resting content of IMTG in both type I and II fibres, which may also contribute to enhanced utilization after training (for review see van Loon, 2004).

9.5.3 Protein metabolism

In contrast to CHO and lipid metabolism, the effects of endurance exercise and training on the regulation of protein metabolism is less well understood. The fate of the muscle free amino acid pool is summarized in Figure 9.38 and generally involves **transamination**, **deamination** or oxidation (these reactions have been discussed in Chapter 4). The amino acids actually oxidized during exercise are primarily the BCAAs and, most notably, leucine (for a review, see Rennie *et al.*, 2006). Regulation of BCAA oxidation is under the control of branched chain keto-acid dehydrogenase (**BCKAD**) located in the mitochondria.

In response to endurance training, leucine oxidation is reduced during acute exercise (McKenzie *et al.*, 2000), and this reduction is probably due to reduced activation of BCKAD, as is evident when exercise is undertaken at either the same absolute or relative intensity post-training (see Figure 9.39).

The attenuated activation of BCKAD following endurance training may be due to training-induced increases in the muscle content of **BCKAD kinase**, the protein responsible for phosphorylation (and de-activation) of BCKAD. Indeed, Howarth *et al.*, (2007) observed BCKAD to be increased after six weeks of sprint interval and endurance training (see Figure 9.40).

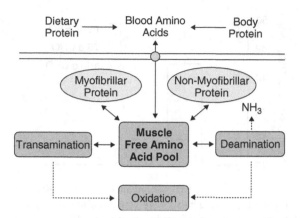

Figure 9.38 Potential fate of the free amino acid pool present in skeletal muscle (adapted from Gibala, 2001)

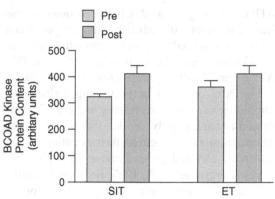

Figure 9.40 BCKAD kinase content pre- and post-6 weeks of sprint interval (ST) or endurance training (ET) (adapted from Howarth *et al.*, 2007)

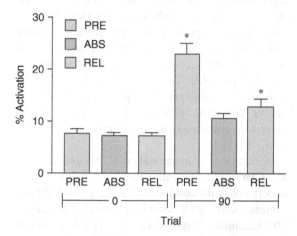

Figure 9.39 Percentage activation of BCKAD during 90 minutes of exercise at 65% VO_{2max} (0 = resting levels and 90 = after 90 min of exercise) undertaken prior to training (PRE) or post-training undertaken at the same absolute (ABS) or relative intensity (REL) (adapted from McKenzie *et al.*, 2000)

The apparent down-regulation of protein oxidation with endurance training could be interpreted as meaning that athletes do not need to consume extra dietary protein. However, given that the capacity to oxidize protein is enhanced with training (as reflected by increases in the maximal activity of BCKAD – McKenzie *et al.*, 2000) and that athletes are often engaged in intensive training programmes with high volume and intensity, it is possible that endurance-based

athletes do, in fact, require additional protein in their diet, especially during times when energy intake is restricted. This remains a contentious issue, and interested readers are directed to the review of Tarnapolsky (2004).

9.6 Mechanisms of fatigue

Fatigue is undoubtedly a complex process which, in the case of endurance exercise, may be due to combined influences of reduced central drive, dehydration and increased circulatory strain, all of which could be augmented by altering the environmental conditions such as increasing ambient temperature or altitude. However, because the focus of this text is on *muscle*, we will limit our discussion to the local factors originating in muscle and, furthermore, those factors which are considered the *primary* fatiguing agents.

In this regard, there is considerable evidence that reduced CHO availability may be the predominant underlying mechanism of fatigue induced by prolonged endurance exercise. Such a theory makes physiological sense, given that race pace is usually around intensities greater than 75% VO_{2max}, which can only be sustained by the combined utilization of muscle glycogen and blood glucose. While a reduction in energy availability not only reduces the rate at which

ATP can be re-generated, CHO depletion can also lead to metabolic disturbances with the peripheral processes involved in muscle contraction, such as EC coupling and the regulation of the Na^+/K^+ ATPase and SERCA pumps (Karelis *et al.*, 2010).

The role of CHO in preventing fatigue and improving exercise performance and capacity was demonstrated as early as the 1960s and 1970s, when investigators focused their attention on the effects of elevated pre-exercise muscle glycogen stores (Bergstrom *et al.*, 1967; Karlsson & Saltin, 1971). These early studies paved the way for the development of CHO-loading strategies which modern athletes still adopt today.

Although not always consistent, the general consensus from the wealth of studies undertaken since that time is that CHO-loading can improve performance and capacity, especially when the exercise is greater than 90 minutes in duration (Hawley *et al.*, 1997). Although we briefly alluded to the role of glycogen depletion in interfering with the peripheral processes of contraction, the enhanced performance effect is likely to be *initially* mediated by a delay in the time-point at which energy availability becomes limiting to the maintenance of the desired workload. In the case of *race pace*, this is dependent on sustained and high rates of CHO oxidation.

Whereas the studies of the 1960s and 1970s focused on CHO-loading studies, research in the next two decades examined the effects of pre-exercise feeding as well as consuming additional CHO during exercise. Pre-exercise feeding (i.e. 3–4 hours before competition) is advantageous not only because it can lead to further elevations in muscle glycogen content, but also because it can restore liver glycogen content, which is usually depleted after an overnight fast. The latter is particularly important, given that liver glycogen content is related to exercise capacity (Casey *et al.*, 2000).

Sherman *et al.* (1991) observed that time trial performance after 90 minutes of steady state exercise at 70% VO_{2max} was greater when 150 g of CHO was consumed before exercise, compared with 75 g of CHO, both of which were greater than no meal (see Figure 9.41). The enhanced performance effect was associated with

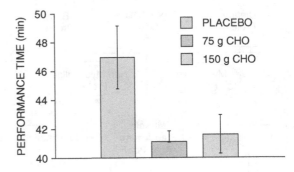

Figure 9.41 Time trial performance when no CHO meal (PLACEBO) or CHO meals were consumed one hour prior to exercise (adapted from Sherman *et al.*, 1991)

maintenance of blood glucose concentration late during the exercise, which is important because liver glucose production and muscle uptake and oxidation become more important when muscle glycogen concentrations begin to decline (see Figure 9.42). In a further study, the same authors also observed that performance can be further increased when CHO is ingested during exercise in addition to a pre-exercise meal (Wright *et al.*, 1991).

In addition to maintenance of plasma glucose and CHO oxidation rates, there is some evidence (albeit not consistent) that CHO ingestion during exercise may spare muscle glycogen utilization. For example, Tsintzas *et al.* (1995) observed that CHO ingestion during 60 min of running at 70% VO_{2max} reduced muscle glycogen utilization, which was largely due to a sparing in type I fibres. In a further study, the same group also showed that CHO ingestion attenuated the reduction in muscle PCr content in type I fibres, and therefore suggested that the reduced accumulation of ADP, AMP and P_i would reduce the post-transformational activation of phosphorylase, thereby explaining reduced glycogenolysis (Tsintzas *et al.*, 2001).

As a result of decades of research on CHO and endurance performance, it is now common practice for athletes to consume high CHO diets in the days leading up to performance, as well as a pre-exercise meal that is supplemented with CHO ingestion during exercise – the latter commonly in

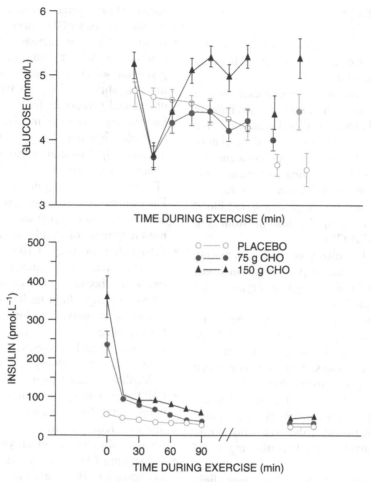

Figure 9.42   Plasma glucose and insulin during exercise when no CHO meal (PLACEBO) or CHO meals were consumed one hour prior to exercise (adapted from Sherman *et al.*, 1991)

the form of drinks, gels and energy bars, etc. While the reduction in substrate may be the initial signal contributing to fatigue, CHO depletion can lead to *secondary* processes relevant to the contractile process itself.

In this regard, recent data has demonstrated that glycogen depletion is associated with impaired Ca^{2+} release from the SR (Ortenblad *et al.*, 2011). In addition, the **Na+/K+ ATPase pump** also appears sensitive to CHO availability (Green *et al.*, 2007; Stewart *et al.*, 2007) and may therefore result in reduced propagation of the action potential along the sarcolemma. Taken together, these data provide a mechanistic

role of CHO availability in attenuating fatigue beyond that of a substrate for ATP resynthesis *per se*.

Finally, we acknowledge that race pace in endurance events is never normally constant, as athletes may increase intensity at stages (e.g. a push for the front or sprint finish) or may deliberately decrease their power output as a result of a pacing strategy. These subtle alterations in intensity can lead to further disturbances in the muscle but, because this fluctuation in intensity is characteristic of intermittent exercise, we will discuss mechanisms of fatigue in this instance in the final chapter.

9.7 Key points

- Endurance exercise typically refers to steady-state exercise performed for durations between five minutes and four hours.
- Metabolic regulation in endurance exercise can be achieved by modifying substrate availability (controlled by diet and hormonal regulation), the abundance of transport proteins and regulatory enzymes and, moreover, through covalent and allosteric regulation of existing enzyme activity.
- Increasing exercise intensity increases CHO utilization (from both muscle glycogen and blood glucose) and reduces lipid oxidation (from both plasma FFA and IMTG).
- Increased CHO utilization with increasing exercise intensity is due to post-transformational allosteric regulation of phosphorylase and transformation of PDH.
- Decreased lipid oxidation with increasing exercise intensity is likely to be due to reduced plasma FFA delivery to muscle (but not as a result of reduced lipolysis) as well as reduced FFA import into the mitochondria.
- Reduced FFA import into the mitochondria with increasing exercise intensity is restricted to LCFAs and is probably due to a reduction in free carnitine availability, thus limiting CPTI activity.
- Increasing exercise duration increases lipid oxidation but reduces CHO oxidation, as reflected by reduced glycogen and blood glucose utilization.
- Increased lipid oxidation with increasing exercise duration is largely due to increased plasma FFA availability due to continual lipolysis in adipose tissue, whereas reduced CHO oxidation is likely to be due to reduced glycogen and glucose availability.
- Reduced glyolytic flux with increasing exercise duration also decreases PDH activity and increases PDH kinase activity.
- CHO-loading increases muscle glycogen concentration and utilization during exercise due to increased phosphorylase activity as a result of increased substrate provision.
- Increased pre-exercise muscle glycogen concentration increases PDH activity and vice versa.
- Lipid oxidation is increased when exercise is commenced with reduced pre-exercise muscle glycogen, which may be due to increased carnitine availability and hence CPTI activity because of reduced glycolytic flux.
- Fat-loading protocols involving high fat diets followed by one day of CHO restoration increases lipid oxidation and reduces CHO oxidation during exercise, despite the restoration of high muscle glycogen concentration.
- Fat-loading may increase lipid oxidation due to increased rates of lipolysis as well as increased muscle content of IMTG and HSL activity.
- Fat-loading reduces CHO oxidation during exercise due to reduced PDH activation (probably because of increased PDH kinase activity during a high fat-low CHO diet), which would be negative for high-intensity exercise performance.
- Pre-exercise and during-exercise CHO ingestion reduces FFA availability and lipid oxidation due to insulin-mediated reductions in lipolysis.
- CHO ingestion before exercise also limits LCFA uptake into the mitochondria, which may be due to a reduction in free carnitine availability because of enhanced glycolytic flux.
- Consuming LGI carbohydrates before exercise, as opposed to HGI carbohydrates, attenuates the insulin-mediated reduction in lipolysis and FFA availability during exercise, thereby increasing lipid oxidation rates.
- Increasing pre-exercise plasma FFA availability (most notably through intralipid and heparin infusion) attenuates glycogenolysis, glycolysis and CHO oxidation, most likely due to reduced activation of phosphorylase, PFK and PDH.
- Endurance training results in increased lipid oxidation and decreased CHO utilization during exercise at the same absolute workload.
- Reduced CHO oxidation following training is due to reduced glycogenolysis (in turn regulated by reduced allosteric modulation of phosphorylase) and PDH activity (likely due to reduced pyruvate production).

- Liver glycogenolysis is reduced following training, as is muscle glucose uptake, the latter most likely due to reduced translocation of GLUT4, despite the fact that training enhances total muscle GLUT4.
- Lipid oxidation is increased following training, but this is not likely due to increased adipose tissue lipolysis, given that catecholamine release is decreased in the trained state.
- Muscle FFA uptake may increase with training, due to increased content of FAT/CD36 and FABPpm.
- IMTG oxidation probably represents the main source of increased lipid oxidation following training, which may be due to increased content of adipose tissue triglyceride lipase (a recently discovered lipase which also regulates IMTG lipolysis in skeletal muscle) and not HSL.
- Training also increases the capacity for mitochondrial LCFA uptake and oxidation, likely due to increased CPTI activity and enzymes of β-oxidation and the TCA cycle, such as β-HAD, CS and SDH.
- Training reduces protein oxidation, probably due to reduced activation of BCKAD and increased content of BCKAD kinase.
- The main cause of fatigue in prolonged endurance exercise is likely reduced muscle glycogen and blood glucose availability, which reduces the availability of substrate required to maintain the high CHO oxidation rates necessary to sustain high power outputs.
- CHO reduction may not only reduce substrate availability *per se* but may also regulate peripheral processes involved with contraction, such as Ca^{2+} release from the SR and maintenance of Na^+/K^+ ATPase activity.

10

High-intensity intermittent exercise

Learning outcomes

After studying this chapter, you should be able to:

- list the key reactions which could potentially contribute to ATP production during intermittent exercise;
- critically evaluate the regulatory processes contributing to energy provision during intermittent exercise;
- critically evaluate the impact of manipulating components of the intermittent protocol (such as duration/intensity of work and rest periods) on regulation of energy provision during exercise;
- critically evaluate the effects of CHO provision on substrate utilization and performance during intermittent exercise;
- critically evaluate the effects of intermittent exercise training on skeletal muscle adaptations depending on the characteristics of the training protocol;
- critically evaluate the effects of intermittent exercise training on metabolic regulation of substrate utilization during sub-maximal exercise;
- critically discuss potential metabolic causes of fatigue during intermittent exercise.

Key words

adenylate kinase reaction	glycogen depletion
ADP	glycogenolysis
aerobic system	glycolysis
aerobic training	glycogenolysis
allosteric effectors	glycolytic flux
AMP	H^+
anaerobic glycolysis	high intensity aerobic training
anaerobic system	high intensity interval training (HIT)
antioxidants	hydrogen peroxide
Ca^{2+} phosphate	intracellular lactate shuttle
cell-to-cell lactate shuttle	K^+
CHO	lactate
CHO oxidation	LCFA oxidation
Cori cycle	lipid oxidation
creatine supplementation	MCT1
energy continuum	MCT4
extracellular K^+	metabolic acidosis
FABPpm	molecular biology
FAT/CD36	Na^+ H^+ exchanger isoform 1 protein (NHE1)
free radicals	
GLUT4	
glycemic index	

Biochemistry for Sport and Exercise Metabolism, First Edition. Don MacLaren and James Morton.
© 2012 John Wiley & Sons, Ltd. Published 2012 by John Wiley & Sons, Ltd.

N-acetylcysteine (NAC)	PGC1α
	PFK
Na⁺ K⁺ ATPase	phosphorylase
NHE1	potassium
NAC	ROS
nutritional status	SIRT1
oxidative stress	speed
PCr depletion	speed endurance
PCr hydrolysis	superoxide
PCr resynthesis	temporary fatigue
PDH	Tfam

10.1 Overview of energy production in intermittent exercise

10.1.1 Definition and models of intermittent exercise

High-intensity intermittent exercise (HIE) refers to periods of exercise that are characterized by fluctuations in exercise intensity over a given time. Typically, HIE consists of repeated periods of high-intensity activity (near maximal or supra-maximal) interspersed with exercise of low to moderate intensity or, in some cases, complete inactivity (i.e. rest). This activity profile is, of course, characteristic of the exercise patterns of some of the world's most popular sports, such as soccer, basketball, rugby, tennis, boxing and hockey, etc.

Despite the relevance of HIE to the sporting world, research examining the metabolic responses to HIE has been limited compared with that carried out on either high-intensity or endurance exercise. Furthermore, given that HIE is essentially exercise consisting of both high-intensity (Chapter 8) and steady state (Chapter 9) activity, you can appreciate that the metabolic regulation of energy provision in this instance is more complex.

Researchers investigating metabolic regulation during HIE have traditionally used cycling protocols, knee extensor models or non-motorized treadmills. The use of these models is advantageous, as power output can be accurately

quantified and, as such, an accurate picture of how repeated bouts of high-intensity activity also affect the muscle's capacity to continually produce high force can be studied. Unfortunately, much of the research which has examined HIE have used exercise protocols involving work-rest ratios that are not entirely relevant to those sports mentioned above.

For example, most of the studies examine responses of skeletal muscle to short periods of maximal activity (ranging from 6–30 seconds), followed by a number of further maximal sprints (ranging from 2–12 seconds), interspersed with resting periods consisting of 30 seconds to four minutes of low-intensity activity or complete rest. In these protocols, the power outputs generated during the work period may be up to four times greater than that which is induced by VO_{2max}. Nevertheless, these protocols have proved useful, as *clamping* the protocols in this way allows for muscle biopsies to be obtained at relevant time-points, and thus an assessment of energy provision can be made during and between maximal efforts (Parolin *et al.*, 1999).

In addition to the above, several researchers have developed both laboratory- (Drust *et al.*, 2000) and field-based protocols (Nicholas *et al.*, 2000) which are designed to simulate the activity profile of team sports characterized by intermittent activity profiles such as soccer. In such instances, distance ran is often greater than 10 km and protocol duration is usually 75 minutes or more, as opposed to the protocols discussed above, which are only minutes in duration.

Given that the exact activity profile of team sports can vary from match to match (dependent on tactics, skill level, etc.) it is difficult to understand fully the regulation of energy provision during these types of sports. Nevertheless, these models are also advantageous as they provide a controlled experimental model that is more representative of the duration and intensity of activity inherent to sport (as opposed to the laboratory). They also allow for assessment of how nutritional and environmental influences may affect regulation of metabolism as well as outlining potential causes of fatigue.

10.1.2 Energy systems utilized in intermittent exercise

Given that HIE consists of both high-intensity (i.e. near maximal or supra-maximal activity) as well as low to moderate intensity activity, ATP production is fuelled by both the **anaerobic (*PCr hydrolysis, adenylate kinase reaction, anaerobic glycolysis*)** and **aerobic system**, where in the case of the latter, **CHO** is the predominant substrate. *Lipid oxidation* is also important, however, especially in the recovery periods between high-intensity efforts and also when the exercise period becomes more prolonged.

An overview of the energy producing reactions is shown below, where anaerobic reactions are shown in blue and aerobic reactions are shown in red.

$$ATP \leftrightarrow ADP + P_i$$
$$PCr + ADP + H^+ \leftrightarrow ATP + Cr$$
$$Glycogen + 3ADP + 3\ P_i \rightarrow 3ATP$$
$$+ 2Lactate^- + 2H^+$$
$$ADP + ADP \leftrightarrow ATP + AMP$$

$$C_6H_{12}O_6\ (glucose) + 6O_2 + 32(ADP + P_i)$$
$$\rightarrow 6CO_2 + 38H_2O + 32ATP$$
$$C_{16}H_{32}O_2\ (palmitate) + 23O_2 + 106(ADP + P_i)$$
$$\rightarrow 16CO_2 + 122H_2O + 106ATP$$

It is a common misconception that HIE is mainly fuelled by the anaerobic system (with no substantial input from oxidative metabolism) and, specifically, by anaerobic glycolysis. However, both the aerobic and anaerobic systems are activated from the *onset* of contraction, and in fact the contribution of the aerobic system becomes more important as the duration of the exercise increases. The interaction of metabolic pathways during exercise is often taught as an *energy continuum*, where the resulting perception is that there is an immediate switching *off* of one pathway and an immediate switching *on* of another pathway as exercise duration progresses. In reality, however, there is a switching on of *all* energy pathways at the onset of contractile activity and it is simply the percentage contribution of a specific pathway to ATP production which varies as the exercise bout progresses. The metabolic processes that regulate which metabolic pathway is most active at a given time are discussed in the next section.

10.2 Metabolic regulation in intermittent exercise

Given that CHO metabolism is integral to the high-intensity periods inherent to HIE, it is important to refresh ourselves with the regulation of the key enzymes involved in **glycogenolysis**, **glycolysis** and **CHO oxidation**. A schematic of these reactions is shown in Figure 10.1 along with some of the positive and negative **allosteric effectors** which can regulate **phosphorylase**, **PFK** and **PDH** activity. In the subsequent text, we review some of the key research studies which have examined metabolic regulation during HIE, and Figure 10.1 should be used as a reference point to help with understanding enzyme regulation during HIE.

In one of the classic studies of metabolic regulation during HIE, Gaitanos *et al.* (1993) quantified anaerobic energy provision in male subjects during 10×6-second maximal sprints on a cycle ergometer, interspersed with 30 seconds of rest. Muscle biopsies were obtained from the vastus lateralis before and after the first and tenth sprint. These authors observed a progressive decrease in both peak and mean power during each sprint throughout the duration of the exercise protocol (see Figure 10.2).

On the basis of calculations from muscle metabolite data, the rate of ATP production during sprint 1 was $14.9\ \mathrm{mmol.kg\ dw^{-1}.s^{-1}}$, where degradation of PCr accounted for 49% of ATP resynthesis and the remainder was largely accounted for by glycolysis (see Figure 10.3). In contrast, in sprint 10, anaerobic ATP production was reduced by 35% and had fallen to $5.3\ \mathrm{mmol.kg\ dw^{-1}.s^{-1}}$, and the contribution of glycolysis had markedly fallen to 16%. The 30-second recovery periods were not sufficient for complete *PCr resynthesis*, and glycogenolysis was also reduced in sprint 10 compared with sprint 1 (see Table 10.1). The latter occurred despite high plasma adrenaline concentrations which would be expected to sustain glycogen breakdown.

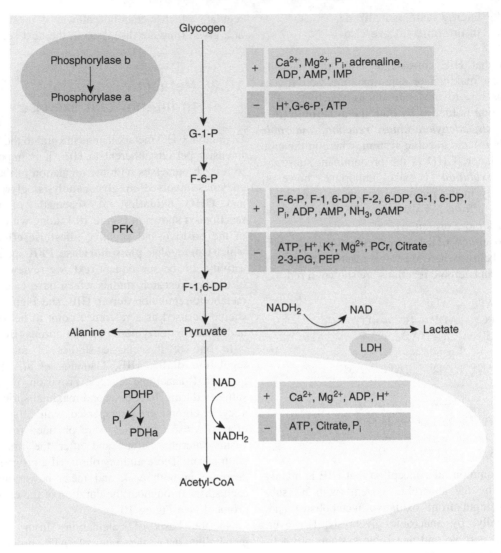

Figure 10.1 Schematic overview of the regulation of key components of CHO metabolism (adapted from Bangsbo, 1996)

The reduction in glycogenolysis with repeated sprints therefore suggests that aerobic metabolism becomes more important as HIE progresses although, in this study, oxidative energy provision was not assessed. Nevertheless, other studies have shown that both whole body (see Figure 10.4) and local oxygen uptake (see Figure 10.5) increases with repeated bouts of intense exercise.

In order to provide a mechanistic insight into the apparent shift in energy system utilization,

Parolin *et al.* (1999) conducted a study where male subjects performed three 30-second maximal sprints interspersed with four minutes of rest. This study was unique in that muscle biopsies were obtained *during* the first and third sprint (at 0, 6, 15 and 30 seconds) and, as such, a time-course of the metabolic responses and enzyme activation could be obtained.

Consistent with earlier observations discussed above, glycogen utilization was lower during

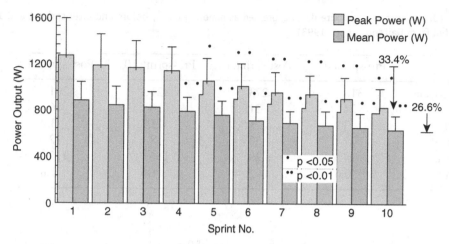

Figure 10.2   Peak and mean power output for each of the 10 × 6-second sprints (adapted from Gaitanos *et al.*, 1993)

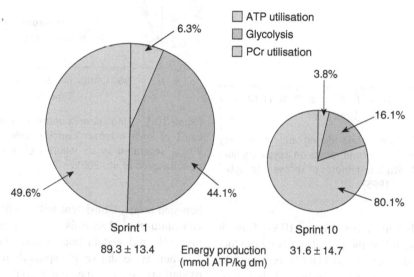

Figure 10.3   Total anaerobic ATP production and percentage contribution from ATP, PCr and glycolysis during sprint 1 and 10. The smaller pie chart for sprint 10 reflects a smaller anaerobic ATP production (adapted from Gaitanos *et al.*, 1993)

sprint 3 compared with sprint 1, and neither muscle lactate nor pyruvate increased in sprint 3, whereas a marked increase was observed in sprint 1 (see Figure 10.6). In accordance with reduced rates of glycogenolysis (see Figure 10.7), pyruvate production and lactate accumulation was reduced in sprint 3 compared with sprint 1 (see Figure 10.8).

When examining enzyme activation, phosphorylase activation (as expressed by percentage in the *a* form) increased during the first 15 seconds of bout 1, then declined thereafter and also did not show any further increase in bout 3. PDH activation was progressively increased during bout 1 and also displayed greater activation at the onset of bout 3

Table 10.1   Muscle metabolite data, expressed as mmol.kg dw^{-1}, before and after sprint 1 and 10 (adapted from Gaitanos *et al.*, 1993)

	Pre-sprint 1	Post-sprint 1	Pre-sprint 10	Post-sprint 10
Glycogen	316	273	221	201
ATP	24	21	16	16
ADP	3	3.5	2.7	3.2
PCr	77	32	38	12
Lactate	4	29	116	112
Pyruvate	0.6	2	1.6	1.8

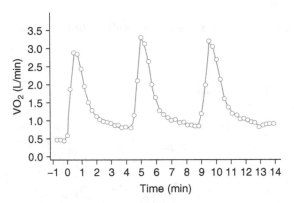

Figure 10.4   Oxygen uptake during and in recovery from three maximal 30-second sprints on a cycle ergometer interspersed with four minutes of recovery (adapted from Putman *et al.*, 1995)

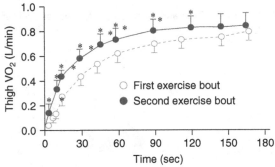

Figure 10.5   Thigh oxygen uptake during 2 × 3-minute bouts of knee extensor exercise undertaken at 120% VO$_{2max}$ separated by six minutes of recovery (adapted from Bangsbo *et al.*, 2001)

compared with bout 1 (see Figure 10.9). Thus, it becomes apparent that the rate of pyruvate production during bout 1 exceeded PDH activity, resulting in lactate accumulation. In bout 3, however, pyruvate oxidation was more closely matched to pyruvate production (thus resulting in minimal further lactate accumulation), owing to the reduced rates of glycogenolysis and greater PDH activity.

The calculated contribution of PCr hydrolysis, glycolysis and oxidative phosphorylation during sprints 1 and 3 are shown in Figure 10.10. In accordance with a decline in average power output between sprints, ATP turnover rate was reduced

between bouts. Consistent with earlier studies, the contribution of glycolysis to ATP turnover was significantly reduced in bout 3 compared with bout 1, whereas oxidative phosphorylation (i.e. CHO oxidation) became the major contributor to ATP production after only six seconds of sprinting in bout 3. In order to catalyze the high rates of glycogen breakdown in bout 1, both transformational and post-transformational regulation of phosphorylase activity was likely needed.

Transformational regulation of phosphorylase in bout 1 was likely mediated by **Ca^{2+}** release and its effects on phosphorylase kinase, whereas post-transformational regulation was likely achieved by

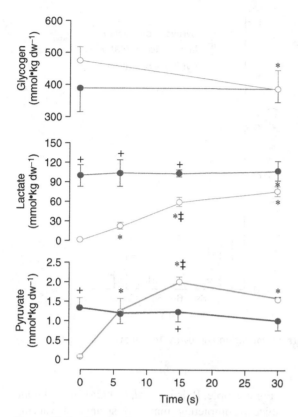

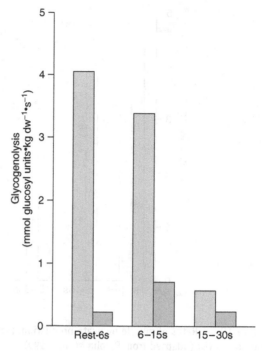

Figure 10.7   Rates of muscle glycogenolysis during bout 1 (blue bars) and bout 3 (pink bars) (adapted from Parolin *et al.*, 1999)

Figure 10.6   Muscle glycogen, lactate and pyruvate at rest and during bout 1 (green symbols) and bout 3 (red symbols) (adapted from Parolin *et al.*, 1999)

increased substrate provision of P_i (provided from *PCr hydrolysis*) as well as the presence of positive allosteric modulators such as **AMP**. The reduced rates of glycogenolysis in the second half of bout 1, as well as throughout bout 3, coincided with the reversion of phosphorylase *a* to *b*. These data suggest that the Ca^{2+} mediated phosphorylase transformation was being overridden by other factors, potentially H^+-induced inhibition of phosphorylase kinase.

The progressive increase in PDH activation during bout 1 was likely mediated by Ca^{2+}-induced activation of PDH phosphatase, as well as pyruvate-induced inactivation of PDH kinase, thereby collectively rendering PDH

active. Increased pyruvate production would, of course, also serve as a substrate for the PDH reaction. Furthermore, whereas increased H^+ may down-regulate phosphorylase transformation, in the case of PDH regulation it serves to increase transformation. The increased presence of these metabolites at the onset of bout 3 therefore likely contributed to the more rapid increase in PDH activation during this sprint.

The authors therefore postulated that H^+ production serves an important regulatory function, by which it may spare glycogen stores and limit further lactate accumulation but also stimulate aerobic metabolism. Indeed, the enhanced activity of PDH ensures that pyruvate production is more closely matched to oxidation, thus increasing acetyl-CoA provision for the TCA cycle.

In reviewing these data, you should now appreciate (and contrary to common perception) that the

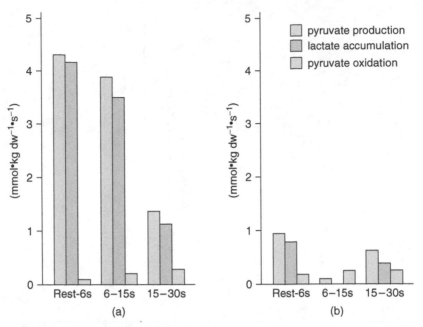

Figure 10.8   Rates of muscle pyruvate production, lactate accumulation and pyruvate oxidation during bout 1 (a) and bout 3 (b) (adapted from Parolin *et al.*, 1999)

aerobic system is very important during HIE. In fact, depending on the actual intensity and duration of both the interval and recovery period, as well as the work : rest ratio (see next section), *oxidative phosphorylation* may become the predominant contributor to ATP production, especially for prolonged HIE. For this reason, it is essential that athletes involved in HIE sports have well-developed aerobic systems and high maximal oxygen uptakes in order to ensure high rates of oxygen delivery and utilization by the exercising muscles.

10.3 Effects of manipulating work-rest intensity and ratio

While we have covered some of the underlying principles of metabolic regulation during HIE, it is important to appreciate how subtle differences in the intensity and duration of both the interval and recovery periods, as well as the work-rest ratio, can affect the metabolic responses to the exercise protocol.

For example, Balsom *et al.* (1992a) studied male subjects completing maximal sprints of varying distance of 15, 30 or 40 m in an indoor running track. Each sprint was separated by 30 seconds and the subjects completed sprints until a total distance of 600 m had been ran. In this way, the 15, 30 and 40 m protocols consisted of 40, 20 or 15 sprints, respectively.

However, despite the fact that recovery between sprints was always 30 seconds, and the same distance was ran in each protocol, the metabolic and performance responses were markedly different between protocols. Indeed, the 15 m sprints (which typically took 2.5 seconds to complete) could be performed with minimal decrements in sprint time (see Figure 10.11) and metabolic stress, as indicated by plasma hypoxanthine and uric acid (see Figure 10.12) and lactate (see Figure 10.13), whereas performance appeared to decline and the metabolic stress was greater in the longer sprint conditions. It appears, therefore, that simply increasing sprint duration from 2.5 seconds to 5–6 seconds can significantly alter the pattern of energy system utilization.

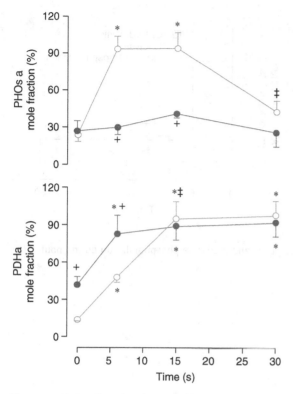

Figure 10.9 Phosphorylase and PDH activity (expressed as per cent in the active *a* form) during bout 1 (green symbols) and bout 3 (red symbols) (adapted from Parolin *et al.*, 1999)

In a subsequent study, the same group examined the effects of recovery duration on the ability to repeatedly perform 15 × 40 m maximal sprints (Balsom *et al.*, 1992b). In this instance, recovery between sprints was 30, 60 or 120 seconds. The decline in sprint performance was greatest with 30 seconds of recovery, and post-exercise blood lactate and plasma hypoxanthine was also greatest in this condition. The authors speculated that the decrement in sprint performance with the 30-second recovery protocol was most likely due to insufficient resynthesis of PCr and/or inability to restore muscle pH to resting values.

In keeping with this theory, recall that Gaitanos *et al.* (1993) observed PCr resynthesis to be incomplete when recovery between six-second sprints was restricted to 30 seconds (see

Table 10.1), whereas Parolin *et al.* (1999) observed that four minutes of recovery between 30-second maximal sprints was sufficient to allow for almost maximal PCr resynthesis. Similarly, Bogdanis *et al.* (1996) observed almost complete PCr resynthesis with four minutes of recovery after a 30-second maximal sprint (see Figure 10.14).

Unfortunately, studies examining the effects of intensity and duration of both the interval and recovery period on PCr hydrolysis and resynthesis are limited in sport-specific contexts (due to the need for continual muscle sampling), but the consensus is that higher intensity activity will cause greater depletion and that greater durations of recovery will lead to greater resynthesis. Furthermore, resynthesis rates are dependent on blood flow and oxygen delivery and, for this reason, trained individuals whom have a well-developed aerobic capacity exhibit greater resynthesis rates (Bogdanis *et al.*, 1996).

In relation to quantifying substrate utilization of CHO and lipids during *prolonged* HIE, Essen *et al.* (1978) demonstrated that CHO and lipid oxidation was not different between 60 minutes of HIE (15 seconds of exercise at 100% VO_{2max} interspersed with 15 seconds of rest) and continuous exercise (90 minutes of exercise at the same average oxygen consumption and power output as the intermittent protocol, i.e. approximately 55% VO_{2max}). In contrast, Christmass *et al.* (1999a) more recently observed that CHO oxidation is greater, and lipid oxidation lower, during HIE (90 minutes of exercise consisting of 12 seconds at 120% VO_{2max} interspersed with 18 seconds of rest), compared with 90 minutes of continuous exercise matched for the same energy expenditure and average intensity as the intermittent protocol, which corresponded to approximately 70% VO_{2max}.

In this instance, the discrepancy between studies is likely to be due to the higher work period intensity (e.g. 120 versus 100% of VO_{2max}) as well as the higher average intensity (e.g. 70 versus 55% of VO_{2max}), especially given the evidence discussed in Chapter 9 on the role of exercise intensity on substrate utilization. Furthermore, Christmass *et al.* observed

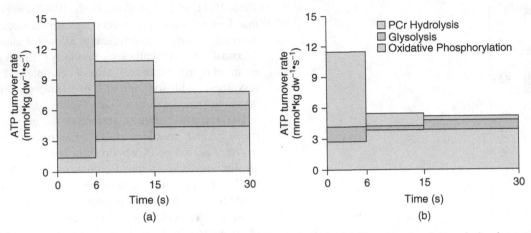

Figure 10.10   ATP turnover rates from PCr hydrolysis, glycolysis and oxidative phosphorylation during bout 1 (a) and bout 3 (b) (adapted from Parolin *et al.*, 1999)

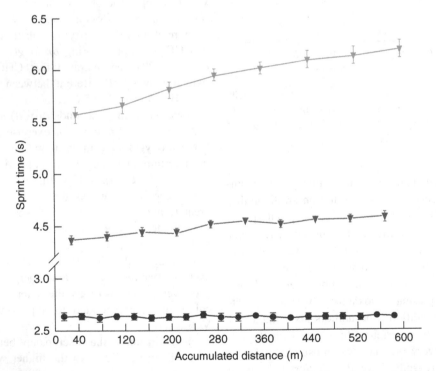

Figure 10.11   Sprint times for 15 m protocol (blue symbols), 30 m protocol (red symbols) and 40 m protocol (green symbols) (adapted from Balsom *et al.*, 1992a)

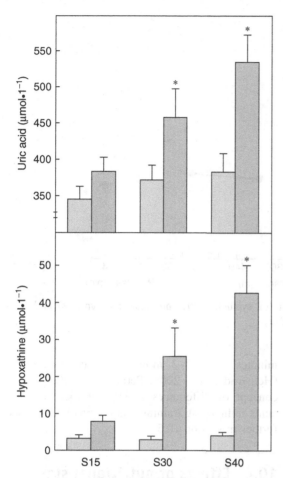

Figure 10.12 Plasma hypoxanthine and uric acid before (blue bars) and after (pink bars) 15 m protocol (S15), 30 m protocol (S30) and 40 m protocol (S40) (adapted from Balsom *et al.*, 1992a)

plasma glycerol to be similar between intermittent and continuous exercise, suggesting that reduced lipolysis did not contribute to the reduced rates of lipid oxidation in intermittent exercise, compared with continuous exercise. Rather, such an attenuation of lipid oxidation was probably peripheral in nature, owing to the effects of high rates of **glycolytic flux** on **LCFA oxidation** within the muscle itself (see Chapter 9).

Indeed, in a subsequent study, Christmass *et al.* (1999b) examined the effects of 40 minutes of intermittent running at 120% VO$_{2max}$ when undertaken as short (6 seconds on, 9 seconds

off) or long (24 seconds on, 36 seconds off) interval exercise protocols. In this instance, CHO oxidation was higher and lipid oxidation lower in the long interval protocol compared with the short, most likely due to the negative effects of accelerated rates of glycolytic flux on limiting lipid metabolism within the muscle. These findings have more recently been confirmed by Price & Halabi (2005) and Price & Moss (2007).

These laboratory models of HIE, however, should not be interpreted to mean that lipid oxidation is not quantitatively important during HIE that is relevant to *sport*. In fact, plasma FFA can rise considerably during sports such as soccer, especially during the second half of games (Krustrup *et al.*, 2006). These findings are most likely due to the combined effects of the lower relative exercise intensity (given that low to moderate intensity activity represent the most frequent form of activity performed) as well as hormonal regulation through adrenaline.

Despite the clear evidence that subtle alterations in the characteristics of the HIE protocol can greatly affect energy system utilization and metabolic regulation (even when total work done is comparable between protocol variations), there are few studies in this area. However, the application of this work is very important, especially in relation to optimizing training programs for the desired goal.

For example, if development of **speed** is the training aim, then clearly the intensity of the sprints should be maximal and their duration less than ten seconds, so as to focus on the utilization of PCr hydrolysis and glycolysis for the main contributors to ATP turnover (Mohr *et al.*, 2007). Similarly, recovery between sprints should be at least 60 seconds, in an attempt to maximize PCr resynthesis and restore muscle pH (Mohr *et al.*, 2007).

Alternatively, if it is the ability to continuously produce high power outputs for sustained periods of time that is to be trained (i.e. **speed endurance**), then the duration of the interval should be increased to approximately 30–90 seconds (with approximately an equal recovery period), so as to tax fully the glycolytic and oxidative system (Mohr *et al.*, 2007).

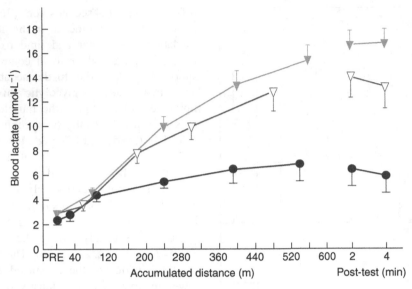

Figure 10.13 Blood lactate during the 15 m protocol (blue symbols), 30 m protocol (red symbols) and 40 m protocol (green symbols) (adapted from Balsom *et al.*, 1992a)

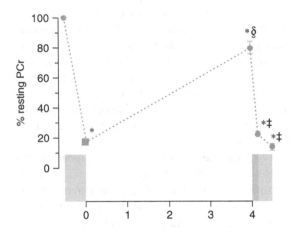

Figure 10.14 PCr concentration during two maximal sprints on a cycle ergometer separated by 4 minutes. Sprint 1 was 30 seconds (first blue bar) and sprint two was either 10 seconds (pink bar) or 30 seconds (second blue bar) (adapted from Bogdanis *et al.*, 1996)

Finally, if maximizing development of the *aerobic system* (both oxygen uptake and oxidative capacity of skeletal muscle) is the training aim, then it is likely that the intensity and duration of the interval should be close to VO_{2max} for 2–4

minutes, with 2–3 minutes of active recovery (Helgerud *et al.*, 2007; Perry *et al.*, 2008). This concept of differences in HIE protocol components influencing training adaptations is discussed further in section 10.5.

10.4 Effects of nutritional status

In contrast to endurance exercise, there are relatively few studies which have examined the influence of **nutritional status** on the regulation of substrate utilization during HIE. Furthermore, most of these studies have largely focused on descriptive responses (such as measuring plasma metabolites and whole-body oxidation rates, etc.), as opposed to detailed measurements within the muscle, where examining the *regulation* of metabolic processes (through measurement of enzyme activity and associated regulatory metabolites) is often the main experimental aim (as discussed in Chapter 9).

In this section, we review studies which have examined the influence of nutritional status on substrate utilization during more prolonged HIE protocols (given their relevance to sport), where

Table 10.2 Plasma metabolites before (pre-game), at 45 min and after a 90 min soccer match (post-game) commenced with normal (N-CHO) or lowered (L-CHO) muscle glycogen (adapted from Balsom *et al.*, 1999a)

	N-CHO Pre-game	N-CHO 45 min	N-CHO Post-game	L-CHO Pre-game	L-CHO 45 min	L-CHO Post-game
FFA(mmol.L^{-1})	0.32	0.53	0.89	0.63	0.91	1.39
Glycerol (μmol.L^{-1})	77	202	266	106	293	366
Glucose (mmol.L^{-1})	4.5	8	7.2	5.1	7.5	5.8
Lactate (mmol.L^{-1})	1.1	4.5	3.9	1.3	3.6	3.0

the focus is on pre-exercise muscle glycogen availability and the provision of carbohydrate in the hours before and during the exercise itself. To our knowledge, there are no studies to date which have examined the effects of fat-loading or high-fat pre-exercise meals on metabolism and performance during HIE.

10.4.1 Muscle glycogen availability

In one of the most practical studies in this area, Balsom *et al.* (1999a) videoed six male soccer players during a 90-minute friendly soccer game that was commenced with either normal (400 mmol.kg dw^{-1}) or reduced (280 mmol.kg dw^{-1}) muscle glycogen stores. Venous blood samples were obtained before the game, at half-time and afterwards (see Table 10.2). Plasma FFA and glycerol were significantly higher and glucose significantly lower when the game was commenced with reduced glycogen stores, compared with normal glycogen levels. Furthermore, the normal glycogen condition was associated with increased percentage of time engaged in high-intensity activity, an important performance parameter for soccer-specific performance.

While the regulatory mechanisms underpinning these responses cannot be elucidated in this study, they are likely to be similar to those outlined in Chapter 9. In a laboratory based study, Balsom *et al.* (1999b) also examined the effects of high (540 mmol.kg dw^{-1}) or low (180 mmol.kg dw^{-1}) muscle glycogen concentration on the ability to

perform repeated 6-second sprints, interspersed with 30-second rest periods. As expected, exercise capacity was significantly longer for the high-glycogen condition (178 minutes) compared to the low condition (67 minutes), and RER values were significantly higher, thus indicating enhanced CHO utilization. For these reasons, it is common practice for athletes engaged in high-intensity team sports to consume a high-CHO diet in the days leading up to games in order to ensure high pre-match muscle glycogen stores.

10.4.2 Pre-exercise CHO ingestion

Recent research in this area has examined the effects of the **glycemic index** (GI) of the pre-exercise meal (Little *et al.*, 2010a) on substrate metabolism during laboratory-based HIE designed to simulate the activity patterns of soccer (Drust *et al.*, 2000). This research is particularly important, given that low-GI pre-exercise meals may alter substrate utilization in favour of lipid oxidation and spare muscle glycogen (as has been observed for moderate-intensity continuous exercise – see Chapter 9) for later utilization, such as in the later stage of competition (e.g. the second half).

Little *et al.* (2010a) observed that lipid oxidation was greater and CHO oxidation lower during fasted conditions, compared with pre-exercise CHO feeding (see Figure 10.15). As discussed in Chapter 9, such findings are likely mediated by the insulin-induced attenuation of lipolysis, thereby reducing plasma FFA availability (see

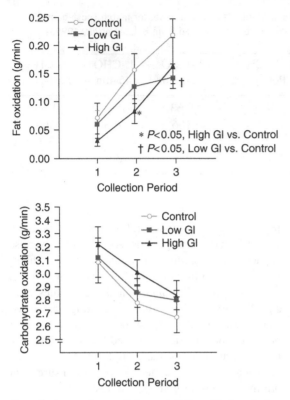

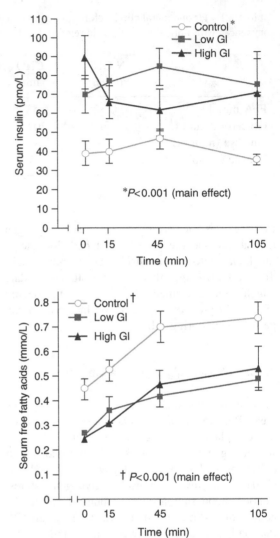

Figure 10.15 Rates of fat and CHO oxidation during 90 minutes of soccer specific exercise undertaken in fasted conditions (control) or when LGI or HGI pre-exercise meal was consumed two hours prior to exercise (adapted from Little *et al.*, 2010a)

Figure 10.16). However, there was no difference in substrate utilization between HGI or LGI meals, suggesting that GI appears to exert minimal influences during HIE exercise, possibly due to an overriding effect of the high-intensity exercise periods associated with HIE against any differences in insulin, glucose or FFA availability between conditions.

These authors also observed that repeated sprint performance undertaken after the 90-minute simulated game (distance ran during 5 × 1-minute sprints interspersed with 2.5 minutes of recovery) was greater in the CHO conditions compared with fasted conditions, though there was no difference between LGI or HGI meals. It was suggested that the enhanced performance with CHO feeding was due to higher muscle glycogen availability prior to

Figure 10.16 Serum insulin and FFA concentrations during 105 minutes of soccer specific exercise undertaken in fasted conditions (control) or when LGI or HGI pre-exercise meal was consumed two hours prior to exercise (adapted from Little *et al.*, 2010a)

the sprint testing in the CHO trials, compared with fasted (>300 versus $200\,\text{mmol.kg}\,\text{dw}^{-1}$, respectively). Such data suggest there are no advantages to consuming LGI versus HGI pre-exercise meals for prolonged HIE in terms of augmenting lipid oxidation, sparing endogenous CHO utilization and also for repeated sprint performance.

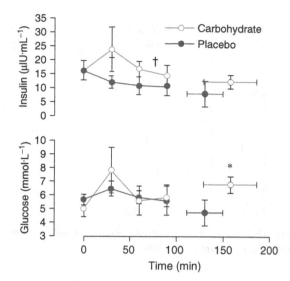

Figure 10.17 Plasma insulin and glucose concentrations during exhaustive soccer specific exercise undertaken with CHO or placebo ingestion prior to and during exercise (adapted from Foskett *et al.*, 2008)

Furthermore, because most athletes in these real-world sporting situations would consume further CHO (usually in the form of HGI drinks or gels) during the game and at half-time, any small advantages to consuming LGI pre-exercise meals (which were perhaps undetectable in the experimental design) are likely to be further negated. Nevertheless, due to the limited data in this area, future research is required before clear practical recommendations can be made.

10.4.3 CHO ingestion during exercise

Similarly to the previous section, research in this area has generally used protocols involving simulations of team sport activity. For example, Nicholas *et al.* (1999) examined the effects of ingesting a 6% CHO solution on metabolism and performance during a prolonged indoor shuttle running protocol. These authors observed that muscle glycogen utilization (when commenced with normal glycogen stores of 350–400 mmol.kg dw^{-1}) during 90 minutes of HIE was reduced when CHO was ingested during exercise, especially in type II fibres. Nearly a decade later,

the same group repeated the study but, on this occasion (Foskett *et al.*, 2008), exercise was commenced with elevated pre-exercise glycogen stores (>500 mmol.kg dw^{-1}), as would be expected following the CHO-loading strategies that team sport athletes are advised to adopt. In this experiment, subjects also continued running until exhaustion after completion of the 90 minute protocol so as to provide a measure of exercise capacity.

As expected, plasma insulin and glucose were higher (see Figure 10.17) and glycerol and FFA lower (see Figure 10.18) in the CHO condition, compared with placebo ingestion. exercise capacity was also greater in the CHO trial, compared with a placebo (158 versus 131 minutes), despite the fact on this occasion mixed muscle glycogen utilization was not different between trials (see Figure 10.19). It was therefore suggested that the enhanced exercise capacity may have been due to the maintenance of plasma glucose availability and high rates of CHO oxidation required to sustain HIE.

Unfortunately, one of the limitations of using this exercise model of shuttle running is that substrate utilization rates cannot be quantified

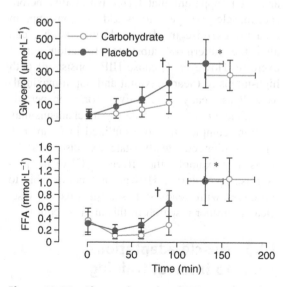

Figure 10.18 Plasma glycerol and FFA concentrations during exhaustive soccer specific exercise undertaken with CHO or placebo ingestion prior to and during exercise (adapted from Foskett *et al.*, 2008)

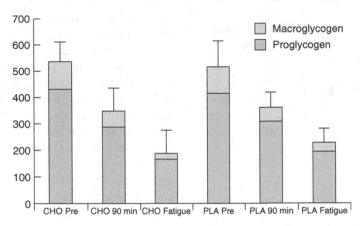

Figure 10.19   Muscle glycogen concentration during exhaustive soccer specific exercise undertaken with CHO or placebo (PLA) ingestion prior to and during exercise (adapted from Foskett *et al.*, 2008)

unless portable gas analysers that can be strapped to the subject are used. Nevertheless, data from our group using a laboratory-based simulation of soccer-specific exercise (Drust *et al.*, 2000) has confirmed that CHO ingestion during HIE augments plasma glucose, insulin and CHO oxidation while attenuating plasma glycerol, FFA and lipid oxidation (Clarke *et al.*, 2008).

In summarizing the limited data available in this area, it is apparent that CHO availability before (i.e. muscle glycogen stores and the consumption of a pre-exercise meal) and during exercise can alter the pattern of substrate utilization during exercise. However, because HIE consists of both high-intensity (near maximal and supra-maximal) as well as steady state activity (or even periods of complete rest), the regulatory mechanisms may be more complex to those outlined in Chapter 9, where prolonged steady state exercise was the focus. For example, the effects of GI of the pre-exercise meal during HIE are not comparable to those seen with steady-state sub-maximal exercise. Clearly, further research in this area is required.

10.5 Muscle adaptations to interval training

Traditional approaches to endurance training normally involve prolonged periods of moderate-intensity exercise. In recent years, however, researchers have become increasingly interested in examining the efficacy of **high-intensity interval training (HIT)** as opposed to continuous training approaches. HIT protocols usually consist of repeated supra-maximal sprints (ranging from 6–30 seconds in duration) interspersed with rest periods from 1–4 minutes or, alternatively, longer interval durations such as 1–4 minutes that are undertaken at near maximal intensity (i.e. 90% VO_{2max}). Dependent on the specifics of the training protocol, these interventions could be further classified as *speed/sprint, speed endurance* or *high-intensity aerobic interval training*.

When taken together, these protocols have proved successful in inducing the typical skeletal muscle adaptations that are normally associated with traditional high-volume endurance training. In some instances, researchers have observed that HIT is in fact a more time-efficient and potent training stimulus, compared with continuous approaches, despite the fact that the training volume is markedly reduced. The use of HIT is particularly useful for athletes engaged in intermittent-type sports, given that it has the capacity to develop components of the anaerobic and aerobic systems (MacDougall *et al.*, 1998), both of which are heavily utilized in this type of sporting activity.

Some researchers have also shown that HIT can improve aspects of metabolic health such as insulin sensitivity (Babraj *et al.*, 2009; Whyte *et al.*, 2010; Richards *et al.*, 2010), thus demonstrating the relevance of this training stimulus beyond that of the sporting domain.

The most informative studies undertaken thus far are those which have directly compared HIT to moderate-intensity continuous training protocols. In this regard, Gibala and colleagues have conducted two studies testing Wingate type training protocols (i.e. $4 - 6 \times 30$-second maximal sprints on a cycle ergometer interspersed with four minutes of recovery) versus traditional endurance training (1–2 hours of cycling at 65% VO_{2max}).

In the first of these studies, subjects performed six training sessions over 14 days, such that training time commitment was 2.5 hours for the HIT group and 10.5 hours for the endurance training (ET) group (Gibala *et al.*, 2006). Training decreased the time required to complete 50 and 750 kJ time trials, though there was no difference between groups. Similarly, training increased cytochrome C oxidase (COX) activity, COXII and COXIV protein content as well muscle buffering capacity and resting glycogen content, with comparable improvements between training groups.

In their subsequent study, the authors extended the duration of training to six weeks such that total training times were nine hours for the HIT group and 27 hours for the ET group (Burgomaster *et al.*, 2008). In terms of adaptations in resting muscle, training induced comparable increases in maximal activity of CS and β-HAD as well as total protein content of PDH and **PGC1α**. The latter protein is of particular interest as it is thought to be a *master regulator* of mitochondrial biogenesis. In this study, the subjects also performed 60 minutes of sub-maximal exercise at 65% of pre-training VO_{2max} before and after training in order to assess training-induced shifts in substrate utilization. Training decreased CHO oxidation, muscle glycogen utilization and PCr hydrolysis, and increased lipid oxidation during exercise, again with comparable magnitudes of change between training protocols. The ability of HIT to alter substrate utilization during exercise was consistent with earlier observations from the same researchers'

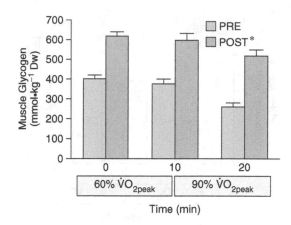

Figure 10.20 Muscle glycogen content at rest and after 10 minutes of exercise at 60 and 90% VO_{2max} before and after 2 weeks of HIT (adapted from Burgomaster *et al.*, 2006)

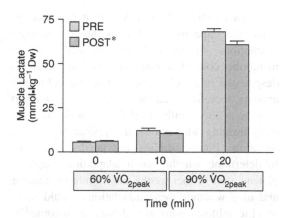

Figure 10.21 Muscle lactate content at rest and after 10 minutes of exercise at 60 and 90% VO_{2max} before and after 2 weeks of HIT (adapted from Burgomaster *et al.*, 2006)

laboratory, although in this case HIT was studied in the absence of an ET control group (Burgomaster *et al.*, 2006). On this occasion, glycogenolysis (see Figure 10.20) and lactate accumulation (see Figure 10.21) during moderate to high-intensity exercise were reduced following training. A contributing factor to this may be training-induced increases in PDH activity during exercise (see Figure 10.22), such that there was a closer matching between pyruvate production and oxidation.

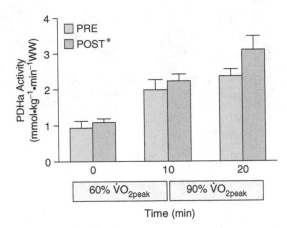

Figure 10.22 Muscle PDH activity at rest and after 10 minutes of exercise at 60 and 90% VO$_{2max}$ before and after 2 weeks of HIT (adapted from Burgomaster *et al.*, 2006)

Taken together, these series of studies demonstrate the capacity of HIT to induce oxidative adaptations of skeletal muscle and improve metabolic control during sub-maximal exercise, despite the relatively reduced training volume. It appears, therefore, that increased *training intensity* may be a more influential factor in determining early training adaptations, as opposed to *training duration*. Future studies are needed, however, to determine whether such adaptations begin to plateau after further weeks and months of training, and also whether these adaptations would occur in elite athletes who are already accustomed to the demands of intense training.

In this regard, Iaia *et al.* (2009) observed that when endurance-trained runners replaced their normal endurance training routine (approximately 45 km of continuous running per week) with four weeks of speed endurance training (8 − 12 × 30-second sprints interspersed with three minutes of rest), muscle oxidative capacity (as reflected by CS and β-HAD activity), capillarization, VO$_{2max}$ and 10 km time trial did not decline, despite the reduced training volume. Furthermore, running economy was improved in the speed endurance training group, whereas those runners who maintained their normal training programme showed no improvement.

In a similar study, the same researchers showed that four weeks of speed endurance training improved exercise capacity during progressive high-intensity intermittent shuttle running, as well as during constant load supra-maximal exercise at 130% VO$_{2max}$ (Iaia *et al.*, 2008). These changes in performance were accompanied by training-induced increases in the muscle content of the α_1 and α_2 subunits of **Na$^+$ K$^+$ ATPase** pump protein, as well as the *Na$^+$ H$^+$ exchanger isoform 1 protein* (**NHE1**). None of these changes were observed in the endurance training group. Interestingly, venous K$^+$ during exhaustive exercise was lower after training, thus suggesting a role of the Na$^+$ K$^+$ ATPase pump in maintaining K$^+$ homeostasis in the aetiology of fatigue during repeated intense exercise. This concept is discussed further in Section 10.6.

The observation of increased Na$^+$ K$^+\alpha_2$ subunit and NHE1 content after speed endurance training was also observed by Mohr *et al.* (2007). However, when the interval training protocol was altered to 15 × 6-second sprints with one minute of recovery, so as to reflect *speed*-type training, these adaptations were not apparent. The specific muscle adaptations induced by speed endurance training (that were not evident with speed training) were suggested as a potential mechanism underpinning the improved exercise capacity during an exhaustive treadmill test as well as high-intensity intermittent shuttle running. In contrast, subjects in the speed training group displayed improved 50 m sprint time, which was associated with increased muscle CK activity, while these changes did not occur in the speed endurance training group. These data provide further support for the training principle of *specificity*, surmising that training adaptations are highly specific to the physiological stimulus.

We discussed earlier in this chapter how subtle alterations in components (duration and intensity of interval and recovery period) of the HIE protocol can alter the metabolic responses to exercise. This study provides further support for the application of this concept in terms of modulating training adaptation (see Figure 10.23).

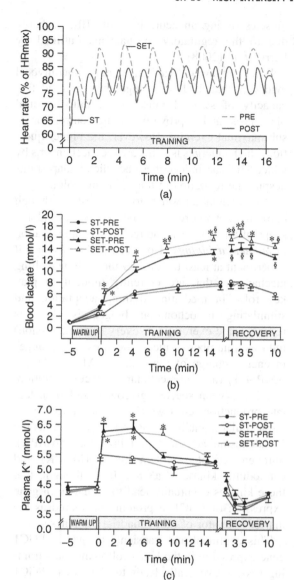

Figure 10.23 Heart rate (a), blood lactate (b) and blood potassium (c) during a sprint training (ST) and speed endurance training (SET) session undertaken before (PRE) and after (POST) the training period (adapted from Mohr *et al.*, 2007)

In addition to HIT protocols with work intervals from 6–30 seconds, several researchers have investigated the effect of HIT training which are more reflective of *high-intensity aerobic training*, i.e. intervals lasting 1–4 minutes performed at 90–100% VO_{2max}

For example, Little *et al.* (2010b) observed that six sessions of $8 - 12\times$ one-minute bouts of cycling at 100% VO_{2max}, interspersed with 75 seconds of recovery (performed over a two-week period) increased resting muscle glycogen content, CS and COX activity and total protein content of COXII, COXIV, CS, **GLUT4**, mitochondrial transcription factor A (**Tfam**), silent information regulator T1 (**SIRT1**) and nuclear abundance of PGC1α. The adaptive responses of the latter three proteins, especially the *nuclear localization* of PGC1α, is particularly interesting, considering their role as signalling proteins in regulating mitochondrial biogenesis.

Perry *et al.* (2008) have also examined the effect of HIT on muscle adaptation and metabolism by studying a training model consisting of longer durations of intervals (ten repeated four-minute intervals at 90% VO_{2max} separated by two minutes of rest). After a six-week training period, there was increased activity of muscle CS, β-HAD and PDH, and increased content of COXIV protein and glycogen. Training also increased the content of the metabolic transport proteins involved in glucose (GLUT4), lipid (**FAT/CD36, FABPpm**) and lactate (**MCT1, MCT4**) transport.

Increased GLUT4 content is consistent with studies using 30-second interval-type training protocols (Burgomaster *et al.*, 2007; Little *et al.*, 2010b), while some (Burgomaster *et al.*, 2007) but not others (Iaia *et al.*, 2008) have also observed increased content of the lactate transport proteins. More importantly, these authors observed training-induced improvements in the lipid transport proteins, which has not been observed after the Wingate training protocols, even after six weeks of training (Burgomaster *et al.*, 2007). Taken together, such data suggest that longer durations of intervals may be needed to induce the signal (which may be simply to increase the flux through the relevant metabolic pathway) required to stimulate up-regulation of some of the transport proteins involved in metabolic regulation, especially for those involved in lipid metabolism.

In terms of substrate utilization during intense exercise, Perry *et al.* (2008) also observed that HIT

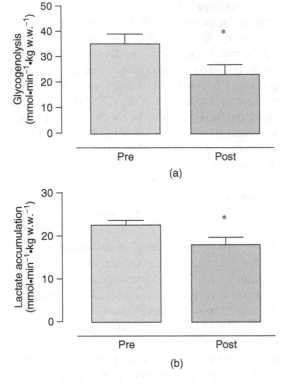

Figure 10.24   Muscle glycogen utilization (a) and lactate accumulation (b) during 5 min of exercise at 90% VO_{2max} undertaken pre- and post- 6 weeks of HIT (adapted from Perry *et al.*, 2008)

reduced rates of PCr degradation, glycogenolysis and muscle lactate accumulation during five minutes of exercise at 90% VO_{2max} (see Figure 10.24), the latter of which is likely due to smaller increases in **ADP, AMP** and P_i, thus providing conditions that favour reduced activation of phosphorylase (see Table 10.3). Consistent with classic adaptations to endurance training, HIT also increased and decreased whole body rates of lipid and CHO oxidation, respectively, during 60 minutes of sub-maximal exercise at 60% VO_{2max}.

Data from our laboratory using similar types of HIT protocols and running as the exercise mode (Morton *et al.*, 2009) have also showed reduced glycogen utilization after six weeks of training in both the vastus lateralis and gastrocnemius

muscles during an acute bout of HIE, probably due to the regulatory mechanisms outlined by Perry *et al.* (2008).

When reviewed together, there is unequivocal evidence that HIT can augment the oxidative capacity of skeletal muscle (i.e. mitochondrial biogenesis) and improve metabolic control during sub-maximal exercise. However, the bigger question which emerges is, what are the mechanisms by which HIT can induce these beneficial adaptations despite the reduction in total training volume?

The potential answer(s) to this question (though currently not entirely understood) is beyond the scope of this textbook and requires an appreciation of ***molecular biology***. However, in this instance it is pertinent at least to consider the early signalling mechanisms that are currently thought to play key roles in mediating training adaptation and stimulating mitochondrial biogenesis. In this regard, acute exercise (i.e. every training session) induces a number of metabolic stressors (changes in energy charge of the cell, i.e. ATP : ADP + AMP + P_i ratio, intracellular Ca^{2+} concentration, reactive oxygen species, glycogen depletion, lactate production, etc.) which activate a variety of intracellular signalling protein kinases such as the 5' adenosine activated protein kinase (AMPK), mitogen activated protein kinase (MAPK) and calmodulin kinase (CaMK). It is thought that these kinases eventually lead to a change in gene expression of PGC1, a protein considered as the master regulator of mitochondrial biogenesis.

This continual and transient changes in PGC1 gene expression in the hours following each training session eventually leads to changes in PGC1 protein which, in turn, acts as a transcriptional co-activator to increase expression of those proteins which modulate mitochondrial biogenesis downstream of these initial signalling events (Perry *et al.*, 2010). In the context of HIT, it has been shown that the supra-maximal intensity of the interval exercise periods are capable of activating these early signalling pathways, even though they may only involve 30 seconds of contractions (Gibala *et al.*, 2009). It therefore seems that the training adaptations observed with HIT are a result of

Table 10.3 Muscle metabolites, expressed as mmol.kg dw^{-1}, at rest and after five minutes of exercise at 90% VO$_{2max}$ undertaken pre- and post- six weeks of HIT. Note that ADP and AMP are expressed as μmol.kg.dw^{-1}. (adapted from Table 1, Perry *et al.*, 2008)

	Pre-training rest	Pre-training 5 min	Post-training rest	Post-training 5 min
Cr	49.8	114.1	49.3	101.7
PCr	76.1	13.6	76.5	24.2
ATP	23.6	20.5	22.8	22.6
ADP	83.9	366	78.8	265.4
AMP	0.29	6.79	0.27	3.39
P$_i$	10.8	80.9	10.8	68.2

the repeated activation of early signalling events, which are largely driven by the intensity of the contraction, given that high-intensity activity will induce a greater a degree of cellular stress in the first instance, compared with prolonged exercise of lower intensity.

The precise molecular mechanisms and signalling pathways underpinning muscle adaptation to exercise training now represent one of the major research areas within sport and exercise sciences and, with the advancement in molecular biology techniques, this is a rapidly changing and advancing field. Interested readers are directed to several recent reviews and research papers for current opinion (Ljubricic *et al.*, 2010; Uguccioni *et al.*, 2010; Perry *et al.*, 2010).

10.6 Mechanisms of fatigue

Given that HIE is characterized by periods of both high-intensity effort interspersed with periods of reduced intensity, the study of the mechanisms of *fatigue* in this instance is extremely complex. Furthermore, the typical laboratory models of HIE which we have discussed so far in this chapter (i.e. 2–12 intervals ranging in duration from six seconds to four minutes) are not usually representative of the metabolic demands that are placed on athletes in the sporting situation.

For example, a 90-minute game of soccer is characterized by an average intensity of 70% VO$_{2max}$, but there is also considerable anaerobic energy production, owing to the fact that 150–250 intense actions are performed (Bangsbo *et al.*, 2006). In addition, time-motion analysis studies have demonstrated that while players become progressively fatigued towards the end of a game, there also instances in which soccer players exhibit *temporary fatigue*, where the ability to perform high-intensity running is reduced in the minutes following the most intense periods (Mohr *et al.*, 2003). Clearly, the contributing factors to fatigue are therefore likely to vary at specific time-points of the HIE protocol and are dependent on the *total* duration of the exercise, as well as the nature of the exercise which was undertaken in the minutes prior to the onset of performance decrements.

In this section, we outline potential causes of fatigue and pay particular reference to prolonged models of HIE that are relevant to sport (much of this research has been conducted in reference to soccer). Where appropriate, we also integrate findings from laboratory models of fatigue which may help explain the aetiology of fatigue in sporting situations. It is important to appreciate, however, that the variety of experimental models employed in the literature (from both human and animal studies) offer a number of advantages and disadvantages, and these should be taken

Table 10.4   Advantages and disadvantages of various experimental approaches to study mechanisms of fatigue (adapted from Allen *et al.*, 2008)

Muscle in vivo	Advantages	All physiological mechanisms present Fatigue can be central or peripheral All types of fatigue can be studied Stimulation patterns appropriate for fiber types and stage of fatigue
	Disadvantages	Mixture of fiber types Complex activation patterns Produces correlative data; hard to identify mechanisms Experimental interventions very limited
Isolated muscle	Advantages	Central fatigue eliminated Dissection simple
	Disadvantages	Mixture of fiber types Inevitable extracellular gradients of O_2, CO_2, K^+, lactic acid Mechanisms of fatigue biased by presence of extracellular gradients Drugs cannot be applied rapidly because of diffusion gradients
Isolated single fiber	Advantages	Only one fiber type present Force and other changes (ionic, metabolic) can be unequivocally correlated Fluorescent measurements of ions, metabolites, membrane potential, etc. possible Easy and rapid application of extracellular drugs, ions, metabolities, etc.
	Disadvantages	Dissection difficult Environment different to in vivo K^+ accumulation and other in vivo changes absent Prone to damage at physiological temperatures Small size makes analysis of metabolities difficult
Skinned single	Advantages	Precise solutions can be applied Possible to study myofibrillar properties, SR release and uptake, AP/Ca^{2+} release coupling Metabolic and ionic changes associated with fatigue can be studied in isolation
	Disadvantages	Relevance to gatigue can be questionable May lose important intracellular constituents Relevant metabolites to study must be identified in other systems

into consideration when reviewing these data (see Table 10.4).

10.6.1   Carbohydrate availability

Although muscle glycogen is not likely to be limiting in the Wingate-type models of HIE, there is substantial evidence that *glycogen depletion* may contribute to fatigue in prolonged HIE. Indeed, whereas mixed muscle glycogen (as assessed from whole muscle homogenates) is only depleted by around 40–50% after a soccer game (Krustrup *et al.*, 2006), examination of individual fibres revealed that 50% of individual fibres were classified as completely empty or almost empty (see Figure 10.25 and 10.26). This complete depletion of glycogen, especially in type II fibres, could explain the inability to perform high-intensity exercise during the second half of a game.

The role of glycogen depletion in contributing to fatigue in this instance is not only likely related to a reduction in substrate to fuel high rates of ATP production, but also in impairing Ca^{2+} release from the SR (see Chapter 9). Support for the role of glycogen in limiting HIE performance is also provided by the experimental studies reviewed in section 10.4.

Although blood glucose is unlikely to decline to levels associated with hypoglycaemia during prolonged HIE, there is evidence to suggest that maintaining or elevating glucose levels through

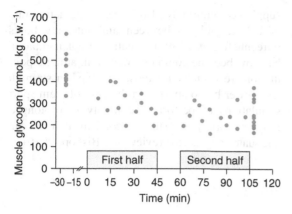

Figure 10.25   Muscle glycogen at rest and at various stages throughout the first and second halves of a 90-minute soccer match as well as immediately after the game. Each dot represents individual values (adapted from Krustrup *et al.*, 2006)

the consumption of sports drinks can improve intermittent shuttle running capacity, likely due to maintaining high rates of CHO oxidation when glycogen availability becomes limiting to performance (Foskett *et al.*, 2008).

10.6.2   PCr depletion

You are now well familiar with the fact that PCr hydrolysis is essential to ATP turnover during maximal activity <10 seconds in duration. It has been suggested that **PCr depletion** may be one of the contributing factors to the occurrence of *temporary* fatigue, where the capacity to perform high-intensity running is reduced in the minutes following intense periods of activity (Mohr *et al.*, 2003).

Given that elite soccer players in the English Premier League can perform 40 maximal sprints per game, and that recovery time between high-intensity efforts is limited to around 70 seconds (Bradley *et al.*, 2009; refer back to Section 10.3 for a discussion on the role of recovery duration in influencing PCr resynthesis), it is conceivable that there would be considerable PCr depletion throughout a game. Indeed, data from games where biopsies (from whole-muscle homogenates) have been obtained approximately 30 seconds after an intense period have revealed individual values as low as 45 mmol.kg dw^{-1} (Krustrup *et al.*, 2006).

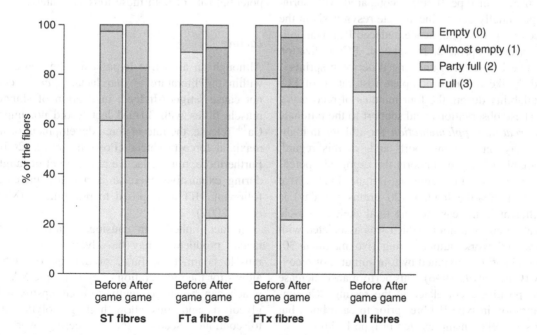

Figure 10.26   Relative glycogen content in type I, IIa and IIx fibres as well as all fibres before and after a soccer game (adapted from Krustrup *et al.*, 2006)

It is, of course, inappropriate to perform the multiple biopsies required to fully map the time-course of PCr depletion and resynthesis in such instances. However, based on findings from laboratory models of HIE, it is likely that PCr depletion may be greater in *individual* fibre populations. Indeed, both glycogen and PCr utilization is greater in type II fibres compared with type I fibres during 30 seconds of treadmill sprinting (Greenhaff *et al.*, 1994).

The role of PCr depletion as a metabolic factor involved in fatigue during HIE is supported by the observation that the restoration of power output following a maximal 30-second sprint is paralleled by the resynthesis of PCr, despite the fact that muscle pH remains low (Bogdanis *et al.*, 1995). Furthermore, four minutes of recovery after a 30-second maximal sprint is still not sufficient for PCr resynthesis in type II fibres, whereas resynthesis is almost complete in type I fibres (Casey *et al.*, 1996). When a subsequent sprint was performed after the four-minute recovery period, performance was reduced by comparison with the first sprint, which may be due to reduced PCr utilization in type II fibres compared with sprint 1, potentially due to incomplete resynthesis in the recovery period and, hence, reduced PCr availability prior to sprint 2. In contrast, PCr utilization in type I fibres was unchanged between sprints 1 and 2, likely due to complete restoration of PCr availability during the four minutes of recovery.

These observations lend support to the rationale for **creatine supplementation** for athletes in high-intensity intermittent sports and, in this regard, available evidence supports the ergogenic potential of creatine in attenuating fatigue. Indeed, five days of creatine loading (20 grams per day) is sufficient to increase resting total skeletal muscle creatine concentration, which was associated with improved work output during two maximal 30-second sprints separated by four minutes of recovery (Casey *et al.*, 1996). This performance increase was positively correlated to the resting PCr concentration in type II fibres prior to each bout, but no such relationship existed in type I fibres.

Data also demonstrate that, in addition to increased resting PCr concentration, creatine supplementation may also increase the actual rate of PCr resynthesis between high-intensity bouts (Greenhaff *et al.*, 1994). Creatine supplementation has now become common practice in athletic populations (especially for those involved in strength and power based sports). In the case of team sport simulations of performance involving prolonged HIE, a variety of studies confirm that it can attenuate fatigue (for review see Bishop, 2010).

10.6.3 Acidosis

Increases in muscle *lactate* and H^+ have long been cited as a possible cause of fatigue in both single and repeated bouts of high-intensity exercise. Indeed, this research area remains one of the most hotly debated areas within the sport and exercise sciences, and it was the subject of point-counterpoint debate in the *Journal of Applied Physiology* in 2006 (Lamb *et al.*, 2006; Bangsbo & Juel, 2006). During high-intensity exercise, the lactic acid that is produced disassociates into lactate anions and H^+, so we will discuss the potential role of both these ions separately.

Lactate

Although an attractive hypothesis, the consensus within the literature is that lactate *per se* does not cause fatigue. Indeed, incubation of skinned muscle fibres with 30 mM lactate did not impair Ca^{2+} release, the rate of force development or the maximal force produced (Posterino *et al.*, 2001). Furthermore, muscle lactate at the point of fatigue during exhaustive exercise is actually increased following HIT as opposed to pre-training (Mohr *et al.*, 2007).

In fact, rather than causing negative effects, lactate production may be advantageous during muscle contraction. First, production of lactate allows for the regeneration of cytoplasmic NAD^+, which can be subsequently re-used upstream in glycolysis and thus allow high glycolytic rates to continue. Second, the pioneering work of George Brooks has demonstrated the presence of **cell-to-cell lactate shuttles**, whereby lactate that

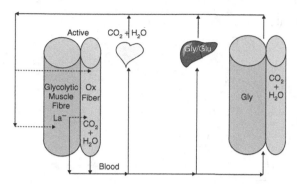

Figure 10.27   Schematic illustration of the cell to cell lactate shuttle (adapted from Gladden, 2008)

is predominantly produced in glycolytic fibres can be shuttled to other cells such as oxidative muscle fibres (either active or inactive), the heart or the liver for use as an additional energy substrate (see Figure 10.27). In the case of the latter, lactate can be transported to the liver to serve as a glucogenic precursor (a process is known as the *Cori cycle*), whereby the glucose produced from lactate can help to maintain plasma glucose levels. In this way, lactate is more than an inevitable by-product of anaerobic metabolism (in fact lactate is also produced in fully oxygenated conditions), as it appears that the product of one pathway serves as a substrate for another.

More recent data surrounding lactate metabolism has suggested the presence of an *intracellular lactate shuttle*, whereby lactate produced in the cytoplasm can be oxidized by mitochondria of the same cell (Brooks, 2009). The presence of such a shuttle would be advantageous, as not only would it generate an additional substrate in the form of lactate for conversion to pyruvate, but it would also generate reducing equivalents (i.e. NADH), thus supporting the role of the malate-aspartate and glycerol-phosphate shuttles. Furthermore, lactate has also emerged as a putative signalling molecule capable of inducing aspects of mitochondrial biogenesis (for a review, see Brooks, 2009). Clearly, the field of lactate metabolism has advanced considerably since the traditional belief that it was a metabolic waste product responsible for muscle fatigue!

Reduced pH

The H^+ ions which disassociate from lactate during intense muscle contraction can reduce muscle pH by approximately 0.5 pH units, and the resulting **metabolic acidosis** is often postulated to be a major cause of fatigue. Acidosis could impair muscle contraction by reducing Ca^{2+} release, voltage sensor activation and Ca^{2+} binding to troponin C, as well as reducing enzyme activity, thereby impairing ATP turnover (Allen *et al.*, 2008).

However, there are several lines of evidence which suggest that acidosis may not be as big a contributor to fatigue as initially thought. Indeed, the recovery of force following a single 30-second maximal sprint occurs much more rapidly than does muscle pH (Bogdanis *et al.*, 1995). Furthermore, the negative effect of pH on contractile force of isolated fibres is less apparent when cell temperature is increased to physiological temperatures (see Figure 10.28). Finally, in the case of prolonged HIE (such as soccer), muscle pH is only moderately reduced (>6.8), and muscle temperature is approximately 40°C, thus suggesting that acidosis is not a major contributor to fatigue in these types of sports (Krustrup *et al.*, 2006).

Lactate and H^+ transport

Although the above discussion suggests that pH regulation may not be the major contributor to fatigue, it is important to note that exercise training (especially when performed at high intensity) enhances the capacity to transport lactate and H^+. Co-transport of these ions is facilitated by a family of monocarboxylate transport (MCT) proteins, of which the *MCT1* and *MCT4* isoforms seem to be the most important.

In general, MCT1 appears to be more prevalent in type I fibres, whereas MCT4 is expressed more so in type II fibres (Pilegaard *et al.*, 1999). On the basis of the lactate shuttle principle, it is possible that MCT4 is largely responsible for lactate transport out of glycolytic cells (where it has mainly been produced) and MCT1 is responsible for lactate uptake into oxidative cells.

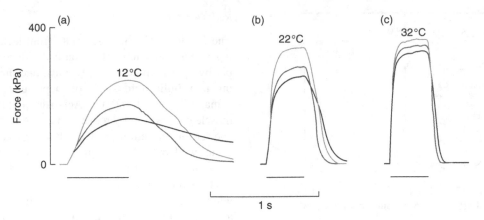

Figure 10.28 Force produced during an isometric contraction when fibre temperature was 12°C (a), 22°C (b) or 32°C (c) when alkaline (green line), neutral (red line) or acidic (blue line) (adapted from Westerblad *et al.*, 1997)

Endurance training of steady state nature has been shown to increase muscle MCT1 content (but not MCT4 – Dubouchard *et al.*, 2000), whereas HIT appears to increase MCT1 (Mohr *et al.*, 2007) and both MCT1 and MCT4 (Burgomaster *et al.*, 2007; Perry *et al.*, 2008; Juel *et al.*, 2004). Accordingly, lactate and H$^+$ release from contracting muscle is increased during exhaustive incremental exercise when performed after eight weeks of HIT (see Figures 10.29 and 10.30) and exercise capacity is also improved (Juel *et al.*, 2004). Training also increased the content of NHE1 and this protein, together with MCT1 and MCT4, may have collectively contributed to improved H$^+$ release. In such instances, training-induced increases in muscle blood flow is also likely to have contributed to the enhanced release (Juel, 2008).

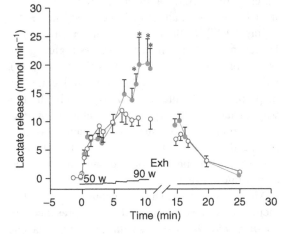

Figure 10.29 Muscle lactate release from an untrained (red symbols) and trained leg (green symbols) during incremental exercise performed until the point of fatigue. (adapted from Juel *et al.*, 2004)

10.6.4   Extracellular potassium

There is now strong evidence suggesting that the accumulation of **extracellular K$^+$** accumulation is of considerable importance in the development of fatigue during HIE. During exercise, K$^+$ is released from contracting muscles and, when it accumulates in the extracellular space, it can lead to depolarization of the membrane potential, thus causing membrane inexcitability and a reduction

in force (Sejersted & Sjogaard, 2000). In order to maintain high rates of power output, this loss in excitability has to be counterbalanced by rapid restoration of Na$^+$ and K$^+$ gradients, and this is the major role of the Na$^+$ K$^+$ ATPase pumps located on both the muscle membrane and T-tubules (Clausen, 2003).

In one of the earlier studies in this area, using a unilateral training model, Nielsen *et al.* (2004) observed that HIT reduces muscle interstitial K$^+$

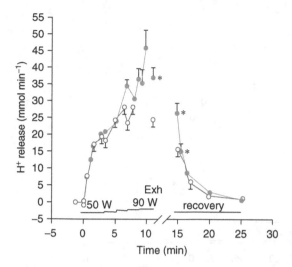

Figure 10.30 Muscle H$^+$ release from an untrained (red symbols) and trained leg (green symbols) during incremental exercise performed until the point of fatigue (adapted from Juel *et al.*, 2004)

during both steady state sub-maximal exercise as well as during incremental exercise (see Figure 10.31). Given that the release of K$^+$ was the same between both trained and untrained legs, it was suggested that the reduced levels of interstitial K$^+$ following training was due to enhanced re-uptake of K$^+$ by contracting muscle cells, which was facilitated by training-induced increases in the activity of the Na$^+$ K$^+$ ATPase α_1 and α_2 subunits.

Since this initial finding using knee extensor exercise, the same group (as reviewed in Section 10.5) later showed that speed endurance training elevates the expression of the Na$^+$ K$^+$ ATPase α subunits, which is associated with decreased accumulation of venous plasma K$^+$ and increased performance repeated bouts of high-intensity exercise (Iaia *et al.*, 2008; Bangsbo *et al.*, 2009). This imbalance in muscle K$^+$ homeostasis and impaired excitation of the sarcolemma may therefore be a potential cause of the temporary fatigue that is observed during intermittent sports, where the capacity to perform intense exercise is reduced for several minutes following a brief period of high-intensity exercise.

Finally, it is important to note that metabolic acidosis appears to enhance K$^+$ efflux from the muscle to the interstitium (Street *et al.*, 2005). In this regard, HIT-induced increases in NHE1, coupled with increased content of the Na$^+$ K$^+$ ATPase α_2 subunit, has been put forward as a mechanism to explain the reduced extracellular K$^+$ accumulation and improved performance that is observed following speed endurance training (Mohr *et al.*, 2007).

10.6.5 Reactive oxygen species (ROS)

Muscle contraction (especially when high-intensity and exhaustive) can lead to the production of *free radicals*, defined as atoms or molecules which contain one or more unpaired electrons capable of independent existence. The term *ROS* not only refers to oxygen-centred radicals (e.g. *superoxide*) but also reactive derivatives such as *hydrogen peroxide* (H_2O_2). A detailed discussion of redox biology is beyond the scope of this text, and the reader is directed to the recent review of Powers & Jackson (2008).

Although our muscles possess a variety of enzymatic and non-enzymatic **antioxidants** to protect against ROS production, exercise can create conditions of *oxidative stress*, whereby ROS production overwhelms the antioxidant system. In such instances, ROS are capable of attacking a variety of biomolecules, causing them to lose function. In the context of fatigue, the relevant biomolecules are likely to be a variety of key proteins involved in the contractile process.

Studies implicating ROS in the aetiology of fatigue are based on the observations that exogenous antioxidant compounds enhance force production and exercise performance. Most of these studies have been conducted in isolated muscles, either in single fibres or skinned fibres (for a review see Allen *et al.*, 2008), though there are instances supporting ROS-mediated fatigue in exercising humans. This is especially apparent for those studies which have administered *N-acetylcysteine* (**NAC**), a compound capable of supporting the resynthesis of the non-enzymatic antioxidant glutathione.

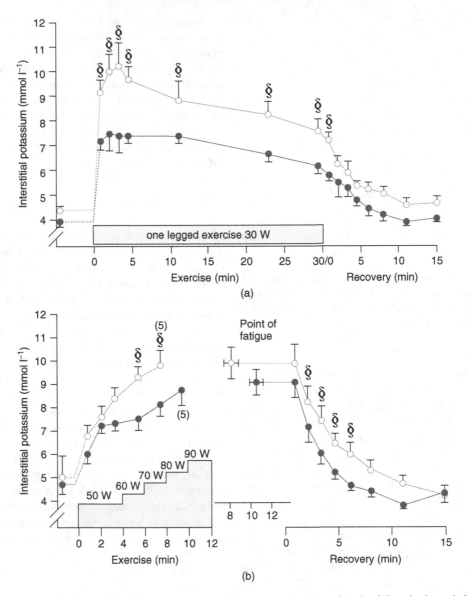

Figure 10.31 Muscle interstitial K^+ in an untrained (green symbols) and trained leg (red symbols) during sub-maximal exercise (a) and incremental exercise (b) performed until the point of fatigue (adapted from Nielsen *et al.*, 2004)

For example, McKenna *et al.* (2006) observed that infusion of NAC attenuated the decline in the activity of $Na^+ K^+$ ATPase pump during 45 minutes of cycling at 70% VO_{2max} and reduced the rise in plasma K^+. Exercise capacity at 90% VO_{2max} was also enhanced with NAC infusion.

We have also recently shown that NAC, when administered orally, can improve high-intensity intermittent shuttle running capacity (Cobley *et al.*, 2011).

Contraction-induced ROS may therefore contribute to the role of extracellular K^+

accumulation (as discussed previously) in fatigue during HIE, given the negative effects they can induce on Na^+ K^+ ATPase activity. In addition to this protein, it is also possible that ROS can reduce SERCA activity, thereby attenuating the re-uptake of Ca^{2+} into the SR and thus Ca^{2+} release and availability for contraction (Allen et al., 2008). Other regulatory proteins related to Ca^{2+} release, such as the ryanodine receptor, may also be altered by ROS production.

Finally, ROS also have the capacity to modify the structure and function of the myofilaments themselves, which would of course reduce force production (Ferrerira & Reid, 2008). Clearly, the role of ROS in mediating fatigue is at an exciting stage and further studies are required, especially in relation to whole body exercise and specifically, prolonged HIE.

10.6.6 P_i accumulation and impaired Ca^{2+} release

Data from isolated muscle models have consistently shown that impaired Ca^{2+} release is characteristic of fatigue. As reviewed above, it has been suggested that ROS-induced impairments in SERCA activity and modification of the ryanodine receptor may contribute to reduced Ca^{2+} release. However, one other mechanism is precipitation of Ca^{2+} with P_i (owing to high rates of PCr hydrolysis during high-intensity periods of activity) in the SR to produce *Ca^{2+} phosphate*, thereby reducing the amount of free available for release (Westerblad et al., 2002). Indeed, studies from mice that have been genetically modified so that they lack creatine kinase (and thus do not display marked P_i accumulation) do not display the pattern of fatigue induced by intermittent contractions in wild type mice.

In addition to Ca^{2+} P_i precipitation, P_i may impair force production through acting directly on the myofibrils, and reduce Ca^{2+} sensitivity as well as reducing SERCA activity, thereby reducing Ca^{2+} re-uptake into the SR (Westerblad et al., 2002). A further discussion of mechanisms of impaired Ca^{2+} release with fatigue, as well as the

impact of P_i on crossbridge function, is provided by the recent reviews of Allen et al. (2008) and Fitts (2008).

In summarizing the potential causes of fatigue in HIE, it is clear that fatigue is an extremely complex process, but one that it is further complicated by the fluctuations in exercise intensity characteristic of HIE. In the case of prolonged HIE that is relevant to sport, fatigue could be due to reduced substrate availability (e.g. PCr and glycogen) required to fuel high rates of ATP production, as well as a number of metabolic disturbances which can impair force production. For example, extracellular accumulation of K^+ can impair membrane excitability, which may be due to a ROS induced impairment of Na^+ K^+ ATPase function. Contraction-induced ROS may also impair SERCA and the ryanodine receptor, thereby reducing Ca^{2+} release available for contraction. ROS could also impair Ca^{2+} sensitivity of the contractile proteins, as well as alter the structure of the myofibrillar proteins, thereby impairing function. The reduced Ca^{2+} release which is characteristic of fatigue could be due to precipitation with P_i in the SR, the latter of which is produced from high rates of PCr hydrolysis. Although lactate *per se* is not likely to cause fatigue, the reduction in muscle pH due to H^+ accumulation may, in some situations, lead to reduced force production through interfering with the contractile apparatus, reducing activity of key enzymes and increasing K^+ efflux from contracting muscle.

Unfortunately, *direct* evidence for these theories in human skeletal muscle is lacking, due to the limitations of establishing cause and effect in an intact human being performing whole-body exercise, as opposed to data from animal models using isolated intact or skinned fibres. However, supporting evidence from human studies is provided by those experiments which have utilized interventions such as nutritional manipulations or, more importantly, exercise training. The use of the latter is particularly informative, given that training appears to interact with all of the potential fatiguing processes outlined above, while simultaneously improving performance – e.g. reduced glycogenolysis, PCr hydrolysis, increased content and activity of the oxidative, antioxidant and ion transport proteins, etc.

Finally, it is important to note that in the context of HIE relevant to sport, the factors outlined above do not operate in isolation but, rather, are likely to contribute collectively to the onset of fatigue.

As sport and exercise scientists, ultimately we are left with the task of critically evaluating our own and others' research of exercise metabolism in the hope of integrating training and nutritional strategies which maximize performance. At the end of this, our final chapter in the study of *Biochemistry for Sport and exercise Metabolism*, we hope that we have now provided you with the appropriate platform for which to do so!

10.7 Key points

- High-intensity intermittent exercise (HIE) is characterized by brief periods of high-intensity activity (near maximal or supra-maximal) interspersed with periods of low- to moderate-intensity exercise or periods of inactivity (i.e. rest). HIE is representative of the activity profiles of some of the world's most popular sports, e.g. soccer, rugby, basketball, etc.
- Unfortunately, many of the laboratory models studied in the literature are not representative of the activity profile of HIE, in terms of intensity and duration of the exercise, that is relevant to sport.
- Energy production during HIE may be fuelled by both anaerobic (PCr hydrolysis, adenylate kinase, anaerobic glycolysis) and aerobic metabolism of both carbohydrate and lipids, though the precise contribution of each is dependent on the characteristics of the protocol.
- It is a common misconception that anaerobic metabolism is the most important energy producing pathway during HIE. Indeed, oxidative phosphorylation becomes more important to ATP turnover with each successive bout of high-intensity interval exercise and, in some cases, is the main contributor to ATP production.

- The increased reliance upon oxidative metabolism appears to be due to a down-regulation of glycogenolysis (due to reduced phosphorylase activity) and increased activity of PDH prior to and during each successive interval period.
- Regulation of energy provision during HIE is largely dependent on the exact intensities and duration of both the interval and recovery periods, as well as the work-rest ratio. For example, in the case of PCr, the duration of the recovery period will determine its resynthesis and, therefore, its availability prior to and utilization during the next high-intensity effort.
- The implication of protocol manipulation has applications for training programme design in terms of whether it is speed, speed endurance or high-intensity aerobic training that is the main training goal.
- Commencing HIE with reduced muscle glycogen availability enhances lipid oxidation but has negative effects on exercise capacity.
- CHO ingestion prior to HIE augments plasma insulin, glucose and CHO oxidation and suppresses plasma glycerol, FFA and lipid oxidation. However, unlike steady-state endurance exercise, there appears to be no differences between HGI and LGI carbohydrates.
- CHO ingestion during HIE may spare muscle glycogen utilization, maintain CHO oxidation rates and improve exercise capacity.
- Depending on the specifics of the exercise protocol, high-intensity interval training (HIT) is capable of inducing beneficial anaerobic and aerobic adaptations in skeletal muscle.
- HIT can induce similar oxidative adaptations (as well as inducing shifts in substrate utilization during sub-maximal exercise) in skeletal muscle when compared with traditional endurance training, despite being much lower in training duration and volume.
- Although the exact mechanisms underpinning the adaptations induced by HIT are currently not well defined, it is likely due to the effects of the brief high-intensity exercise periods on the activation of key signalling kinases which modulate

gene expression of those proteins involved in regulating mitochondrial biogenesis.

- Given that HIE consists of high-intensity and moderate-intensity exercise, mechanisms of fatigue are more complex than endurance or high intensity exercise *per se*, and are also influenced by the specific nature of the exercise stimulus, i.e. intensity and duration of the interval and recovery periods and the work-rest ratio.

- In the context of prolonged HIE that is relevant to sport, fatigue may be related to depletion of substrates such as glycogen and PCr, especially in type II fibres.

- Metabolic disturbances within the muscle during HIE may also lead to impairment in the ability to generate an action potential, to release Ca^{2+} from the SR and also to form crossbridges. In such situations, increased ROS production, extracellular K^+ accumulation, intracellular P_i accumulation and reduced muscle pH are all likely, either directly or indirectly, to *collectively* contribute to the development of fatigue.

References and suggested readings

Achten, J. & Jeukendrup, A. (2004) Optimising fat oxidation through exercise and diet. *Nutrition* **20**, 716–727.

Allen, D.G., Lamb, G.D. & Westerblad, H. (2008) Skeletal muscle fatigue: cellular mechanisms. *Physiological Reviews* **88**, 287–332.

Alsted, T.J., Nybo, L., Schweiger, M., Fledelius, C., Jacobsen, P., Zimmermann, R., Zechner, R. & Kiens, B. (2009) Adipose triglyceride lipase in human skeletal muscle is upregulated by exercise training. *American Journal of Physiology* **296**, E445–E453.

Arkinstall, M.J., Bruce, C.R., Nikolopoulos, V., Garnham, A.P. & Hawley, J.A. (2001) Effect of carbohydrate ingestion on metabolism during running and cycling. *Journal of Applied Physiology* **91**, 2125–2134.

Arkinstall, M.J., Bruce, C.R., Clark, S.A., Rickards, C.A., Burke, L.M. & Hawley, J.A. (2004) Regulation of fuel metabolism by pre–exercise muscle glycogen content and exercise intensity. *Journal of Applied Physiology* **97**, 2275–2283.

Armstrong, L.E., Costill, D.L. & Fink, W.J. (1985) Influence of diuretic-induced dehydration on competitive running performance. *Medicine and Science in Sports and Exercise* **17**, 456–461.

Babraj, J.A., Vollaard, N.B.J., Keast, C., Guppy, F.M., Cottrell, G. & Timmons, J.A. (2009) Extremely short duration high intensity interval training substantially improves insulin action in young healthy males. *BMC Endocrine Disorders* **9**, 3.

Ball, D., Greenhaff, P.L. & Maughan, R.J. (1996) The acute reversal of a diet-induced metabolic acidosis does not restore endurance capacity during high intensity exercise in man. *European Journal of Applied Physiology* **66**, 49–54.

Balsom, P.D., Sejer, J.Y., Sjodin, B. & Ekblom, B. (1992a) Physiological responses to maximal intermittent exercise. *European Journal of Applied Physiology* **65**, 144–149.

Balsom, P.D., Sejer, J.Y., Sjodin, B. & Ekblom, B. (1992b) Maximal intensity intermittent exercise: effect of recovery duration. *International Journal of Sports Medicine* **13**, 528–533.

Balsom, P.D., Wood, K., Olsson, P. & Ekblom, B. (1999a) Carbohyrate intake and multiple sprint sports: with special reference to football (soccer). *International Journal of Sports Medicine* **20**, 48–52.

Balsom, P.D., Gaitanos, G.C., Soderlund, K. & Ekblom, B. (1999b) High-intensity exercise and muscle glycogen availability in humans. *Acta Physiologica Scandinavica* **165**, 337–345.

Bangsbo, J. (1996) Regulation of muscle glycogenolysis and glycolysis during intense exercise: in vivo studies using repeated intense exercise. In *Biochemistry of Exercise IX*, Human Kinetics, Champaign, IL.

Bangsbo, J. (1997) Quantification of anaerobic energy production during intense exercise. *Medicine & Science in Sports & Exercise* **30**, 47–52.

Bangsbo, J. & Juel, C. (2006) Lactic acid accumulation is an advantage/disadvantage during muscle activity. *Journal of Applied Physiology* **100**, 1412–1413.

Bangsbo, J., Mohr, M. & Krustrup, P. (2006) Physical and metabolic demands of training and match play in the elite football player. *Journal of Sports Sciences* **24**, 665–674.

Bangsbo, J., Graham, T.E., Kiens, B. & Saltin, B. (1992) Elevated muscle glycogen and anaerobic energy production during exhaustive exercise in man. *Journal of Physiology* **451**, 205–227.

Bangsbo, J., Krustrup, P., Gonzalez-Alonso, J. & Saltin, B. (2001) ATP production and efficiency of human skeletal muscle during intense exercise: effect of previous exercise. *American Journal of Physiology* **280**, E956–E964.

Bangsbo, J., Gunnarsson, T.P., Wendell, J., Nybo, L. & Thomassen, M. (2009) Reduced volume and increased training intensity elevate muscle Na^+K^+ pump alpha 2 subunit expression as well as short and long term work capacity in humans. *Journal of Applied Physiology* **107**, 1171–1180.

Bangsbo, J., Gollnick, P.D., Graham, T.E., Juel, C., Kiens, B., Mizuno, M. & Saltin, B. (1990) Anaerobic energy production and the O_2 deficit-debt relationship during exhaustive exercise in humans, *Journal of Physiology* **422**, 539–559.

Bergman, B.C., Butterfield, G.E., Wolfel, E.E., Lopaschuk, G.D., Casazza, G.A., Horning, M.A. & Brooks, G.A. (1999) Muscle net glucose uptake and glucose kinetics after endurance training in men. *American Journal of Physiology* **277**, E81–E92.

Bergstrom, J., Hermansen, L., Hultman, E., & Saltin, B. (1967) Diet, muscle glycogen and physical performance. *Acta Physiologica Scandinavica* **71**, 140–150.

Bezaire, V., Heigenhauser, G.J. & Spriet, L.L. (2004) Regulation of CPTI activity in

intermyofibrillar and subsarcolemmal mitochondria from human and rat skeletal muscle. *American Journal of Physiology* **286**, E85–E91.

Bigland-Ritchie, B. & Woods, J.J. (1984) Changes in muscle contractile properties and neural control during human muscular fatigue. *Muscle & Nerve* **7**, 691–699.

Bishop, D. (2010) Dietary supplements and team sport performance. *Sports Medicine* **40**, 995–1017.

Bogdanis, G.C., Nevill, M.E., Boobis, L.H. & Lakomy, H.K. (1996) Contribution of phosphocreatine and aerobic metabolism to energy supply during repeated sprint exercise. *Journal of Applied Physiology* **80**, 876–884.

Bogdanis, G.C., Nevill, M.E., Boobis, L.H., Lakomy, H.K. & Nevill, A.M. (1995) Recovery of power output and muscle metabolites following 30 s of maximal sprint cycling in man. *Journal of Physiology* **482**, 467–480.

Boobis, L.H., Williams, C. & Wootton, S.A. (1983) influence of sprint training on muscle metabolism during brief maximal exercise in man. *Journal of Physiology* **342**, 36P–37P.

Booth, F.W. & Laye, M.J. (2009) Lack of adequate appreciation of physical exercise's complexities can pre-empt appropriate design and interpretation in scientific discovery. *Journal of Physiology* **587**, 5527–5539.

Bradley, P.S., Sheldon, W., Wooster, B., Olsen, P., Boanas, P. & Krustrup, P. (2009) High intensity running in English FA Premier league soccer matches. *Journal of Sports Sciences* **15**, 159–168.

Brooks, G.A. (1985) Lactate: glycolytic product and oxidative substrate during sustained exercise in mammals the lactate shuttle. *Comparative Physiology and Biochemistry: Current Topics and Trends*, vol. A, Respiration-Metabolism-Circulation, 208–218.

Brooks, G.A. (2009) Cell-cell and intracellular lactate shuttles. *Journal of Physiology* **587**, 5591–5600.

Brosnan, J.T. & Brosnan, M.E. (2006) Branched amino acids: enzymes and substrate regulation. *Journal of Nutrition* **136**, 207S–211S.

Burgomaster, K.A., Heigenhasuer, G.J.F. & Gibala, M.J. (2006) Effect of short term interval training on humans skeletal muscle carbohydrate metabolism during exercise and time trial performance. *Journal of Applied Physiology* **100**, 2041–2047.

Burgomaster, K.A., Hughes, S.C., Heigenhauser, G.J.F., Bradwell, S.N. & Gibala, M.J. (2005) Six sessions of sprint interval training increases muscle oxidative potential and cycle endurance capacity in humans. *Journal of Applied Physiology* **98**, 1985–1990.

Burgomaster, K.A., Cermak, N.M., Phillips, S.M., Benton, C.R., Bonen, A. & Gibala, M.J. (2007) Divergent response of metabolite transport proteins in human skeletal muscle after sprint interval training and detraining. *American Journal of Physiology* **292**, R1970–R1976.

Burgomaster, K., Howart, K.R., Phillips, S.M., Rakobowchuk, M., MacDonald, M.J., McGee, S.L. & Gibala, M.J. (2008) Similar metabolic adaptations during exercise after low volume sprint interval and traditional endurance training in humans. *Journal of Physiology* **586**, 151–156.

Burgomaster, K.A., Howarth, K.R., Phillips, S.M., Rakobowchuk, M., Macdonald, M.J., McGee, S.L. & Gibala, M.J. (2008) Similar metabolic adaptations during exercise after low volume sprint interval and traditional endurance training in humans. *Journal of Physiology* **586**: 151–160.

Burke, L.M., Claassen, A., Hawley, J.A. & Noakes, T.D. (1998) Carbohydrate intake during prolonged cycling minimises effect of glycemic index of preexercise meal. *Journal of Applied Physiology* **85**, 2220–2226.

Burke, L.M., Angus, D.J., Cox, G.R., Cummings, N.K., Febbraio, M.A., Gawthorn, K., Hawley, J.A., Minehan, M., Martin, D.T. & Hargreaves, M. (2000) Effect of fat adaptation and carbohydrate restoration on metabolism and performance during prolonged cycling. *Journal of Applied Physiology* **89**, 2413–2421.

Calbet, J.A., De Paz, J.A., Garatachea, N., Cabeza de Vaca, S. & Chavarren, J. (2003) Anaerobic energy provision does not limit Wingate exercise performance in endurance-trained cyclists. *Journal of Applied Physiology* **94**, 668–676.

Casey, A., Constantin-Teodosiu, D., Howell, S., Hultman, E. & Greenhaff, P.L. (1996) Metabolic responses of type I and II muscle fibres during repeated bouts of maximal exercise in humans. *American Journal of Physiology* **271**, E38–E43.

Casey, A., Mann, R., Banister, K., Fox, J., Morris, P.G., Macdonald, I.A. & Greenhaff, P.L. (2000) Effect of carbohydrate ingestion on glycogen resynthesis in human liver and skeletal muscle, measured by (13) C MRS. *American Journal of Physiology* **278**, E65–E75.

Castell, L.M., Burke, L.M., Stear, S.J., McNaughton, L.R. & Harris, R.C. (2010) *BJSM* reviews: A–Z of nutritional supplements: dietary supplements, sports nutrition foods and ergogenic aids for health and performance Part 5: Buffers: sodium bicarbonate and sodium citrate; β-alanine and carnosine. *British Journal of Sports Medicine* **44**, 77–78.

Centers for Disease Control and Prevention (1998) Hyperthermia and dehydration related deaths associated with intentional rapid weight loss in three collegiate wrestlers. *Journal of the American Medical Association* **279**, 824–825.

Cheetham, M.E., Boobis, L.H., Brooks, S. & Williams, C. (1986) Human muscle metabolism during sprint running in m man. *Journal of Applied Physiology* **61**, 54–60.

Chesley, A., Hultman, E. & Spriet, L.L. (1995) Effects of epinephrine infusion on muscle glycogenolysis during intense aerobic exercise. *American Journal of Physiology* **268**, E127–E134.

Chesley, A., Heigenhauser, G.J. & Spriet, L.L. (1996) Regulation of glycogen phosphorylase activity following short term endurance training. *American Journal of Physiology* **270**, E328–E325.

Chester, N (2011) Caffeine in *Drugs in Sport: 5th Edition* (edited by David R Mottram), pp 274–293. Routledge, London.

Christmass, M.A, Dawson, B., Passeretto, P. & Arthur, P.G. (1999a) A comparison of skeletal muscle oxygenation and fuel use in sustained continuous and intermittent exercise. *European Journal of Applied Physiology* **80**, 423–435.

Christmass, M.A, Dawson, B., Goodman, C. & Arthur, P.G. (1999b) Brief intense exercise followed by passive recovery modifies the pattern of fuel use in humans during subsequent sustained intermittent exercise. *Acta Physiologica Scandinavica* **172**, 39–52.

Clarke, N.D., Drust, B., MacLaren, D.P. & Reilly, T. (2008) Fluid provision and metabolic responses to soccer-specific exercise. *European Journal of Applied Physiology* **104**, 1069–1077.

Clausen, T. (2003) Na^+–K^+ pump regulation and skeletal muscle contractility. *Physiological Reviews* **83**, 1269–1324.

Cobley, J.N., McGlory, C., Morton, J.P. & Close, G.L. (2011) N-acetylcysteine attenuates fatigue following repeated bouts of intermittent exercise: practical implications for tournament situations. *International Journal of Sport Nutrition and Exercise Metabolism*, in press.

Coffey, V.G. & Hawley, J.A. (2007) The molecular bases of training adaptation. *Sports Medicine* **37**, 737–63.

Coggan, A.R., Swanson, S.C., Mendenhall, L.A., Habash, D.L. & Klein, C.L. (1995) Effect of endurance training on hepatic glycogenolysis and gluconeogenesis during prolonged exercise in men. *American Journal of Physiology* **268**, E375–E383.

Coggan, A.R., Rguso, C.A., Gastaldelli, A., Sidossis, L.S. & Yeckel, C.W. (2000) Fat metabolism during high intensity exercise in endurance trained and untrained men. *Metabolism* **49**, 122–128.

Constantin-Teodosiu, D., Greenhaff, P.L., McIntyre, D.B. Round, J.M., & Jones, D.A. (1997) Anaerobid energy production in human skeletal muscle in intense contraction: a comparison of ^{31}P magnetic resonance spectroscopy and biochemical techniques. *Experimental Physiology* **82**, 593–601.

Costill, D.L., Daniels, J., Evans, W., Fink, W., Krahenbuhl, G. & Saltin, B. (1976) Skeletal muscle enzymes and fiber composition in male and female track athletes. *Journal of Applied Physiology* **140**, 149–154.

Coyle, E.F., Jeukendrup, A., Wagenmakers, A.J. & Saris, W.H. (1997) Fatty acid oxidation is directly regulated by carbohydrate metabolism during exercise. *American Journal of Physiology* **273**, E268–E275.

Drummond, M.J., Dreyer, H.C., Fry, C.R., Glynn, E.L. & Rasmussen, B.B. (2009) Nutritional and contractile regulation of human skeletal muscle protein synthesis and mTORC1 signalling. *Journal of Applied Physiology* **106**, 1374–1384.

Drust, B., Reilly, T. & Cable, N.T. (2000) Physiological responses to laboratory based soccer specific intermittent and continuous exercise. *Journal of Sports Sciences* **18**, 885–892.

Drust, B., Rasmussen, P., Mohr, M., Nielsen, B. & Nybo, L. (2005) Elevations in muscle temperature impairs sprint performance. *Acta Physiologica* **183**, 181–190.

Dubouchard, H., Butterfield, G.E., Wolfel, E.E., Bergman, B.C. & Brooks, G.A. (2000) Endurance training, expression and physiology of LDH, MCT1 and MCT4 in human skeletal muscle. *American Journal of Physiology* **278**, E571–E579.

Dyck, D.J., Peters, S.J., Wendling, P.S., Chesley, A., Hultman, E. & Spriet, L.L. (1996) Regulation of glycogen phosphorylase activity during intense aerobic cycling with elevated FFA. *American Journal of Physiology* **270**, E116–E125.

Enoka, R.M. & Duchateau, J. (2008) Muscle fatigue: what, why and how it influences muscle function. *Journal of Physiology* **586**, 11–23.

Essen, B., Hagenfedlt, L. & Kaijser, L. (1978) Utilisation of blood borne and intramuscular substrates during continuous and intermittent exercise in man. *Journal of Physiology* **265**, 489–506.

Faulkner, J.A. (2003) Terminology for contractions of muscles during shortening, while isometric and during lengthening. *Journal of Applied Physiology* **95**, 455–459.

Ferreira, L.F. & Reid, M.B. (2008) Muscle derived ROS and thiol regulation in muscle fatigue. *Journal of Applied Physiology* **104**, 853–860.

Fitts, R.H. (2008) The cross bridge cycle and skeletal muscle fatigue. *Journal of Applied Physiology* **104**, 551–558.

Foskett, A., Williams, C., Boobis, L. & Tsintzas, K. (2008) Carbohydrate availability and muscle energy metabolism during intermittent running. *Medicine & Science in Sports & Exercise* **40**, 96–103.

Frayn, K.N. (2010) Fat as a fuel: emerging understanding of the adipose tissue skeletal muscle axis. *Acta Physiologica* **199**, 509–518.

Gaitanos, G.C., Williams, C., Boobis, L.H. & Brooks, S. (1993) Human muscle metabolism during intermittent maximal exercise. *Journal of Applied Physiology* **75**, 712–719.

Gandevia, S.C. (2001) Spinal and supra-spinal factors in human muscle fatigue. *Physiological Reviews* **81**, 1725–1789.

Gibala, M.J (2001) Regulation of skeletal muscle amino acid metabolism during exercise. *International Journal of Sport Nutrition and Exercise Metabolism* **11**, 87–108.

Gibala, M.J. (2009) Molecular responses to high-intensity interval exercise. *Applied Physiology, Nutrition, and Metabolism* **34**, 428–432.

Gibala, M.J., & McGee, S. (2008) Metabolic adaptations to short term high-intensity interval training: a little pain for a lot of gain? *Exercise and Sport Science Reviews* **36**, 58–63.

Gibala, M.J., McGee, S.L., Garnham, A.P., Howlett, K.F., Snow, R.J. & Hargreaves, M. (2009) Brief intense interval exercise activates AMPK and p38 MAPK signalling and increases the expression of PGC-1α in human skeletal muscle. *Journal of Applied Physiology* **106**, 929–934.

Gibala, M.J., Little, J.P., van Essen, M., Wilkin, G.P., Burgomaster, K.A., Safdar, A., Raha, S., Tarnopolsky, M.A. (2006) Short-term sprint interval versus traditional endurance training: similar initial adaptations in human skeletal muscle and exercise performance. *Journal of Physiology* **575**, 901–911.

Gladden, B. (2008) A 'lactatic' perspective on metabolism. *Medicine & Science in Sports & Exercise* **40**, 477–485.

Gollnick, P.D., Piehl, K. & Saltin, B (1974) Selective glycogen depletion pattern in human muscle fibres after exercise of varying intensity and at varying pedalling rates. *Journal of Physiology* **241**, 45–57.

Gollnick, P.D., Armstrong, R.D., Saltin, B., Saubert, C.W., Sembrowich, W.L. & Shepherd, R.E. (1973) Effects of training on enzyme activity and fibre composition in human skeletal muscle. *Journal of Applied Physiology* **34**, 107–111.

Graham, T.E., Battram, D.S., Dela, F., El-Sohemy, A. & Thong, F.S. (2008) Does caffeine alter muscle carbohydrate and fat metabolism during exercise. *Applied Physiology, Nutrition, and Metabolism* **33**, 1311–1318.

Green, H.J. (1990) Manifestations and sites of neuromuscular fatigue. In, *Biochemistry of Exercise*, VII. International Series on Sports Science **21**, 13–35.

Green, H.J., Duhamel, T.A., Foley, K.P., Ouyang, J., Smith, I.C. & Stewart, R.D. (2007) Glucose supplements increase human muscle in vitro N+K+ATPase activity during prolonged exercise. *American Journal of Physiology* **293**, R354–R362.

Greenhaff, P.L., Gleeson, M. & Maughan, R.J. (1987a) The effects of dietary manipulation on blood acid-base status and the performance of high-intensity exercise. *European Journal of Applied Physiology*, **56**, 331–337.

Greenhaff, P.L., Gleeson, M. & Maughan, R.J. (1988) The effects of a glycogen loading regimen on acid-base status and blood lactate concentration before and after a fixed period of high intensity exercise in man. *European Journal of Applied Physiology*, **57**, 254–259.

Greenhaff, P.L., Gleeson, M., Whiting, P.H. & Maughan, R.J. (1987b) Dietary composition and acid-base status: limiting factors in the performance of maximal exercise in man. *European Journal of Applied Physiology*, **56**, 444–450.

Greenhaff, P.L., Nevill, M.E., Soderlund, K., Bodin, K., Boobis, L.H., Williams, C. & Hultman, E. (1994) The metabolic response of human type I and II muscle fibres during maximal treadmill sprinting. *Journal of Physiology* **478**, 149–155.

Hargreaves, M., McConell, G. & Proietto, J. (1995) Influence of muscle glycogen on glycogenolysis and glucose uptake during exercise in humans. *Journal of Applied Physiology* **78**, 288–292.

Hargreaves, M., McKenna, M.J., Jenkins, D.G., Warmington, S.A., Li, J.L., Snow, R.J. & Febbraio, M.A. (1998) Muscle metabolites and performance during high-intensity intermittent exercise. *Journal of Applied Physiology* **84**, 1687–1691.

Hargreaves, M., Finn, J.P., Withers, R.T., Halbert, J.A., Scroop, G.C., Mackay, M., Snow, R.J. & Carey, M.F. (1997). Effect of muscle glycogen availability on maximal exercise performance. *European Journal of Applied Physiology* **75**, 188–192.

Hawke, T.J. & Garry, D.J. (2001) Myogenic satellite cells: physiology to molecular biology. *Journal of Applied Physiology*, 91, 534–541.

Hawley, J.A. & Burke, L.M. (2010) Carbohydrate availability and training adaptation: effects on cell metabolism. *Exercise and Sport Sciences Reviews* **38**, 152–160.

Hawley, J.A., Schabort, E.J., Noakes, T.D. & Dennis, S.C. (1997) Carbohydrate loading and exercise performance. *Sports Medicine* **24**, 73–81.

Helge, J.W., Biba, T.O., Galbo, H., Gaster, M. & Donsmark, M. (2006) Muscle triacylglycerol and hormone sensitive lipase activity in untrained and trained human muscles. *European Journal of Applied Physiology* **97**, 566–572.

Helgerud J, Hoydal K, Wang E, Karlsen T, Berg P, Bjerkaas M, Simonsen T, Helgesen C, Hjorth N, Bach R. & Hoff J. (2007) Aerobic high intensity intervals improve VO$_{2max}$ more than moderate training. *Medicine & Science in Sports & Exercise* **39**, 665–671.

Henriksson, J. (1977) Training induced adaptation of skeletal muscle and metabolism during submaximal exercise. *Journal of Physiology* **270**, 661–675.

Holloszy, J.O. & Coyle, E.F. (1984) Adaptations of skeletal muscle to endurance exercise and their metabolic consequences. *Journal of Applied Physiology* **56**, 831–838.

Horowitz, J.F. & Klein, S. (2000) Lipid metabolism during endurance exercise. *American Journal of Clinical Nutrition* **72**, 558S–563S.

Horowitz, J.F., Mora-Rodriguez, R., Byerley, L.O. & Coyle, E.F. (1997) Lipolytic suppression following carbohydrate ingestion limits fat oxidation during exercise. *American Journal of Physiology* **273**, E768–E775.

Houston, M.E. (2006) *Biochemistry Primer for Exercise Science*. Human Kinetics, Champaign, IL.

Howarth, K.R., Burgomaster, K.A., Phillips, S.M. & Gibala, M.J. (2007) Exercise training increases branched chain oxoacid dehydrogenase kinase content in human skeletal muscle. *American Journal of Physiology* **293**, R1335–1341.

Howlett, R.A., Parolin, M.L, Dyck, D.J., Jones, N.L., Heigenhauser, G.J. & Spriet, L.L. (1998) Regulation of skeletal muscle glycogen phosphorylase and PDH at varying exercise power outputs. *American Journal of Physiology* **275**, R418–R425.

Hultman, E., Sahlin, K. & Sjoholm, H. (1981) Glycolytic and oxidative energy metabolism and contraction characteristics of intact human muscle. *Journal of Clinical Chemistry and Clinical Biochemistry* 19, 705–705.

Hultman, E., Bergstrom, M., Spriet, L.L. & Soderlund, K (1990) Energy metabolism and fatigue. *Biochemistry of Exercise VII*, **21**, 73–92.

Hurley, B.F., Nemeth, P.M., Martin, W.H., Hagberg, J.M., Dalsky, G.P. & Holloszy, J.O. (1986) Muscle triglyceride utilisation during exercise: effect of training. *Journal of Applied Physiology* **60**, 562–567.

Iaia, F.M. & Bangsbo, J. (2011) Speed endurance training is a powerful stimulus for physiological adaptations and performance improvements of athletes. *Scandinavian Journal of Medicine and Science in Sports* **20** (Suppl. 2), 11–23.

Iaia, M.F., Hellsten, Y., Nielsen, J.J., Fernstorm, M., Sahlin, K. & Bangsbo, J. (2009) Four weeks of speed endurance training reduces energy expenditure during exercise and maintains muscle oxidative capacity despite a reduction in training volume. *Journal of Applied Physiology* **106**, 73–80.

Iaia, F.M., Thomassen, M., Kolding, H., Gunnarsson, T., Wendell, J., Rostgaard, T., Nordsborg, N., Krustrup, P., Nybo, L., Hellsten, Y. & Bangsbo, J. (2008) Reduced volume but increased training intensity elevates muscle Na1-K1 pump alpha1-subunit and NHE1 expression as well as short-term work capacity in humans. *American Journal of Physiology – Regulatory, Integrative and Comparative Physiology* **294**, R966–R974.

Insel, P., Turner, R.E. & Ross, D. (2010) *Discovering Nutrition*. Jones & Bartlett, London.

Jensen, T.E., Wojtaszewski, J.F.P. & Richter, E.A (2009) AMP-activated protein kinase in contraction regulation of skeletal muscle metabolism: necessary and/or sufficient? *Acta Physiologica* **196**, 155–174.

Jones, N.L., McCartney, N., Graham, T., Spriet, L.L., Kowalchuk, J.M., Heigenhauser, G.J.M. & Sutton, J.R. (1985) Muscle performance and metabolism at slow and fast speeds. *Journal of Applied Physiology* **59**, 132–136.

Jong-Yeon, K., Hickner, R.C., Dohm, G.L. & Houmard, J.A. (2002) Long and medium chain fatty acid oxidation is increased in exercise trained humans skeletal muscle. *Metabolism* **51**, 460–464.

Joyner, M. & Coyle, E.F. (2008) Endurance exercise performance: the physiology of champions. *Journal of Physiology* **586**, 35–44.

Juel, C. (2008) Regulation of pH in human skeletal muscle: adaptations to physical activity. *Acta Physiologica* **193**, 17–24.

Juel, C., Klarskov, C., Nielsen, J.J., Krustrup, P., Mohr, M. & Bangsbo, J. (2004) Effect of high intensity intermittent training on lactate and H+ release from humans keletal muscle. *American Journal of Physiology* **286**, E245–E251.

Karelis, A.D., Smith, J.W., Passe, D.H. & Peronnet, F. (2010) Carbohydrate administration and exercise performance: what are the potential mechanisms involved. *Sports Medicine* **40**, 747–763.

Karlsson, J, & Saltin, B. (1970) Lactate, ATP and CP in working muscles during exhaustive exercise in man. *Journal of Applied Physiology* **29**, 596–602.

Karlsson, J. & Saltin, B. (1971) Diet, muscle glycogen and endurance performance. *Journal of Applied Physiology* **31**, 203–206.

Katz, A., Broberg, S., Sahlin, K. & Wahren, J. (1986) Leg glucose uptake during maximal dynamic exercise in humans. *American Journal of Physiology* **251**, E65–E70.

Kiens, B. (2006) Skeletal muscle lipid metabolism in exercise and insulin resistance. *Physiological Reviews* **86**, 205–243.

Kiens, B., Roemen, T.H. & van der Vusse, G.J. (1999) Muscular long chain fatty acid content during graded exercise in humans. *American Journal of Physiology* **276**, E352–E357.

Kiens, B., Essen-Gustavsson, B., Christensen, N.J. & Saltin, B. (1993) Skeletal muscle substrate utilisation during submaximal exercise in man: effect of endurance training. *Journal of Physiology* **469**, 459–478.

Kiens, B., Kristiansen, S., Jensen, P., Richter, E.A. & Turcotte, L.P. (1997) Membrane associated fatty acid binding protein (FABPpm) in human skeletal muscle is increased by endurance training. *Biochemical and Biophysical Research Communications* **231**, 463–465.

Kiens, B., Roepstorff, C., Glatz, J.F., Bonen, A., Schjerling, P., Knudson, J. & Nielsen, J.N. (2004) Lipid binding proteins and lipoprotein lipase activity in human skeletal muscle: influence of physical activity and gender. *Journal of Applied Physiology* **97**, 1209–1218.

Kiilerich, K., Gudmundsson, M., Birk, J.B., Lundby, C., Taudorf, S., Plomgard, P., Saltin, B., Pedersen, P.A., Wojtaszewski, J.F.P. & Pilegaard, H. (2010) Low muscle glycogen and elevate dplasma free fatty acid modify but do not prevent exercise-induced PDH activation in human skeletal muscle. *Diabetes* **59**, 26–32.

Klein, S., Coyle, E.F. & Wolfe, R.R. (1994) Fat metabolism during low intensity exercise in endurance trained and untrained men. *American Journal of Physiology* **267**, E934–E940.

Kraniou, G.N., Cameron-Smith, D. & Hargreaves, M. (2006) Acute exercise and GLUT4 expression in human skeletal muscle: influence of exercise intensity. *Journal of Applied Physiology* **101**, 934–937.

Krustrup, P., Mohr, M., Steensberg, A., Bencke, J., Kjaer, M. & Bangsbo, J. (2006) Muscle and blood metabolites during a soccer game: implications for sprint performance. *Medicine & Science in Sports & Exercise* **38**, 1165–1174.

Kumar, V., Atherton, P., Smith, K. & Rennie, M.J. (2009) Human muscle protein synthesis and breakdown during and after exercise. *Journal of Applied Physiology* **106**, 2026–2039.

Kunkel, L.M. (1986) Analysis of deletions in DNA from patients with Becker & Duchenne muscular dystrophy. *Nature* **322**, 73–77.

Lamb, G.D. & Stephenson, G. (2006) Lactic acid accumulation is an advantage/disadvantage during muscle activity. *Journal of Applied Physiology* **100**, 1410–1412.

Langfort, J., Zarzeczny, R., Pilis, W. & Nazar, K. (1997) The effect of a low-carbohydrate diet on performance, hormonal and metabolic responses to a 30-s bout of supramaximal exercise. *European Journal of Applied Physiology* **76**, 128–133.

LeBlanc, P.J., Howarth, K.R., Gibala, M.J. & Heigenhauser, G.J. (2004) Effects of 7 weeks of endurance training on human skeletal muscle metabolism during submaximal exercise. *Journal of Applied Physiology* **97**, 2148–2153.

Little, J.P., Safdar, A., Wilkin, G.P., Tarnapolosky, M.A. & Gibala, M.J. (2010b) A practical model of low volume high intensity interval training induces mitochondrial biogenesis in human skeletal muscle: potential mechanisms. *Journal of Physiology* **588**, 1011–1022.

Little, J.P., Chilibeck, P.D., Ciona, D., Forbes, S., Rees, H., Vandenberg, A. & Zello, G.A. (2010a) Effect of low and high glycemic index meals on metabolism and performance during high-intensity intermittent exercise. *International Journal of Sport Nutrition and Exercise Metabolism* **20**, 447–456.

Ljubicic, V., Joseph, A-M., Saleem, A., Uguccioni, G., Collu-Marchese, M., Lai, R.Y.J., Nguyen, L.M.D. & Hood, D.A. (2010) Transcriptional and post-transriptional regulation of mitochondrial biogenesis in skeletal muscle: effects of exercise and ageing. *Biochimica et Biophysica Acta*, **1800**, 223–234.

MacDougall, J.D., Hicks, A.L., MacDonald, J.R., McKelvie, R.S., Green, H.J. & Smith, K.M. (1998) Muscle performance and enzymatic adaptations to sprint interval training. *Journal of Applied Physiology* **84**, 2138–2142.

MacLaren, D. (2011) Supplements for high intensity exercise: creatine and other ergogenic aids. In *Drugs in Sport:* 5th Edition (Mottram, R.D., ed.), pp 247–261. Routledge; London.

MacLaren, D.P.M., Gibson, H, Parry-Billings, M. & Edwards R.H.T. (1989) A review of metabolic and physiological factors in fatigue. *Exercise and Sports Science Reviews* **17**, 29–66.

MacLaren, D.P.M., Reilly, T., Campbell, I.T. & Hopkin, C. (1999) Hormonal and metabolic responses to maintained hyperglycaemia during prolonged exercise. *Journal of Applied Physiology* **87**, 124–131.

Martin, I.K., Katz, A. & Wahren, J. (1995) Splanchnic and muscle metabolism during exercise in NIDDM patients. *American Journal of Physiology* **269**, E583–E590.

Martin, W.H., Dalsky, G.P., Hurley, B.F., Matthews, D.E., Bier, D.M., Hagberg, J.M., Rogers, M.A., King, D.S. & Holloszy, J.O. (1993) Effect of endurance training on plasma free fatty acid turnover and oxidation during exercise. *American Journal of Physiology* **265**, E708–E714.

Maughan, R.J. & Poole, D.C. (1981) The effects of a glycogen-loading regimen on the capacity to perform anaerobic exercise. *European Journal of Applied Physiology* **46**, 211–219.

Maughan, R.J., Greenhaff, P.L., Leiper, J.B., Ball, D., Lambert, C.P. & Gleeson, M. (1997) Diet composition and the performance of high-intensity exercise. *Journal of Sports Sciences* **15**, 265–275.

McCartney, N., Spriet, L.L., Heigenhauser, G.J.F., Kowalchuk, J.M., Sutton, J.R. & Jones, N.L. (1986) Muscle power and metabolism in maximal intermittent exercise. *Journal of Applied Physiology* **60**, 1164–1169.

McKee, T. & McKee, J.R. (2003) *Biochemistry: The Molecular Basis of Life*. McGraw Hill, London.

McKenna, M.J., Medved, I., Goodman, C.A., Brown, M.J., Bjorksten, A.R., Murphy, K.T., Petersen, A.C., Sostarc, S. & Gong, X. (2006) N-acetylcysteine attenuates the decline in muscle Na+K+ pump acitivty and delays fatigue during prolonged exercise in humans. *Journal of Physiology* **576**, 279–288.

McKenzie, S., Phillips, S.M., Carter, S.L., Lowther, S., Gibala, M.J. & Tarnapolsky, M.A. (2000) Endurance exercise training attenuates leucine oxidation and BCOAD activation during exercise in humans. *American Journal of Physiology* **278**, E580–E587.

Messonnier, L., Kristensen, M., Juel, C. & Denis, C. (2007) Importance of pH regulation and lactate/H$^+$ transport capacity for work production during supramaximal exercise in humans. *Journal of Applied Physiology* **102**, 1936–1944.

Mitchell, P. (1961) Coupling of phosphorylation to electron and hydrogen transfer by a chemi-osmotic type of mechanism. *Nature* **191**, 144–148.

Mohr, M., Krustrup, P. & Bangsbo, P. (2003) Match performance of high standard soccer players with special reference to the development of fatigue. *Journal of Sports Sciences* **21**, 439–449.

Mohr, M., Krustrup, P., Nybo, L., Nielsen, J.J. & Bangsbo, J. (2004) Muscle temperature and sprint performance during soccer matches – beneficial effect of re-warm-up at half-time. *Scandinavian Journal of Medicine and Science in Sports* **14**. 156–162.

Mohr, M., Krustrup, P., Nielsen, J.J., Nybo, L., Rasmussen, M.K., Juel, C. & Bangsbo, J. (2007) Effect of two different intense training regimens on skeletal muscle ion transport proteins and fatigue development. *American Journal of Physiology – Regulatory, Integrative and Comparative Physiology* **292**, R1594–R1602.

Montain, S.J., Hooper, M.K., Coggan, A.R. & Coyle, E.F. (1991) Exercise metabolism at different time intervals after a meal. *Journal of Applied Physiology* **70**, 882–888.

Morton, J.P., MacLaren, D.P.M., Cable, N.T., Bongers, T., Griffiths, R., Campbell, I.T., Evans, L., Kayani, A., McArdle, A. & Drust, B. (2006) Time-course and differential expression of the major heat shock protein families in human skeletal muscle following acute non-damaging treadmill exercise. *Journal of Applied Physiology* **101**, 176–182.

Morton, J.P., Doran, D.A. & MacLaren, D.P.M. (2008) Common student misconceptions in exercise physiology and biochemistry. *Advances in Physiology Education* **32**, 142–146.

Morton, J.P., Croft, L., Bartlett, J., MacLaren, D.P.M., Reilly, T., Evans, L., McArdle, A. & Drust, B. (2009) Reduced carbohydrate availability does not modulate training-induced heat shock protein adaptations but does up-regulate oxidative enzyme activity in human skeletal muscle. *Journal of Applied Physiology* **106**, 1513–1521.

Morton, J.P., Sutton, L., Robertson, C. & MacLaren, D.P.M. (2010) Making the weight: a case-study from professional boxing. *International Journal of Sports Nutrition and Exercise Metabolism* **20**, 80–85.

Nevill, M.E., Boobis, L.H., Brooks, S. & Williams, C. (1989) Effect of training on muscle metabolism during treadmill sprinting. *Journal of Applied Physiology* **67**, 2376–2382.

Nicholas, C.W., Nutall, F.E. & Williams, C. (2000) The Loughborough intermittent shuttle test: a field test that simulates the activity pattern of soccer. *Journal of Sports Sciences* **18**, 97–104.

Nicholas, C.W., Tsintzas, K., Boobis, L. and Williams, C. (1999) Carbohydrate-electrolyte ingestion during intermittent high-intensity running. *Medicine & Science in Sports & Exercise* **31**, 1280–1286.

Nielsen, J.J., Mohr, M., Klarskov, C., Kristensen, M., Krustrup, P., Juel, C. & Bangsbo, J. (2004) Effects of high-intensity intermittent training on potassium kinetics and performance in human skeletal muscle. *Journal of Physiology* **554**, 857–870.

Nye, C.K., Hanson, R.W. & Kalhan, S.C. (2008) Glyceroneogenesis is the dominant pathway for triglyceride glycerol synthesis in vivo in the rat. *The Journal of Biological Chemistry* **283**, 27565–27574.

Odland, L.M., Heigenhauser, G.J. & Spriet, L.L. (2000) Effects of high fat provision on muscle PDH activation and malonyl CoA content in moderate exercise. *Journal of Applied Physiology* **89**, 2352–2358.

Odland, L.M., Hollidge-Horvat, M., Heigenhauser, G.J.F. & Spriet, L.L. (1998b) Effects of increased fat availability on fat-carbohydrate interaction during prolonged aerobic exercise in men. *American Journal of Physiology – Regulatory, Integrative and Comparative Physiology* **274**, R894–R902.

Odland, L.M., Howlett, R.A., Heigenhauser, G.J., Hultman, R. & Spriet, L.L. (1998a) Skeletal muscle malonyl CoA content at the onset of exercise at varying power output in humans. *American Journal of Physiology* **274**, E1080–E1085.

Ortenblad, N., Nielsen, J., Saltin, B. & Holmberg, H.C. (2011) Role of glycogen availability in sarcoplasmic reticulum Ca2+ kinetics in human skeletal muscle. *Journal of Physiology* **589**, 711–725.

Parolin, M.L., Chesley, A., Matsos, M.P., Spriet, L.L., Jones, N.L. & Heigenhauser, G.J.F. (1999) Regulation of skeletal muscle glycogen phosphorylase and PDH during maximal intermittent exercise. *American Journal of Physiology* **277**, E890–E900.

Parra, J., Cadefau, J.A., Rodas, G., Amigo, N. & Cusso, R. (2000) The distribution of rest periods affects performance and adaptations of energy metabolism induced by high-intensity training in human muscle. *Acta Physiologica Scandinavica* **169**, 157–165.

Pathare, N., Walter, G.A., Stevens, J.E., Yang, Z., Okerke, E., Gibbs, J.D., Esterhai, J.L., Scarborough, M.T., Gibbs, C.P., Sweeney, H.L. & Vandenborne, K. (2005). Changes in inorganic phosphate and force production in human skeletal muscle after cast immobilization. *Journal of Applied Physiology* **98**, 307–314.

Periasamy, M. & Kalyanasundaram, A. (2007) SERCA pump isoforms: their role in calcium transport and disease. *Muscle and Nerve* **35**, 430–442.

Perry, C.G.R., Heigenhauser, G.J.F., Bonen, A. & Spriet, L.L. (2008) High-intensity aerobic interval training increases fat and carbohydrate metabolic capacities in human skeletal muscle. *Applied Physiology, Nutrition, and Metabolism* **33**, 1112–1123.

Perry, C.G., Lally, J., Holloway, G.P., Heigenhauser, G.J., Bonen, A., Spriet, L.L. (2010) Repeated transient mRNA bursts precede increases in transcriptional and mitochondrial proteins during training in human skeletal muscle. *Journal of Physiology* **588**, 4795–4810.

Peters, S.J., St Amand, T.A., Howlett, R.A., Heigenhauser, G.J.F. & Spriet, L.L. (1998) Human skeletal muscle pyruvate dehydrogenase kinase activity increases after a low carbohydrate diet. *American Journal of Physiology* **275**, E980–E986.

Philips, S.M., Glover, E.I. & Rennie, M.J. (2009) Alterations of protein turnover underlying disuse atrophy in human skeletal muscle. *Journal of Applied Physiology* **107**, 645–654.

Phillips, S.M., Green, H.J., Tarnapolsky, M.A., Heigenhauser, G.J., Hill, R.E. & Grant, S.M. (1996) Effects of training duration on substrate turnover and oxidation during exercise. *Journal of Applied Physiology* **81**, 2182–2191.

Pilegaard, H., Terzis, G., Halestrap, A. & Juel, C. (1999) Distribution of the lactate/H+ transporter isoforms MCT1 and MCT4 in human skeletal muscle. *American Journal of Physiology* **276**, E843–E848.

Posterino, G.S., Dutka, T.L. & Lamb, G.D. (2001) L(+) lactate does not affect twitch and tetanic responses in mechanically skinned mammalian muscle fibres. *Pflügers Archiv: European Journal of Physiology* **442**, 197–203.

Powers, S.K. & Jackson, M.J. (2008) Exercise-induced oxidative stress: cellular mechanisms and impact on force production. *Physiological Reviews* **88**, 1243–1276.

Price, M. & Halabi, K. (2005) The effects of work-rest duration on intermittent exercise and subsequent performance. *Journal of Sports Sciences* **23**, 835–842.

Price, M. & Moss, P. (2007) The effects of work-rest duration on physiological and perceptual responses during intermittent exercise and performance. *Journal of Sports Sciences* **25**, 1613–1621.

Putman, C.T., Jones, N.L., Lands, L.C., Bragg, T.M., Hollidge-Horvat, M.G. & Heigenhauser, G.J.F. (1995) Skeletal muscle pyruvate dehydrogenase activity during maximal exercise in humans. *American Journal of Physiology* **269**, E458–E468.

Reid, M.B. (2005) Response of the ubiquitin-proteasome pathway to changes in muscle activity. *American Journal of Physiology* **288**, R1423–1431.

Rennie, M.J., Bohe, J., Smith K., Wackerhage, H. & Greenhaff, P.L. (2006) Branched chain amino acids as fuels and anabolic signals in human muscle. *Journal of Nutrition* **136**, 264S–268S.

Richards, J.C., Johnson, T.K., Kuzma, J.N., Lonac, M.C., Schweder, M.M., Voyles, W.F. & Bell, C. (2010) Short-term sprint interval training increases insulin sensitivity in healthy adults but does not affect the thermogenic response to beta-adrenergic stimulation. *Journal of Physiology* **588**, 2961–2972.

Richter, E.A. & Ruderman, N.B. (2009) AMPK and the biochemistry of exercise: implications for human health and disease. *Biochemical Journal* **418**, 261–275.

Richter, E.A., Jensen, P., Kiens, B. & Kristiansen, S. (1998) Sarcolemmal glucose transport and GLUT4 translocation during exercise are diminished by endurance training. *American Journal of Physiology* **274**, E89–E95.

Robergs, R.A., Ghiasvand, F. & Parker, D. (2004) Biochemistry of exercise-induced metabolic acidosis *American Journal of Physiology – Regulatory, Integrative and Comparative Physiology* **287**, R502–R516.

Roberts, A.D., Billeter, R. & Howald, H. (1982) Anaerobic muscle enzyme changes after interval training. *International Journal of Sports Medicine* **3**, 18–21.

Rodas, G., Ventura, J.L., Cadefau, J.A., Cusso, R. & Parra, J. (2000) A short training programme for the rapid improvement of both aerobic and anaerobic metabolism. *European Journal of Applied Physiology* **82**, 480–486.

Roepstorff, C., Halberg, N., Hillig, T., Saha, A.K., Ruderman, N.B., Wojtaszewski, J.F.P., Richter, E.A. & Kiens, B. (2005) Malonyl CoA and carnitine in regulation of fat oxidation in human skeletal muscle during exercise. *American Journal of Physiology* **288**, E133–E142.

Romijn, J.A., Coyle, E.F., Sidossis, L.S., Zhang, X.J. & Wolfe, R.R. (1995) Relationship between fatty acid delivery and fatty acid oxidation during strenuous exercise. *Journal of Applied Physiology* **79**, 1939–1945.

Romijn, J.A., Sidossis, L.S., Gastaldelli, A., Horowitz, J.F., Endert, E. & Wolfe, R.R. (1993) Regulation of endogenous fat and carbohydrate metabolism in relation to exercise intensity and duration. *American Journal of Physiology* **265**, E380–E391.

Rose, A.J. & Richter, E.A. (2005) Skeletal muscle glucose uptake during exercise: how is it regulated. *Physiology* **20**, 260–270.

Rose, A.J. & Richter, E.A. (2009) Regulatory mechanisms of skeletal muscle protein turnover during exercise. *Journal of Applied Physiology* **106**, 1702–1711.

Ross, A. & Leveritt, M. (2001) Long-term metabolic and skeletal muscle adaptations to short-sprint training: implications for sprint training and tapering. *Sports Medicine* **31**, 1063–1082.

Salter, H. (1967) McArdle's syndrome: a review and a preliminary report of four further cases. *Postgraduate Medical Journal* **43**, 365–371.

Saltiel, A.R. & Pessin, J.F. (2007) *Mechansims of Insulin Action*. New York, Springer Science.

Saris, W.H.M., van Erp-Baart, M.A., Brouns, F., Westerterp, K.R. & ten Hoor, F. (1989) Study on food intake and energy expenditure during extreme sustained exercise: the Tour de France. *International Journal of Sports Medicine* **10**, S26–S31.

Schneiter, P., Di Vetta, V., Jequier, E. & Tappy, L. (1995) Effect of physical exercise on glycogen turnover and net substrate utilisation according to nutritional state. *American Journal of Physiology* **269**, E1031–E1036.

Sejersted, O.M. & Sjogaard, G. (2000) Dynamics and consequences of potassium shifts in skeletal muscle and heart during exercise. *Physiological Reviews* **80**, 1411–1481.

Serresse, O., Lortie, G., Bouchard, C. & Boulay, M.R. (1988) Estimation of the contrivbution of the various energy systems during maximal work of short duration. *International Journal of Sports Medicine* **9**, 456–460.

Shepley, B., MacDougall, J.D., Cipriano, N., Sutton, J.R., Tarnopolsky, M.A. & Coates, G. (1992) Physiological effects of tapering in highly trained athletes. *Journal of Applied Physiology* **72**, 706–711.

Sherman, W.M., Peden, M.C. & Wright, D.A. (1991) Carbohydrate feedings 1h before exercise improves cycling performance. *American Journal of Clinical Nutrition* **54**, 866–870.

Sidossis, L.S., Wolfe, R.R. & Coggan, A.R. (1998) Regulation of fatty acid oxidation in untrained vs trained men during exercise. *American Journal of Physiology* **274**, E510–E515.

Sidossis, L.S., Gastaldelli, A., Klein, S. & Wolfe, R.R. (1997) Regulation of plasma fatty acid oxidation during low and high intensity exercise. *American Journal of Physiology* **272**, E1065–E1070.

Silverthorn, D.U. (2008) *Human Physiology An Integrated Approach*, (5th Edition), Benjamin Cummings, San Francisco.

Smith, J.C. & Hill, D.W. (1991) Contribution of energy systems during a Wingate power test. *British Journal of Sports Medicine* **25**, 196–199.

Soderlund, K. & Hultman, E. (1986) Effects of delayed freezing on content of phosphagens in human skeletal muscle biopsy samples. *Journal of Applied Physiology* **61**, 832–835.

Soderlund, K., Greenhaff, P.L. & Hultman, E. (1992) Energy metabolism in type I and II human muscle fibres during short term electrical stimulation at different frequencies. *Acta Physiologica Scandinavica* **144**, 15–22.

Spriet, L.L. (2007) Regulation of substrate use during the marathon. *Sports Medicine* **37**, 332–336.

Spriet, L.L. & Watt, M.J. (2003) Regulatory mechanisms in the interaction between carbohydrate and lipid oxidation during exercise. *Acta Physiologica Scandinavica* **178**, 443–452.

Spriet, L.L., Soderlund, K., Bergstrom, M., Hultman, E. (1987) Skeletal muscle glycogenolysis, glycolysis, pH during electrical stimulation in men. *Journal of Applied Physiology* **62**, 616–621.

Spriet, L.L., Lindinger, M.I., McKelvie, R.S., Heigenhauser, G.J.F. & Jones, N.L. (1989) Muscle glycogenolysis and H^+ concentration during maximal intermittent cycling. *Journal of Applied Physiology* **66**, 8–13.

Spurway, N. & Wackerhage, H. (eds.) (2006) *Genetics and Molecular Biology of Muscle Adaptation*. Churchill Livingstone Elsevier, London.

Stear, S.J., Castell, L.M., Burke, L.M. & Spriet, L.L. (2010) BJSM reviews: A–Z of nutritional supplements: dietary supplements, sports nutrition foods and ergogenic aids for health and performance Part 6: Caffeine. *British Journal of Sports Medicine* **44**, 297–298.

Stellingwerff, T., Spriet, L.L., Watt, M.J., Kimber, N.E., Hargreaves, M., Hawley, J.A. & Burke, L.M. (2006) Decreased PDH activation and glycogenolysis during exercise following fat adaptation with carbohydrate restoration. *American Journal of Physiology* **290**, E380–E388.

Stephens, F.B., Constantin-Teodosiu, D. & Greenhaff, P.L. (2007) New insights concerning the role of carnitine in the regulation of fuel metabolism in skeletal muscle. *Journal of Physiology* **581**, 431–444.

Stewart, R.D., Duhamel, T.A., Foley, K.P., Ouyang, J., Smith, I.C. & Stewart, R.D. (2007) Protection of muscle membrane excitability during prolonged cycle exercise with glucose supplementation. *Journal of Applied Physiology* **103**, 331–339.

Street, D., Nielsen, J.J., Bangsbo, J. & Juel, C. (2005) Metabolic alkalosis reduces exercise-induced acidosis and potassium accumulation in human skeletal muscle interstitium. *Journal of Physiology* **566**, 481–489.

Tarnapolsky, M. (2004) Protein requirements for endurance athletes. *Nutrition* **20**, 662–668.

Tortora, G.J. & Grabowski, S.R. (2003) *Principles of Anatomy of Physiology* (10th Edition), John Wiley & Sons, New York.

Tsinztas, K., Williams, C., Boobis, L., & Greenhaff, P. (1995) Carbohydrate ingestion and glycogen utilization in different muscle fibre types in man. *Journal of Physiology* **489**, 243–250.

Tsinztas, K., Williams, C., Constantin-Teodosiu, D., Hultman, E., Boobis, L., Clarys, P. & Greenhaff, P. (2001) Phosphocreatine degradation in type I and II muscle fibres during submaximal exercise in man: effect of carbohydrate ingestion. *Journal of Physiology* **537**, 305–311.

Tunstall, R.J., Mehan, K.A., Wadley, G.D., Collier, G.R., Bonen, A., Hargreaves, M. & Cameron-Smith, D. (2002) Exercise training increases lipid metabolism gene expression in human skeletal muscle. *American Journal of Physiology* **283**, E66–E72.

Turcotte, L.P., Richter, E.A. & Kiens, B. (1992) Increased plasma FFA uptake and oxidation during prolonged exercise in trained vs untrained humans. *American Journal of Physiology* **262**, E791–E799.

Uguccioni, G., D'souza, D. & Hood, D.A. (2010) Regulation of PPAR gamma coactivator 1 alpha function and expression in muscle: effect of exercise. *PPAR Research*, in press.

van Loon, L.J. (2004) Use of intramuscular triaglycerol as a substrate source during exercise in humans. *Journal of Applied Physiology* **97**, 1170–1187.

van Loon, L.J., Greenhaff, P.L., Constantin-Teodosiu, D., Saris, W.H. & Wagenmakers, A.J. (2001) The effects of increasing exercise intensity on muscle fuel utilisation in humans. *Journal of Physiology* **536**, 295–304.

Vandenberghe, K., Hespel, P., Eynde, B.V., Lysens, R. & Richter, E.A. (1995). No effect of glycogen level on glycogen metabolism during high intensity exercise. *Medicine and Science in Sports and Exercise* **27**, 1278–1283.

Wackerhage, H. & Ratkevicius, A. (2008) Signal transduction pathways that regulate muscle growth. *Essays in Biochemistry* **44**, 99–108.

Watt, M.J. & Spriet, L.L. (2010) Triacylglycerol lipses and metabolic control:implications for health and disease. *American Journal of Physiology* **299**, E162–E168.

Watt, M.J., Heigenhauser, G.J., Dyck, D.J. & Spriet, L.L. (2002) Intramuscular triacglycerol, glycogen, and acetyl group metabolism during 4h of moderate exercise in man. *Journal of Physiology* **541**, 969–978.

Watt, M.J., Heigenhauser, G.J., LeBlanc, P.J., Inglis, J.G., Spriet, L.L. & Peters, S.J. (2004) Rapid upregulation of pyruvate dehydrogenase kinase activity in human skeletal muscle during prolonged exercise. *Journal of Applied Physiology* **97**, 1261–1267.

Wee, L.-S., Williams, C., Tsintzas, K. & Boobis, L. (2005) Ingestion of a high glycemic index meal increases muscle glycogen storage at rest but augments its utilization during subsequent exercise. *Journal of Applied Physiology* **99**, 707–714.

Westerblad, H., Bruton, J.D. & Lannergren, J. (1997) The effect of intracellular pH on contractile function of intact, single fibres of mouse muscle declines with increasing temperature. *Journal of Physiology* **500**, 193–204.

Westerblad, H., Allen, D.G. & Lannergren, J. (2002) Muscle fatigue: lactic acid or inorganic phosphate the major cause? *News in Physiological Sciences* **17**, 17–21.

Whitley, H.A., Humphreys, S.M., Campbell, I.T., Keegan, M.A., Jayanetti, T.D., Sperry, D.A., MacLaren, D.P., Reilly, T. & Frayn, K.N. (1998) Metabolic and performance responses during endurance exercise after high fat and high carbohydrate meals. *Journal of Applied Physiology* **85**, 418–424.

Whyte, G. (2006) *The Physiology of Endurance Training*. Churchill Livingstone: Elsevier, Edinburgh.

Whyte, L.J., Gill, J.M., & Cathcart, A.J. (2010) Effect of 2 weeks of sprint interval training on health-related outcomes in sedentary overweight/obese men. *Metabolism* **59**, 1421–1428.

Wilmore, J.H., Costill, D.L. & Kenny, W.L. (2008) *Physiology of Sport and Exercise* (4th Edition), Human Kinetics, Wrisberg, CA.

Winter, E.M. & MacLaren, D.P.M. (2009) *Assessment of maximal intensity exercise*. In: Eston, R. & Reilly, T. (eds.) Kinanthropometry and Exercise Physiology Laboratory Manual. *Vol 2: Physiology*. Routledge, London

Wright, D.A., Sherman, W.M. & Dernbach, A.R. (1991) Carbohydrate feedings before, during or in combination improve cycling endurance performance. *Journal of Applied Physiology* **71**, 1082–1088.

Yeo, W.K., Carey, A.L., Burke, L., Spriet, L.L. & Hawley, J.A. (2011) Fat adaptation in well trained athletes: effects on cell metabolism. *Applied Physiology, Nutrition, and Metabolism* **36**, 12–22.

Yeo, W.K., Lessard, S.J., Chen, Z.P., Garnham, A.P., Burke, L.M., Rivas, D.A., Kemp, B.E. & Hawley, J.A. (2008) Fat adaptation followed by carbohydrate restoration increases AMPK activity in skeletal muscle from trained humans. *Journal of Applied Physiology* **105**, 1519–1526.

Index

Printed in the United States
By Bookmasters